Cultural Profici
Addressing Health Disparities

Edited by

Sade Kosoko-Lasaki, MD, MSPH, MBA

Associate Vice President
Health Sciences–Multicultural and Community Affairs
Professor
Ophthalmology, Preventative Medicine, and Public Health
Creighton University
Omaha, Nebraska

Cynthia T. Cook, PhD

Assistant Professor
Department of Sociology and Criminal Justice
College of Arts and Sciences
Florida A&M University
Tallahassee, Florida

Richard L. O'Brien, MD, FACP

Professor
Center for Health Policy and Ethics
Creighton University
Omaha, Nebraska

JONES AND BARTLETT PUBLISHERS
Sudbury, Massachusetts
BOSTON   TORONTO   LONDON   SINGAPORE

World Headquarters

Jones and Bartlett Publishers	Jones and Bartlett Publishers	Jones and Bartlett Publishers
40 Tall Pine Drive	Canada	International
Sudbury, MA 01776	6339 Ormindale Way	Barb House, Barb Mews
978-443-5000	Mississauga, Ontario L5V 1J2	London W6 7PA
info@jbpub.com	Canada	United Kingdom
www.jbpub.com		

Jones and Bartlett's books and products are available through most bookstores and online book-sellers. To contact Jones and Bartlett Publishers directly, call 800-832-0034, fax 978-443-8000, or visit our website www.jbpub.com.

Substantial discounts on bulk quantities of Jones and Bartlett's publications are available to cor-porations, professional associations, and other qualified organizations. For details and specific discount information, contact the special sales department at Jones and Bartlett via the above contact information or send an email to specialsales@jbpub.com.

This publication is designed to provide accurate and authoritative information in regard to the sub-ject matter covered. It is sold with the understanding that the publisher is not engaged in rendering legal, accounting, or other professional service. If legal advice or other expert assistance is required, the service of a competent professional person should be sought.

Production Credits
Publisher: David Cella
Editorial Assistant: Maro Asadoorian
Production Director: Amy Rose
Production Supervisor: Renée Sekerak
Production Assistant: Jill Morton
Associate Marketing Manager: Lisa Gordon
Manufacturing and Inventory Control Supervisor: Amy Bacus
Cover Design: Brian Moore
Composition: Cape Cod Compositors, Inc.
Cover Image: © Christopher Ursitti/ShutterStock, Inc.
Printing and Binding: Malloy Incorporated
Cover Printing: Malloy Incorporated

Library of Congress Cataloging-in-Publication Data
Cultural proficiency in addressing health disparities / [edited] by Sade
Kosoko-Lasaki, Cynthia Theresa Cook, and Richard L. O'Brien.
    p. ; cm.
  Includes bibliographical references and index.
  ISBN-13: 978-0-7637-5174-6 (pbk.)
  ISBN-10: 0-7637-5174-X (pbk.)
  1. Health services accessibility—United States. 2. Cultural
awareness—United States. 3. Minorities—Health and hygiene-United
States. I. Kosoko-Lasaki, Sade. II. Cook, Cynthia Theresa. III.
O'Brien, Richard L.
  [DNLM: 1. Healthcare Disparities-United States. 2. Cultural
Competency-United States. 3. Minority Health-ethnology-United
States. W 84 AA1 C968 2009]
  RA418.3.U6C85 2009
  362.1089-dc22

                                          2008022734

6048

Printed in the United States of America
13 12 11 10 09   10 9 8 7 6 5 4 3 2

Contents

Chapter 13   Addressing Health Disparities in Immigrant Populations in the United States **247**

Patti Patterson, MD, MPH
Gordon Gong, MD

Chapter 14   Minority Attitudes and Perception of Health Care: A Comparison of Comments from a Cultural Competency Questionnaire and Focus Group Discussion **281**

Cynthia T. Cook, PhD

Chapter 15   Health Disparities: The Nebraska Perspective **311**

Reverend Raponzil L. Drake, DMin
Anthony Zhang, MA
Diane Lowe, BA

Foreword

I congratulate the editors and contributors of this highly needed book on cultural competency and health disparities. It promises to be an important contribution to open and honest discussions of cultural differences, cultural competence, and healthcare delivery.

Disparities in the health of minority communities are a reality. The attitude of minority populations toward healthcare institutions adds to the urgency of this issue. These disparities have become a major concern of healthcare providers, clinical investigators, and policymakers. The Surgeon General's Report, *Healthy People 2010*, makes the reduction of health disparities a major goal. Creighton University has made health disparities research an institutional priority.

I believe our mission and values allow us to speak to these troubling issues. Because Creighton is a faith-based, independent institution, we have, at the core of our mission, a deliberate set of values that speak to service, justice, respect, and dignity of all people. Our students—both undergraduate and professional—are actively engaged in community service. One of Creighton's tag lines is that "we educate our students to be women and men for and with others."

Creighton is fortunate to have within its healthcare professions a Center for Health Policy and Ethics. Consequently, we can teach, discuss, and reflect on ethical issues in health care in a deliberate, focused, and open manner. This collection of chapters echoes that approach.

To deal effectively with disparities and to strive to reduce or eliminate them requires knowledge of the diverse cultures comprising the United States, commitment to the moral imperative of justice, knowledge and skills to relate to persons and communities of diverse cultures in ways that enable and empower them to reduce health risks and to participate effectively with providers and clinical research to reduce those disparities.

It is essential that individual health professionals develop and continuously improve their cultural competence in order to provide compassionate and effective care to those of cultures different from theirs, to relate effectively to communities in which they conduct research, and to relate to the members of those communities who participate in the research. It is equally important that institutions recognize and cultivate cultural competence in their employees and policies. They should engage the communities they serve in the design and implementation of systems of care, research priorities and strategies, and institutional policy formulation and implementation. This book addresses all of these issues and provides accounts of the experiences of a number of professionals who have dedicated themselves to health disparity reduction.

Creighton is an urban institution deeply rooted in its community. A direct consequence of our urban setting is an institutional commitment to provide health care to Omaha's core (downtown) population, which is more diverse and, in terms of income and access to health care, is more needy than other sectors of the city. As an educational institution steeped in the Catholic and Jesuit ethos, we highly value diversity and have an institutional commitment to attract, matriculate, and graduate women and men from underrepresented and underserved groups. That same commitment underlines our healthcare delivery and our outreach to the greater Omaha community.

Let me end by stating that our institutional commitment to undertake health disparities research is very much consonant with the Jesuit Catholic commitment to serve those most in need, to exercise the "preferential option for the poor," and to strive to achieve justice for all. As a university president I am delighted and highly gratified that my faculty are undertaking such research in concert with the mission and identity of Creighton University.

I am honored by the invitation to script the Foreword to this book, *Cultural Proficiency in Addressing Health Disparities*. We, as open, attentive, caring, and discerning people with this book in hand, can seize the opportunity to engage in thoughtful and fruitful conversation on an increasingly important moral challenge for all of our communities.

John P. Schlegel, SJ
President
Creighton University

Acknowledgments

Sade Kosoko-Lasaki, MD, MSPH, MBA

I would like to thank God Almighty for his blessings and for giving me the ability to edit this book. My husband, Dr. Gbolahan Lasaki, PhD, has been a source of encouragement with his unconditional love and support. My children, Adedayo, Adeola, and Abiola, together with my stepchildren, Abimbola, Tolulope, and Folayo, and their families have given me the fortitude and strength both directly and indirectly to continue to aspire to give the best of my ability in all that I do. For this, I am forever grateful.

My parents, Jokotoye and Adebimpe Babalola, together with my sister, Dr. Abimbola Oluremi, and her husband, Engr. Ayotunde Oluremi, pray for me all the time. Thank you.

Ms. Reba Donahue, my administrative assistant at Creighton University, has done an excellent job of copyediting and collating the manuscript. Her efforts are much appreciated.

Finally, I appreciate Creighton University and its leadership, Fr. John Schlegel and Dr. Cam Enarson, for their commitment to diversity. The staff of Health Sciences' Multicultural and Community Affairs (HS-MACA) at Creighton University and the wonderful faculty, staff, and students have helped make this book possible through their comments, challenges, and goodwill.

My co-authors, Dr. Cynthia Cook and Dr. Richard O'Brien, are wonderful people to collaborate with. I have truly enjoyed the experience. Thank you.

Cynthia T. Cook, PhD

I would like to take this opportunity to thank my family, friends, and colleagues for their continued support before, during, and after the completion of this book, and to especially thank Dr. Joyce Williams, my former advisor and former chair of the Department of Sociology at Texas Woman's University. I would like to also acknowledge the continued support and inspiration

I received from my mother, Gloria Cook, while pursuing my graduate work; she passed away in December 2001, a year after I received my doctorate.

Richard L. O'Brien, MD, FACP

I am grateful to my colleagues and the staff at the Center for Health Policy and Ethics for their support and encouragement. Drs. Kosoko-Lasaki and Cook have been pleasures to work with as research and editorial colleagues. And finally I am grateful to my wife Joan, my life's partner for more than 50 years.

Financial support for Chapters 7, 8, 9, and 14: This research was supported by funding from the Nebraska Tobacco Settlement.

Introduction

Sade Kosoko-Lasaki, MD, MSPH, MBA

Health disparities are the results of inequalities in many aspects of life: access to health care, social and economic status, educational opportunity, and environmental conditions. There are also disparities in the training of the healthcare workers who provide the much-needed services to the disadvantaged.

An important contributor to the perpetuation of health disparities is the lack of cultural competence of healthcare personnel. Defined as "a set of congruent behaviors, attitudes, and policies that come together in a system, agency, or among professionals," cultural competence promotes effective service in cross-cultural situations.[1] The current and changing demographics in the United States call for the need for cultural competency training. This training effort will reduce some of the long-standing disparities experienced by individuals from different racial, ethnic, and cultural backgrounds and improve the quality of services and healthcare outcomes.

Cultural competency has been addressed by legislative, accreditation, and regulatory mandates since 1946 (Hill-Burton Act).[2,3] Currently, there are National Standards on Culturally and Linguistically Appropriate Services (CLAS) that are primarily directed at healthcare organizations.[4]

A few years ago, the editors of this book, together with other researchers at Creighton University in Omaha, examined the reasons minorities in the city were reluctant to participate in healthcare research. During the same period, the researchers also examined the perception of healthcare providers at Creighton University about the attitudes of minorities to healthcare institutions in the city. The results from this research were overwhelming and have been detailed.[5-7] There was, however, a great deal of data that has not been previously reported. We attempt to share these results in the first few chapters of this book.

As we continued to plan the publication of this book, we realized that the problem of health disparities and cultural awareness is much larger than we explored in our research and publications. This prompted us to invite other contributors to examine the problem of health disparities in the major racial/ethnic groups in the United States. We recognize that there are other underserved populations—spiritual/religious minorities, patients with stigmatizing diseases like HIV/AIDS, the geriatric population, migrant workers, people with disabilities, to name a few—whose perspectives are not included in this book.

In addition, we invited senior university administrators from Colorado, Tennessee, and Nebraska to share with the readers their perspectives on health disparities. Ethicists and state healthcare leaders from Nebraska and Missouri also reviewed the problem of health disparities. Finally, the economic impact of health disparities is clearly detailed.

The contributors have addressed health disparities through research methodologies, statistical analysis of data, economics, ethical considerations, case studies, and personal experiences. We think the book will be a valuable asset to healthcare providers, students, and anyone interested in providing culturally competent care.

After climbing a great hill, one only finds that there are many more hills to climb.

Nelson Mandela

REFERENCES

1. HHS Office of Disadvantaged Health Culturally and Linguistically Appropriate Services Standards. www.omhrc.gov/assets/pdf/checked/executive.pdf.
2. www.hhs.gov/ocr/hburton.html.
3. http://en.wikipedia.org/wiki/Hill-Burton_Act.
4. http://clas.uiuc.edu/.
5. O'Brien R, Kosoko-Lasaki O, Cook CT, Kissell J, Peak F, Williams EH. Self assessment of cultural attitudes and competence of clinical investigators to enhance recruitment and participation of minority population in research. *Journal of the National Medical Association.* 2006;98:674–682.
6. Cook CT, Kosoko-Lasaki O, O'Brien RL. Satisfaction with and perceived cultural competency of health care providers: The minority experience. *Journal of the National Medical Association.* 2005;97:1–10.
7. Kosoko-Lasaki O, Cook CT, O'Brien RL, Kissell J, Purtilo R, Peak F. Promoting cultural proficiency in researchers to enhance the recruitment and participation of minority populations in research: Part 1, Development and refinement of survey instruments. *Evaluation and Program Planning.* 2006;29:227–235.

List of Contributors

Janet E. Bonet, BA

Genny Carrillo-Zuniga, MD, ScD

Reverend Raponzil L. Drake, DMin

Annette Dula, PhD

Cristina Fernandez, MD

Isidore Flores, PhD

Valda Ford, RN, MPH, MS

Vanessa Gamble, MD, PhD

Gordon Gong, MD

Margaret A. Graham, PhD

Vera Haynatzka, PhD

Gleb Haynatzki, DSc, PhD

Cathy Hudson, MD

Adeola O. Jaiyeola, MD, DOHS, MHSc

Judith Lee Kissell, PhD

Diane Lowe, BA

Nelda Mier, PhD

Ann V. Millard, PhD

Phyllis A. Nsiah-Kumi, MD, MPH

Albert A. Okunade, PhD, MS, MBA

Rubens J. Pamies, MD, FACP

Patti Patterson, MD, MPH

Frank T. Peak, MPA

Michael T. Railey, MD

Karl S. Roth, MD

Esmeralda R. Sánchez, MPH

Reverend John P. Schlegel, SJ

Wehnona Stabler, MPH

John R. Stone, MD, PhD

Chutima Suraratdecha, MBA, PhD

Ethel Williams, PhD

M. Roy Wilson, MD, MS

Anthony Zhang, MA

Chapter 1

Addressing Health Disparities in the 21st Century

Rubens J. Pamies, MD, FACP
Phyllis A. Nsiah-Kumi, MD, MPH

Overview of Health Disparities

Racial and ethnic differences in health status, health care, and health outcomes have existed for centuries. During the slavery era, individuals were considered "property" and suffered unhealthy living conditions and their consequences. When slaves experienced health problems, slave masters often tried many remedies before calling a physician.[1,2] Poor health and health outcomes were also the fate of most new immigrant groups in the United States.

While the dark period of slavery is long over, poor living and working conditions, as well as health and health care, have continued to plague people of color and immigrants.[2,3] While the existence and magnitude of health disparities are well understood, solutions remain elusive.

Definition of Health Disparities

The definition of health disparities has political implications and affects measurements, the actions of government agencies, and the resources committed to address them.[4] Disparities are most often identified along racial and ethnic lines, but they are also associated with income and education. The National Institutes of Health (NIH) prioritizes social and ethnic disparities.[5]

The Institute of Medicine (IOM) distinguishes between health disparities and disparities in health care by emphasizing the differences in health care quality experienced by minority groups.[6] It defines **disparities in health care** as "differences in the quality of health care that are not due to access related factors or clinical needs, preferences, or appropriateness of intervention."[6] (See **Figure 1–1**.) The Surgeon General's report, *Healthy People 2010* (HP2010), sets health objectives for the United States. It defines **disparities in health** as the "unequal burden in disease morbidity and mortality rates experienced by ethnic/racial groups as compared to the dominant group."[7] The Health Resources and Services Administration (HRSA) defines *health disparities* as "population-specific differences in the presence of disease, health outcomes, or access to health care."[8] We will use the definition proposed by the National Institutes of Health in this chapter. **Health disparities** are ". . . the differences in the incidence, prevalence, mortality and burden of diseases and other adverse health conditions that exist among specific groups in the United States."[9]

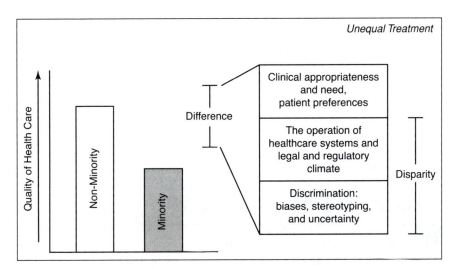

Figure 1–1   *Differences, Disparities, and Discrimination: Populations with Equal Access to Health Care*
Reprinted with permission from the National Academies Press, Copyright 2003, National Academy of Sciences.

Models of Health Disparities

A variety of models have been described to explain the many factors contributing to health disparities. The IOM presents an integrated model of healthcare disparities, emphasizing the role of clinical discretion; social, economic, and cultural differences; and patient input. **Figure 1–2** illustrates the complex interactions of the many factors that contribute to health disparities.

The Integrate Model of Healthcare Disparities (**Table 1–1**) has three dimensions: health before care, access to health care and healthcare delivery.[10]

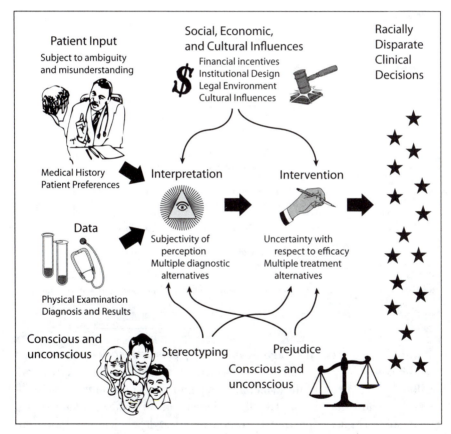

Figure 1–2　*An Integrated Model of Healthcare Disparities*
Reprinted with permission from the National Academies Press, Copyright 2003, National Academy of Sciences.

Table 1–1 *Health Disparities Framework*

Health—Before Care	Access to Care	Healthcare Delivery
Income levels, poverty, and other social conditions	Financial resources	Insurance coverage and type
Safety and adequacy of housing	Availability and proximity of providers	Cultural competency levels
Employment status and type of employment	Access to transportation	Patient–provider communications
Education levels	Insurance coverage	Provider discrimination or bias
Lifestyle choices—diet, exercise, tobacco, and alcohol use	Regular source of care	Differential propensities for certain diseases by racial/ethnic populations
Environmental conditions— air and water quality, pesticide exposure, green space	Language barriers	Patient preferences and adherence to treatment plans
	Legal barriers (e.g., eligibility restrictions, illegal immigrants)	Diversity of the healthcare workforce
	Prior experience with the healthcare system	Appropriateness of care
	Cultural preferences— care-seeking behaviors	Effectiveness of care
	Health literacy levels	Language barriers
	Diversity of the healthcare workforce	

Reprinted with permission from Health Policy Institute of Ohio, "Understanding Health Disparities," November 2004.

An individual's **health care** is affected by personal, socioeconomic, and environmental factors. A number of patient factors influence an individual's health. The aggregate of these factors in a population contributes to the existence of health disparities. Health is dependent on socioeconomic status, employment status, educational attainment, lifestyle choices, and environmental conditions. Employment status and the nature of various jobs play a significant role in health status.[11] Individuals employed in the restaurant industry and in manual labor (e.g. farming and construction) face a variety of occupational exposures and hazards that may negatively affect health and safety. These jobs are disproportionately held by racial and ethnic minorities and immigrants.[12–15]

Healthcare access is affected by an individual's finances, the availability and proximity of providers, access to transportation, insurance status, immigrant status,[16,17] regular source of care,[18,19] language barriers,[20] legal barriers, prior experiences with the healthcare system, and health literacy.[21] The unemployed or those with low income jobs are also more likely to have limited access to care. Workforce distribution also plays a role as it impacts provider availability in and patients' choices of access to health care.

The quality of **healthcare delivery** is affected by insurance coverage, patient–provider communication, language barriers, racial/ethnic predisposition to particular diseases, appropriateness and effectiveness of care, patient preferences and adherence to treatment, diversity of the healthcare workforce, and provider discrimination or bias.

Factors Contributing to Health Disparities

Many factors contribute to disparities in health and health care. Important contributing factors include education, insurance status, segregation, immigration status, healthy behavior and lifestyle choices, healthcare provider behavior, employment, and the nature and operation of the health system.

Education

There is direct correlation between the numbers of years in school and good health outcomes.[22] High school graduates can expect to live 9 years longer than those who do not complete 9th grade. Some of the difference is related to employment and other socioeconomic conditions, but when those factors are controlled for, the difference in health outcomes persists. Educational attainment, however, is insufficient to explain racial differences. African Americans with college educations have poorer health and outcomes than whites with lower education levels.

Insurance Status

Insurance status also is significantly associated with health outcomes. The IOM has reported 18,000 preventable deaths and health care and lost productivity costs of $65 to $130 billion dollars annually. These facts disproportionately affect Hispanics and African Americans; more than a third of Hispanics and almost a quarter of African Americans are uninsured.

Correcting for lack of insurance will have some impact on disparities but will not eliminate them. After adjusting for insurance status and disease severity, minorities receive less comprehensive and lower quality care. Other factors must be addressed to attain equality in health and health care.

Segregation

Segregation is significantly correlated with the existence and persistence of health disparities. Williams and Collins have reported that several American cities are nearly as segregated as South Africa during apartheid.[23] Massey showed that affluent blacks, earning more than $50,000 per year are more segregated than the Latinos or Asians earning less that $15,000 per year. Massey suggests that segregation may lead to an "exodus" of jobs from low-income neighborhoods, further aggravating disparities.[24]

Segregation can result in lack of access to care, poorer quality care, more overcrowded housing, fewer municipal services, greater environmental hazards, fewer resources for schools and recreational facilities, and more exposure to stress and violence, which can all result in unhealthy behaviors. Segregated neighborhoods are also less likely to receive preventive medical services and more likely to use emergency rooms for primary care. Green points out that many residents in poorer neighborhoods live with chronic pain because pharmacies in these areas are not adequately stocked with pain medication.[25] Cities that have a higher percentage of underrepresented minorities, particularly African Americans, tend to have the worst health care of all racial groups. Some exceptions to their findings include the Bronx in New York and Birmingham, Alabama, where the minorities have equal or better health outcomes than the rest of the population.[26]

It is unlikely that the issue of segregated poor neighborhoods will be solved soon. Increasing numbers of immigrant groups arriving in the United States is likely to increase segregation.

Immigration Status

Immigration status is important in health and insurance coverage.[27] Children of immigrants are less likely to have well child care.[17,19] Immigrant Latinas are less likely to have access to breast cancer screening after controlling for acculturation and insurance.[28-31] Undocumented persons tend to have poorer health and are less likely to seek health care if documentation is required.[32,33] Immigrants experience poorer care than those who have better access to care.[19,32,33]

Immigrants will have a significant impact on the healthcare system in this century. By the year 2030, more than one in five children (under the age of

18) in the United States will be a son or daughter of immigrants, with the most common language spoken by those immigrants being Spanish.[6,34]

The jobs that many undocumented immigrants engage in have significant occupational risks (e.g. meat packing, agriculture, outdoor construction, and service industries). Cultural issues, use of alternative or complementary medicine, spiritual and religious beliefs, rare or resistant infectious diseases, mental health concerns (particularly involving trauma or exposure to violence), general lifestyle, and health behaviors all have important effects on immigrant groups.

Lifestyle and Health Behavior

Many Americans behave in ways that are deleterious to their health. Some of these behaviors affect minority populations disproportionately.

Legislation addressing tobacco use, trans-fats in food, school-based health centers, cultural competency training for provider licensure, and seat belt use have been introduced in many states.[35–39] Major companies, such as Union Pacific, will not hire new employees who smoke tobacco, arguing that it is unfair to raise healthcare premiums for everyone because of individuals' bad behavior.[40,41] Airlines have argued that obese customers disproportionately cause them to use more fuel; will they base ticket prices on weight?[42]

Factors contributing to poor health habits include targeted advertising of deleterious products; zoning laws for liquor and junk and fast-food retailers; lack of green space; lack of access to exercise facilities; and other environmental and safety conditions in poorer neighborhoods.[23]

Healthcare Provider Behavior

Health professionals also bear responsibility for health disparities. Physicians are less likely to discuss healthy behavior changes with patients from lower income groups.[43] Healthcare providers frequently lack understanding of cultural, social, psychological, racial, and religious influences on individuals' behaviors and barriers to changing behavior.

Need for Relevant, Effective Interventions

The need to develop, implement, and evaluate effective interventions to reduce and/or eliminate health disparities is imperative. The U.S. population is becoming increasingly multicultural, and we anticipate that groups that currently experience poor health status will grow as a proportion of the total nation's population. By 2048, 50% of the U.S. population will be comprised of racial/ethnic minorities.[6,34] The future health of the nation depends on success in improving the health of racial/ethnic minority populations.[7,44,45]

Historical Perspectives of Health Disparities

Minority Health

The fact that minorities, particularly African Americans, suffer worse health care and health outcomes than whites is well documented. In 1985, the U.S. Secretary of Health and Human Service's Task Force on Black and Minority Health stated that "there is continuing disparity in the burden of death and illness experienced by black and other minority Americans." The Kerner Commission in 1968 and the U.S. Commission on Civil Rights in 1963 both stated, "evidence clearly shows that Negroes do not share the same health benefits as equally as with the white citizens." It went on further to state ". . . the Federal Government, by statute and administration supports racial discrimination in the provision of health facilities." These and other findings have led many legal scholars to view health disparity as a civil rights violation and justification for reparations.[46–51] Past attempts at reparation have been unsuccessful.[52] The African American Slave Descendant litigation was dismissed in July 2005 based on lack of merit, principally because the "crimes were long ago and the statute of limitations has expired."[52] The same reasoning was applied to litigation brought on behalf of victims of the Tulsa race riot.[52] However, the fact that black children today suffer shorter life expectancies than white children provides a new argument for legal scholars.[52] Jack Geiger has pointed out, ". . . the opportunity to maintain a healthy and longer life and to fulfill one's human potential are skewed in the United States by income, education, primary language, race, ethnicity and areas of residence; the injustice is not the consequence of random chance in the distribution of disease. It is injustice by design."[53]

Medical Education

To understand today's health problems, it is useful to look at the past. Where would we be today if the 10 medical colleges that were established shortly after the turn of the century to train black doctors had survived beyond the 1920s? Would we have the access issues? If these colleges had been adequately supported, would research by these institutions yield better solutions to diseases disproportionately affecting African Americans? Would there even be health disparities? With only two medical schools (Howard University and Meharry Medical College) available to train the majority of black physicians for more than 50 years following the 1920s, poor health outcomes in the black community have been inevitable.

Dr. Todd Savitt, a historian of African American medical education, provided an excellent overview of the historical struggles of African American physicians and medical schools in the years following slavery.[1,2] Many of the schools were doomed to failure for lack of financial support and other resources, including faculty and adequate facilities. Early black medical schools were mostly proprietary (entrepreneurial) or missionary (funded by religious organizations). Howard University Medical School, with its federal appropriation, and Meharry Medical School, with better philanthropic and religious organization support, struggled but were better able to weather their financial stresses. The Flexner Report supported these two institutions.[54] However, the reason for this support was to ensure that there were enough black physicians to care for black patients and to prevent the need for these patients to receive care from white physicians. The Report further pointed out that the need for black doctors to treat black patients is important to prevent the spread of disease from blacks to the white population.

Racism and segregation made it difficult for black physicians to obtain continuing education and training. Lack of facilities to care for black patients often forced black physicians to turn over seriously ill patients to white physicians willing to care for them. Some patients mistrusted the black physicians and employed home remedies brought from Africa and the West Indies, which often worsened their conditions. This "separate but equal" approach in the medical establishment lasted several decades and undoubtedly slowed the progress in addressing medical conditions in the African American community.[2]

Contemporary Disparities

In 2003, the IOM released *Unequal Treatment: Confronting Racial and Ethnic Disparities in Health Care*, an eye-opening report that documents disturbing differences in the health and health care of racial/ethnic minorities compared with whites. Based on a vast body of research and the existence of numerous disparities, it documented wide variation in access to care and quality of care provided to racial/ethic minority patients in our nation. Minorities are less likely to receive life-saving interventions but are more likely to receive undesirable procedures such as amputations and radical mastectomy.[6]

The IOM committee recommended increasing awareness to the general public, health care providers, insurance companies, and policy makers about disparities and recommended that "evidence-based" guidelines be used to help providers and health plans to ensure that care is more consistent and equitable. The committee also stressed the need for more minority healthcare providers because they are more likely to serve in minority and underserved communities and of more interpreters to overcome language barriers that may affect the quality of care.[6]

Statistical Overview of Health Disparities

Understanding the state of health disparities in the 21st century is essential to the development of corrective interventions. Throughout the lifespan, racial/ethnic minorities experience poorer health status, poorer health care, and poorer outcomes than whites of European descent. Disparities in prenatal care, birth weight, and infant mortality; differences in pediatric access to care and vaccinations; and disparities in asthma, obesity, and diabetes rates are prevalent in childhood. Disparities in risk-taking behaviors, sexually transmitted infections, teen pregnancy, and mental illness are prevalent in adolescence. Disparities in preventive care; obesity; and diabetes and coronary artery disease, diagnosis, and treatment are also prevalent. Racial/ethnic differences persist in elder health and end-of-life care.

Prenatal Care/Infant Mortality/Low Birth Weight

American Indians/Alaskan Natives are the most likely to have late or no prenatal care (7.9%), followed by African Americans (5.7%), Hispanics (5.4%), Asians (3.0%), and whites (2.2%)—although all groups showed improvement in rates from 1990 to 2004. There are significant differences among Hispanic subgroups; 5.5% of Mexicans but only 2.9% of Cubans had late or no prenatal care.[55]

The frequency of low birth weight children of African-born women (3.6%) more closely resembles that of U.S.-born whites (2.4%) than U.S.-born blacks (7.5%). In both neonatal and post-neonatal periods, black women had higher infant mortality rates than Latina or white women for perinatal conditions,[58] disparities which persist despite early access to prenatal care.[57] Although infant mortality has declined in the past decade, disparities persist for minority populations.[51] In 2003, the infant mortality rate was 13.6 for black newborns, 5.7 for white infants, and 5.65 for Latino infants.[59] Whites are nearing the HP2010 goal of 4.5 deaths per 100 much more rapidly than are African Americans.[60]

Pediatric Preventive Care

Black and Latino children receive less counseling at well child care visits than white children—a finding unexplained by diagnoses or medications dispensed.[61] Latino children are at high risk for behavioral and developmental disorders, school dropout, environmental hazards, obesity, diabetes, asthma, uninsured status, nonfinancial barriers to health care access, and poor quality of care.[62] Latino children are also less likely to receive timely routine care, phone help, and brief wait time compared with whites and African Americans—a finding not explained by language barriers.[63] Minority children also suffer more preventable injuries and fatalities than white children.[64,65]

Pediatric Asthma

Asthma is a prototypic example of disparities in childhood. The asthma burden is greatest in communities of color and low-income communities.[66–71] Black children are more likely to have asthma and to experience emergency department (ED) visits for asthma than white children of comparable socioeconomic status; these disparities are not explained by measurable child or family differences. Children of color benefit from new asthma technologies later than other children,[72] which points to the need for research to determine explanations and remedies.[66,68,73–78]

Adolescence

In adolescents, racial/ethnic disparities exist in risk-taking behaviors such as smoking,[79–81] unsafe driving practices,[82] alcohol use, and illicit drug use.[83,84] Sexually transmitted infections are more common in minority youth.[85,86] Although overall teen pregnancy rates declined between 1990 and 2005, disparities still remain; Hispanic, non-Hispanic black, and American Indian teens have higher rates of pregnancy than their non-Hispanic white counterparts. For 15- to 17-year-olds, the birth rate for whites is 11.5 per 1000, 34.9 per 1000 for non-Hispanic blacks, and 48.9 per 1000 for Hispanics.[59] Disparities also exist in the prevalence and treatment of depression and other mental illnesses in youth.[87–90]

Obesity

Obesity is a growing problem in pediatric and adult populations. This disproportionately affects racial/ethnic minorities of all ages. African American (26.2%) and Mexican American (19.4%) girls are more likely to be obese than white girls (11.6%). Seventeen percent of African American boys, 27.3% of Mexican American boys, and 12.0% of non-Hispanic white boys are obese.[91] Also, 49.7% of African American women, 39.7% of Mexican American women, and 30.1% of non-Hispanic white women were obese. Twenty-eight percent of African American men, 27.3% of Hispanic men and 28.9% of white men are obese.[91] The sequelae of obesity also disproportionately affect minority populations.

Diabetes

Diabetes is an increasingly significant concern of minority populations. It affects an estimated 21 million Americans (approximately 7% of the population).[92,93] Risk for type 2 diabetes is higher among African Americans and Hispanics and those of low socioeconomic status.[91,94-98] Although the cause of these disparities has not been clearly elucidated, a number of factors have been associated with the incidence of diabetes. Excess risk of diabetes is not completely explained by basal metabolic index (BMI), myocardial infarction (MI), physical activity, skinfold thickness, family history of diabetes, income, education, occupational status, age, or sex.[99-101]

There is need for greater understanding of factors (throughout the lifespan) that affect racial/ethnic differences in incident diabetes. The impact of gestational diabetes, the intrauterine environment,[102] prematurity, low birth weight (Barker hypothesis),[103,104] breastfeeding,[105] stress and burnout,[106] diet, sleep/obstructive sleep apnea,[107,108] low vital capacity,[109] autonomic nervous system dysfunction,[110] and symptoms of depression[111] have been implicated. Disparities of environment and lifestyle factors may also play roles in predisposition of racial/ethnic minority populations to diabetes.[112]

Disparities also exist in complications and care of diabetes. Non-Hispanic blacks and Hispanics are less likely than whites to report recent glycosylated hemoglobin testing and retinopathy screening,[113-117] although they are more likely to report high glycosylated hemoglobin values, amputations, renal disease, and MIs than white diabetics.[118-121]

Adults—Preventive Care

The National Health Interview Survey of 2003–2004 showed that among adults aged 18 to 64, Hispanics were most likely to have no usual source of health care, followed by Asians, African Americans, and whites. These differences persist, even when poverty status was considered.[122] The study also demonstrated that Hispanics were most likely not to have had a healthcare visit in the preceding 12 months (27%), followed by Asians (21%), African Americans (18%), and whites (14%).[123] In 2003, Asian women were least likely to have had a mammogram within the past 2 years (42% of 58% who had been screened); 63% of American Indian/Alaskan Natives, 65% of Hispanic women, and 70% of both

African American and white women had been screened in the past two years.[124] The quality of care for dyslipidemia is suboptimal and varies by cardiovascular disease risk group, ethnicity, and gender.[125,126] Colon cancer screening is performed less frequently in Latino and African American populations.[127–129]

Elder Health

Racial/ethnic disparities persist in preventive health care of the elderly despite near-universal coverage by Medicare.[130] Fewer blacks and Latinos receive influenza and pneumococcal vaccines than whites.[131–133] Although similarly insured, whites with ischemic heart disease are more likely than elderly blacks and American Indians to be admitted and are more likely to undergo invasive testing and revascularization. The latter disparity correlates with a 20% reduction in two-year mortality for whites and only an 11% reduction for blacks.[134] Differences also exist in the diagnosis and treatment of late-life depression.[135,136]

Cognitive tests underestimate the abilities of older adults in racial/ethnic minority groups. This may lead to the over-diagnosis of dementia. Population-specific measures or scores should be established for existing measures.[137] Alzheimer's disease has a higher prevalence among racial and ethnic minorities; the reasons are unclear. Risk factors for vascular disease, stroke, and vascular dementia are more prevalent in minority groups. Treatment for dementia varies by racial/ethnic group, which may be related to cultural beliefs.[138] Additional research is needed to further understand these issues. Obtaining informed consent in dementia research is challenging, especially in minority populations. Consent processes should be more culturally appropriate.[139] Health information needs of elders from minority backgrounds should be addressed by community health programs.[140]

End-of-Life Care

Culture plays a significant but complex role in the interplay between patient autonomy and end of life.[141] It is important to respect and attend to patients' values at the end of life, especially spirituality and relationship dynamics. Healthcare professionals should assess patients and their families and provide culturally appropriate end-of-life care, recognizing each patient's individuality.[142,143]

Mortality

Age-adjusted mortality rates of African Americans exceed those of whites. There has been no significant decrease in mortality disparities between blacks and whites since World War II.[144] Heart disease, cancer, and HIV are among the leading causes of death in African Americans.[145] Access to primary care is associated with lower mortality.[146]

It is difficult to say how much excess mortality results from differences in health outcomes, but Satcher and associates calculate that if there were no differences in health outcomes at the turn of this century, 85,000 African American deaths would not have occurred.[147] While there is uncertainty about exactly what fraction of excess mortality is attributable to the healthcare system, 20% to 35% of the differences in mortality have been attributed to the healthcare system.[147]

In addition to disparities in health and health care, there are disparities in disaster preparedness, especially regarding culturally and linguistically appropriate care in emergency situations.[148,149]

Progress on Eliminating Disparities

While this litany of statistics may be disheartening, many interventions have been initiated to address disparities. Progress is being made, but it is sobering to note that despite these efforts, significant disparities persist.

Healthy People 2010 objectives present a framework for comparing disparities between populations as well as changes over time. In 2005 (the midpoint of the *Healthy People 2010* timeline), significant improvement in the nation's overall health had occurred. But health disparities persist and have changed only slightly since the beginning of HP2010. Nearly 60% of objectives were met or progress was made toward them, but 20% were further from the targets.[150]

The 2006 National Health Disparities Report found increasing disparities, especially in chronic disease management. Blacks had 90% more lower extremity amputations for diabetes than whites; Hispanics had 63% more hospitalizations for pediatric asthma. Both of these disparities have increased. According to the Agency for Healthcare Research and Quality (AHRQ), health disparities had increased for 80% of measures for Hispanics and 100% of measures for the poor.[151]

Decreasing disparities in minority populations will require ongoing evaluation of interventions. It is also important to note that measurement of disparities (and therefore detection of improvement) is a challenge.[152–154]

Health Workforce Education

Despite predictions of large demographic shifts in the United States (47% of the population will be underrepresented minorities by 2050), health professions schools have not changed much in the past 30 years. Hispanics make up more than 13% of the population but less than 4% of practicing physicians,[155] 7% of first-year medical school enrollments in 2003–2004,[156] and 5.9% of medical school graduates.[157] African American workforce data are similarly dismal, and the numbers are even worse with respect to the Native American population.[155–157] Arguments for the importance of workforce diversity are abundant in the medical literature, but means to achieve it are not obvious. Given our current knowledge of the pipeline, it is critically important to devise effective means.

There are projections of a 16% increase (5 million) in the number of college-age youth between the ages of 18 and 24 by 2015, and 1.6 million will be attending college. Compared with the baby boom students, 80% of the increase will be non-white, and close to 50% will be Hispanic. Examination of factors affecting college-bound rates for students (family income, race, and participation in college preparation programs) paints a picture that is not bright. Students from low-income households (<$30,000/year) are about 20% less likely to attend college than students from high-income (>$60,000/year) families. Because minorities have disproportionately low socioeconomic status, even with the dramatic increase in the college age group, those actually attending college will be a small fraction of that growth.[158]

Other factors during the K–12 years affect the low rate of college-attendance by minorities. These include stereotyping, lower expectations, fear of not fitting in with peers, lack of minority mentors and teachers, academic segregation (minority students selected to less rigorous curricula), and discrimination by and bias of teachers. Several scholars, including Claude Steele, Geoffrey Cohen, and Richard Sande, have examined these factors, but more research needs to be done to understand better what causes "achievement gaps" between whites and minorities.[159–161]

Another contributor to the paucity of minority health professionals is the many legal challenges to affirmative action in recent years. In states that have had legal challenges, there have been dramatic decreases in medical school enrollment between 1995 and 2001. The decrease was as much as 64.3% in Mississippi.[162,163]

It is not surprising that, while the African American population increased to 12.3% of the total population in 2000, the fraction of African American physicians was 4.4% of the practicing physicians, a 0.9% increase from 1990.[156] In coming decades, we are likely to see several new health professions schools, while existing schools are likely to increase class sizes to meet predicted health workforce shortages. It is critical that schools focus on addressing the shortage of minority healthcare providers. It is also crucial to develop comprehensive approaches to improving K–12 and college programs (including financial aid) to prepare minority students to succeed in the health professions.

Cultural Competence and Trust

Trust and distrust play significant roles in the interactions of racial and ethnic minorities within the healthcare system and the providers. Boulware and colleagues demonstrated that 71% of respondents trusted physicians and 70% trusted hospitals, but only 28% trusted their health insurance plans.[164] Black respondents were less likely to trust physicians than white respondents and more likely to trust their health insurance plans. Blacks were more likely than whites to be concerned about personal privacy and the potential for harmful experimentation in hospitals.[164] A national telephone survey about participation in clinical research revealed that African Americans were less likely than white respondents to trust that their physicians would fully explain research participation and more likely to believe that their physicians could expose them to unnecessary risks.[165] To some degree this may reflect the legacy of the Tuskegee experiment, but other factors play a role as well, including provider's language and patients' perception of racism.[166–168]

Communication and Disparities

Health communication is "the study and use of communication strategies to inform and influence individual and community decisions that enhance health."[169] It is one of the *Healthy People 2010* focus areas. Health communication can influence behavioral changes in individuals, groups, and communities.[170] It has been shown that patients recall as little as half of what providers tell them in clinical encounters.[171–174] Thus, high-quality educational materials that complement and supplement the clinical encounter are essential to patient health promotion and disease self-management. Effective health communication must take many factors into account, including behavior and communication theory, culture, and literacy of the target audience.[175–178] In addition, differences in information-seeking behaviors exist in different populations.[179–182]

Health Literacy

Health literacy is the degree to which individuals have the capacity to obtain, process, and understand health information and services necessary to make appropriate decisions about their health.[183] Individuals of low socioeconomic status and racial/ethnic minority populations are more likely to have limited health literacy skills.[183,184] Estimates from the 1992 Adult Literacy Study suggest that 90 million American adults have literacy skills below high school level and may lack the needed literacy skills to use effectively the U.S. health system.[173,184] There is a need for plain language interventions targeting low literacy populations that teach chronic disease risk factors and promote screening and disease prevention.[170,185,186]

Limited English Proficiency

In our multicultural society, English is often not the primary language spoken in the home. According to the 2005 American Community Survey by the U.S. Census Bureau, 23 million individuals speak English less than "very well." It is essential that important health information be made available in appropriate languages to reach this population.[187] Title VI of the Civil Rights Act states that:

> No person in the United States shall, on the ground of race, color, or national origin, be excluded from participation in, be denied the benefits of, or be subjected to discrimination under any program or activity receiving Federal financial assistance.[188]

Current standards require that healthcare providers provide culturally and linguistically appropriate services to all patients; this has been associated with better patient outcomes.[189,190] With the provision of professional interpreters, hemoglobin A1c values, other laboratory results, and complication rates for non-English-speaking diabetic patients were as good as those for individuals who spoke English.[191] When translating and interpreting material from English to another language, it is essential to ensure accuracy in not only the transmission of words but also in the transmission of cultural messages and analogies. Inaccurate translation and interpretation can be harmful to patients.[192–194]

Health Information Targeting Racial/Ethnic Minority Populations

More information is needed about the presentation of health information in the media, specifically targeting minority populations. Hoffman-Goetz and Friedman found that cancer was covered less frequently and with lower readability in ethnic minority media compared to mainstream print media.[195] Duerksen and colleagues discovered that readers of African American and Hispanic women's magazines are exposed to less health promotion advertising and more health diminishing advertising. They suggest that this may in some way contribute to racial disparities in health behaviors and health status.[196] Social marketing can be effectively used to develop culturally innovative chronic disease interventions.[197-199]

Health Information and Technology

In addition to disparities in health, health care, and health outcomes, disparities exist in how different populations access and use health information and how they use technology to learn about health. With the increasing accessibility of health information on the Internet, it is often assumed that all patients have equal access to information. However, disparities exist in the access of different populations to important health information. The term **digital divide** can be used to describe these disparities in access to health information.[181,200] Several programs and projects have been developed to eliminate these disparities.[170,201-205] One, the National Cancer Institute Digital Divide Project, tests innovative strategies to help underserved populations gain access to and effectively use health information, make informed health-related decisions, prevent disease, and promote health.[179]

Environmental Disparities

There are significant disparities in exposure to harmful environmental factors. These usually occur in urban settings and affect those of low socioeconomic status. A large proportion of those subject to these disparities are ethnic minorities. The "environmental justice" or "environmental equity" movement strives to create cleaner environments for the most polluted communities and diminish disparities of environmental exposures and related health risks suffered by racial/ethnic minorities and/or low-income populations in cities.[206] Morello-Froshch, working with Lopez and Jesdale, determined that estimated cancer risks associated with ambient air toxins were highest in residential tracts of metropolitan areas that are highly segregated and that disparities between racial/ethnic groups were greater in more segregated metropolitan areas.[207,208]

Solutions for the Reduction/Elimination of Health Disparities

Reduction or elimination of health disparities requires effective interventions. Strategies for developing these interventions should identify problems

and context, develop/evaluate solutions and test them in pilot studies of efficacy. When interventions are proven effective, they should be implemented
on a large scale and evaluated by following trends in disparities.

Elimination of health disparities will require interdisciplinary efforts.
Effective interventions must be interwoven into clinical care, health promo-
tion/disease prevention, workforce education, research, and policy.

Successful features of interventions include the use of multifaceted,
intense approaches; culturally and linguistically appropriate methods;
improved access to care; establishment of partnerships with stakeholders;
and community involvement. The usefulness of many studies is limited by
lack of controls, lack of randomization, failure to focus on the most important
contributing factors, measures of appropriateness and quality of care and
health outcomes, and prioritization of dissemination efforts.[209]

Improving Clinical Care

Reduction of disparities in clinical care requires improvement of the quality of care of all patients. Clinical care protocols and algorithms can stan-
dardize care and ensure equal care for racial/ethnic minority patients.
Community-based programs, including faith-based initiatives can play a
significant role in improving the health care received by minority patients.
They can play a role in improved health education and can bridge the
chasm between communities and academic medicine. Health promotion
and disease prevention efforts in community settings can lead to increased
dissemination and implementation of effective interventions.[11,140,209–213]
Improved health literacy and health behaviors (such as those focused on
health communication/patient education) also have a role in improving
clinical patient care.

Improving Health Promotion/Disease Prevention

Community-based health promotion and disease prevention programs can
significantly affect the health of minority populations. Education of minority
communities about the relationships between their behaviors and their health
and strategies to improve preventive care can reduce disparities.[214] Public
health education and health promotion programs must take into account the
characteristics of the communities they target. In its 2002 report, *Speaking
of Health: Assessing Health Communication Strategies for Diverse Populations*, the IOM states "to maximize communication effectiveness, one should
adapt message formats, sources, channels, and frequency of exposure for different audiences. Factors such as age, gender, race/ethnicity, and sexual ori-

entation all draw on different interactions with the world and lead to different understandings regarding what is important and what is appropriate."[170] The associations between health literacy and health behaviors as well as health status are well documented.[215,216] Community interventions should address these as well.

Improving Diversity in the Healthcare Workforce

The proportions of racial/ethnic minority providers and trainees in the health professions and related research is very low compared with their representation in the general population.[217,218] Racial/ethnic minorities are more likely to serve underserved communities once they complete their training.[217,219] To improve access to care for underserved populations, it is imperative to increase the minority workforce in health professions.[220] This requires a focus on early recruitment, retention, and support throughout training and career development.[221-225] Programs that encourage racial/ethnic minorities to consider health professions target children as young as kindergarten and are an important part of efforts to increase the number of minority providers available to care for the growing minority population.[226] Throughout elementary, middle, and high school, children should be exposed to health professionals and experiences in biomedical research. Developing a "pipeline" that fosters the development of minority healthcare professionals is a useful strategy for reducing disparities.[227-230]

Improving Patient–Provider Communication

Cultural differences between providers and patients affect patient–provider relationships. How patients feel about the quality of that relationship is directly linked to patient satisfaction, adherence, and subsequent health outcomes.[231-233] It has been demonstrated that doctors are more likely to ascribe negative racial stereotypes to minority patients, even when differences in minority and nonminority patients' education, income, and personality characteristics were considered.[234] Physicians were also more likely to make negative comments when discussing minority patients' cases during rounds or with other colleagues.[235] In addition, minority patients were more likely to perceive disrespectful treatment in medical encounters.[236] Interventions to improve provider's communication skills with diverse patient populations exist. Programs/education to improve patient–provider education has primarily focused on providers. Interventions targeting patients may also be an effective way to reduce disparities that stem from patient–provider communication issues.

Improving Workforce Cultural Competency

Cultural competency and health disparities education is essential for practicing healthcare professionals and health professions students.[192,237] A variety of models and methods exist to foster this knowledge, but serious challenges remain.[238,239] Effective courses and resources on these issues are essential to train a cadre of health professionals aware of and concerned about the effects of culture and disparities on the health of our nation and their patients.[45] Accrediting bodies can play a useful role by requiring inclusion of cultural competency education in all undergraduate and graduate medical education.

Provision of effective multilingual care is a challenge addressed by the use of interpreters; however, healthcare providers often receive little to no formal training on how to most effectively use the services of interpreters in medical encounters. Proper use of interpreters may improve communication, clinical care, and outcomes in the care of patients in outpatient settings. Training in interpreter use is associated with more frequent use of professional interpreters, comfort level of providers, and greater patient satisfaction with the care provided.[2,8]

A big challenge to the adoption of cultural competency education is that no single method or body of knowledge has been proven to be most effective for educating health professionals and trainees in cultural competency.[238–241]

Research

Health disparities research will be important in eliminating health disparities. The initial phase of descriptive studies describing the existence and magnitude of disparities has reached the point where studies addressing community needs assessment and development of intervention strategies and evaluation are now needed. Effective intervention studies will require the training of a cadre of researchers. Funding agencies must focus on disparities interventions as a priority.

Policy

While sound health services and community-based research are essential in the fight against health disparities, the subject cannot be addressed only through improved care and research. It is imperative that legislators and policy makers address environmental and social structures that contribute to the existence and persistence of racial and ethnic differences in health and health care. Universal health care and additional policy initiatives for social change and the eradication of poverty are essential to bring about fundamental changes that can reduce or eliminate health disparities.

SUMMARY

Poor health and health care disproportionately affect minority populations in the 21st century. The causes of disparities are diverse and include system, patient, and provider-dependent factors. Healthcare providers can play a significant role in improving the health and health care of vulnerable populations. It is important that individuals from all segments of society actively pursue viable solutions so that all members of society can enjoy the best health possible.

In Paul Farmer's book *Pathologies of Power*, he argues that ". . . all who profess even a passing interest in human rights . . . or who wish to be considered humane have ample cause to consider what it means to be sick and poor in the era of globalization and scientific advancement."[242] He went on further to state that "since a physician has access to medicine and supplies he must work on behalf of the victims" (interpreted in his definition as those who suffer from the lack of the most basic human right, the right to survive). He wonders why physicians therefore are not more "deeply involved in pressing for social and economic right." Although Paul Farmer works primarily in developing countries, the same principles apply to our country where many segments of the population have lower life expectancies than citizens of countries that are much poorer. One would think that there would be enough outrage to justify a unified effort from all health professions. Professional organizations and practitioners must unite to seek comprehensive systemic solutions to ensure that everyone—regardless of race, education, or socioeconomic status—will expect that their health care (and the system) provides them the opportunity to achieve their potential for a good and healthy life.

RESOURCES

A vast number of resources exist on health disparities and minority health. A selected list follows.

- U.S. Department of Health and Human Services, Office of Minority Health: http://www.omhrc.gov/
- Agency of Health Research and Quality: http://www.ahrq.gov
- Kaiser Family Foundation: http://www.kff.org/
- The Commonwealth Fund: http://www.cmwf.org/
- Disparities Solution Center, Massachusetts General Hospital: http://www.massgeneral.org/disparitiessolutions/
- Finding Answers: Disparities Research for Change: http://www.solvingdisparities.org/
- Various Disparities Research Centers and EXPORT Centers

REFERENCES

1. Savitt TL. *Medicine and slavery: the diseases and health care of Blacks in antebellum Virginia*. Urbana: University of Illinois Press; 2002.
2. Savitt TL. *Race and medicine in nineteenth- and early-twentieth-century America*. Kent, OH: Kent State University Press; 2007.
3. Randall VR. *Dying while Black*. Dayton, OH: Seven Principles Press; 2006.
4. Braveman P. Health disparities and health equity: concepts and measurement. *Annu Rev Public Health*. 2006;27:167–194.
5. Braveman PA, Cubbin C, Egerter S, et al. Socioeconomic status in health research: one size does not fit all. *JAMA*. 2005;294:2879–2888.
6. Smedley BD, Stith AY, Nelson AR, Institute of Medicine (U.S.). Committee on Understanding and Eliminating Racial and Ethnic Disparities in Health Care. *Unequal Treatment: Confronting Racial and Ethnic Disparities in Health Care*. Washington, DC: National Academy Press; 2003.
7. U.S. Department of Health and Human Services. *Healthy People 2010: National Health Promotion and Disease Prevention Objectives* (conference edition in 2 volumes). Washington, DC: Author; 2000.
8. U.S. Department of Health and Human Services: *Eliminating Health Disparities in the United States*. Rockville, MD: Health Resources Services Administration; 2001.
9. NIH Working Group on Health Disparities. Draft Trans-NIH Strategic Research Plan on Health Disparities. National Institutes of Health. 2000.
10. Health Policy Institute of Ohio. *Understanding Health Disparities*. Columbus, OH: Author; 2004.
11. Krieger N, Barbeau EM, Soobader MJ. Class matters: U.S. versus U.K. measures of occupational disparities in access to health services and health status in the 2000 U.S. National Health Interview Survey. *Int J Health Serv*. 2005;35:213–236.
12. Cartwright E, Schow D, Herrera S, et al. Using participatory research to build effective type 2 diabetes interventions: the process of advocacy among female Hispanic farm workers and their families in Southeast Idaho. *Women Health*. 2006;43:89–109.
13. Taimela S, Läärä E, Malmivaara A, et al. Self-reported health problems and sickness absence in different age groups predominantly engaged in physical work. *Occup Environ Med*. 2007;64:739–746.
14. Treaster C, Hawley SR, Paschal AM, Molgaard CA, St Romain T. Addressing health disparities in highly specialized minority populations: case study of Mexican Mennonite farm workers. *J Community Health*. 2006;31:113–122.
15. Tsai JH, Salazar MK. Occupational hazards and risks faced by Chinese immigrant restaurant workers. *Fam Community Health*. 2007;30:S71–S79.
16. Carrasquillo O, Carrasquillo AI, Shea S: Health insurance coverage of immigrants living in the United States: Differences by citizenship status and country of origin. *Am J Public Health*. 2000;90:917–923.
17. Prudent N, Ruwe M, Meyers A, Capitman J: *Health-Care Access for Children of Immigrants*. New York: McGraw-Hill; 2006.
18. Casey MM, Blewett LA, Call KT: Providing health care to Latino immigrants: Community-based efforts in the rural Midwest. *Am J Public Health*. 2004;94:1709–1711.
19. Guendelman S, Angulo V, Wier M, Oman D. Overcoming the odds: Access to care for immigrant children in working poor families in California. *Matern Child Health J*. 2005;9:351–362.

20. Jacobs EA, Lauderdale DS, Meltzer D, Shorey JM, Levinson W, Thisted RA. Impact of interpreter services on delivery of health care to limited-English-proficient patients. *J Gen Intern Med.* 2001;16:468–474.

21. Sudore RL, Mehta KM, Simonsick EM, et al. Limited literacy in older people and disparities in health and healthcare access. *J Am Geriatr Soc.* 2006;54:770–776.

22. Muennig P. Health returns associated with education interventions targeted at African American Males. In *Symposium on the Social Costs of Inadequate Education.* New York: Columbia University; 2006.

23. Williams DR, Collins C. Racial residential segregation: A fundamental cause of racial disparities in health. *Public Health Rep.* 2001;116:404–416.

24. Massey DS, Denton NA. *American Apartheid: Segregation and the Making of the Underclass.* Boston: Harvard University Press; 1994.

25. Green C. Assessing and managing pain. In: Satcher D, Pamies RJ, Woelfl NN, eds. *Multicultural Medicine and Health Disparities.* New York, McGraw-Hill; 2006: 343–360.

26. Baicker K, Chandra A, Skinner JS. Geographic variation in health care and the problem of measuring racial disparities. *Perspect Biol Med.* 2005;48:S42–S53.

27. Ku L, Matani S. Left out: Immigrants' access to health care and insurance. *Health Aff (Millwood).* 2001;20:247–256.

28. Borrayo EA, Guarnaccia CA. Differences in Mexican-born and U.S.-born women of Mexican descent regarding factors related to breast cancer screening behaviors. *Health Care Women Int.* 2000;21:599–613.

29. Echeverria SE, Carrasquillo O: The roles of citizenship status, acculturation, and health insurance in breast and cervical cancer screening among immigrant women. *Med Care.* 2006;44:788–792.

30. Garbers S, Jessop DJ, Foti H, Uribelarrea M, Chiasson MA. Barriers to breast cancer screening for low-income Mexican and Dominican women in New York City. *J Urban Health.* 2003;80:81–91.

31. Mayo RM, Erwin DO, Spitler HD. Implications for breast and cervical cancer control for Latinas in the rural South: a review of the literature. *Cancer Control.* 2003;10:60–68.

32. Loue S. Access to health care and the undocumented alien. *J Leg Med.* 1992;13: 271–332.

33. Loue S, Faust M, Bunce A. The effect of immigration and welfare reform legislation on immigrants' access to health care, Cuyahoga, and Lorain Counties. *J Immigr Health.* 2000;2:23–30.

34. U.S. Census Bureau. *Populations Projections of the United States, by Age, Sex, Race, and Hispanic Origin: 1993 to 2050.* Washington, DC: Author; 1993.

35. Farrell LV, Cox MG, Geller ES. Prompting safety-belt use in the context of a belt-use law: The flash-for life revisited. *J Safety Res.* 2007;38:407–411.

36. Rivkees SA. No trans fat for you! New York City's bold step. *J Pediatr Endocrinol Metab.* 2007;20:1–3.

37. Ruminski D, Klink H. School-based health centers: a model for delivery of adolescent health care in Portland, Oregon. *J Ambul Care Manage.* 1993;16:29–41.

38. Salas-Lopez D, Holmes LJ, Mouzon DM, Soto-Greene M. Cultural competency in New Jersey: Evolution from planning to law. *J Health Care Poor Underserved.* 2007;18:35–43.

39. Shields M. Smoking bans: Influence on smoking prevalence. *Health Rep.* 2007;18:9–24.

40. Meisler A. All aboard. *Workforce Management*. 2004:30–34. All aboard: Beset by rising insurance costs, the Union Pacific Railroad is saving money by pulling—not yanking—its employees toward better health. It isn't interested in panicking and calling in the Health Police. July 1, 2004.

41. Smerd J. Smokers are being left out in the cold. Some companies won't hire smokers. But should you put it in writing, or not? *Financial Week*. 2007:1. Available at: http://www.financialweek.com/apps/pbcs.dll/article?AID=/20071119/REG/71119 0313. Accessed May 27, 2008.

42. Beaudette M. 2 tickets for large fliers, not new rule; Southwest denies it changed policy. The *Washington Times*. Thursday June 20, 2002. Pg A01.

43. Taira DA, Safran DG, Seto TB, Rogers WH, Tarlov AR. The relationship between patient income and physician discussion of health risk behaviors. *JAMA*. 1997;278:1412–1417.

44. Satcher D. Our commitment to eliminate racial and ethnic health disparities. *Yale J Health Policy Law Ethics*. 2001;1:1–14.

45. Satcher D, Pamies RJ, Woelfl NN. *Multicultural medicine and health disparities*. New York: McGraw-Hill; 2006.

46. Rosenbaum S, Markus S, Darnell J. U.S. Civil Rights Policy and Access to Health Care by Minority Americans: Implications for a Changing Health Care System. *Med Care Res Rev*. 2000;57;236–259.

47. Rosenblatt R, Law S, Rosenbaum S. *Law and the American Health Care System*. Foundation Press. New York. 1997.

48. Smith DB. *Health Care Divided: Race and Healing a Nation*. Ann Arbor, Michigan: University of Michigan Press. 1999.

49. Perez TE. The Civil Rights Dimension of Racial and Ethnic Disparities in Health Status. In Institute of Medicine, *Unequal Medicine*. 2003;626–663.

50. Smith DB. Racial and Ethnic Health Disparities and the Unfinished Civil Rights Agenda. *Health Affairs*. 2005;24(2):317–324

51. U.S. Commission on Civil Rights. The Health Care Challenge: Acknowledging Disparity, Confronting Discrimination, and Ensuring Equality Volume I, The Role of Governmental and Private Health Care Programs and Initiatives. Washington DC: No. 005-902-00062-2. September 1999. Available at: http://www.usccr.gov/pubs/pubsndx.htm

52. Outterson K. Tragedy and remedy: Reparations for disparities in black health. *DePaul J Health Care Law*. 2005;9:735–791.

53. Geiger H. Medical care. In Levy BS, Sidel VW, eds. *Social Injustice and Public Health*. Oxford, UK: Oxford University Press; 2006:207–219.

54. Flexner A. Medical Education in the United States and Canada. Bulletin Number Four (The Flexner Report). 1910. New York: The Carnegie Foundation for the Advancement of Teaching.

55. National Center for Health Statistics. *Table 7, Health, United States, 2006 with Chartbook on Trends in the Health of Americans*. Hyattsville, MD: Author; 2006.

56. Hessol NA, Fuentes-Afflick E. Ethnic differences in neonatal and postneonatal mortality. *Pediatrics*. 2005;115:e44–e51.

57. Healy AJ, Malone FD, Sullivan LM, et al. Early access to prenatal care: Implications for racial disparity in perinatal mortality. *Obstet Gynecol*. 2006;107:625–631.

58. Singh GK, Yu SM. Pregnancy outcomes among Asian Americans. *Asian Am Pac Isl J Health*. 1993;1:63–78.

59. Hamilton BE, Minino AM, Martin JA, Kochanek KD, Strobino DM, Guyer B. Annual summary of vital statistics: 2005. *Pediatrics*. 2007;119:345–360.

60. National Center for Health Statistics. *Health, United States, 2004 with Chartbook on Trends in the Health of Americans*. Washington, DC: U.S. Government Printing Office; 2004.

61. Hambidge SJ, Emsermann CB, Federico S, Steiner JF. Disparities in pediatric preventive care in the United States, 1993–2002. *Arch Pediatr Adolesc Med*. 2007;161:30–136.

62. Flores G, Fuentes-Afflick E, Barbot O, et al. The health of Latino children: Urgent priorities, unanswered questions, and a research agenda. *JAMA*. 2002;288:82–90.

63. Brousseau DC, Hoffmann RG, Yauck J, Nattinger AB, Flores G. Disparities for Latino children in the timely receipt of medical care. *Ambul Pediatr*. 2005;5:319–325.

64. Bernard SJ, Paulozzi LJ, Wallace DL. Fatal injuries among children by race and ethnicity—United States, 1999–2002. *MMWR Surveill Summ*. 2007;56:1–16.

65. Pressley JC, Barlow B, Kendig T, Paneth-Pollak R. Twenty-year trends in fatal injuries to very young children: the persistence of racial disparities. *Pediatrics*. 2007;119:e875–e884.

66. Bai Y, Hillemeier MM, Lengerich EJ. Racial/ethnic disparities in symptom severity among children hospitalized with asthma. *J Health Care Poor Underserved*. 2007;18:54–61.

67. Liu LL, Stout JW, Sullivan M, Solet D, Shay DK, Grossman DC. Asthma and bronchiolitis hospitalizations among American Indian children. *Arch Pediatr Adolesc Med*. 2000;154:991–996.

68. McDaniel M, Paxson C, Waldfogel J. Racial disparities in childhood asthma in the United States: Evidence from the National Health Interview Survey, 1997–2003. *Pediatrics*. 2006;117:e868–e877.

69. Milgrom H. Childhood asthma: breakthroughs and challenges. *Adv Pediatr*. 2006;53:55–100.

70. Pearlman DN, Zierler S, Meersman S, Kim HK, Viner-Brown SI, Caron C. Race disparities in childhood asthma: Does where you live matter? *J Natl Med Assoc*. 2006;98:239–247.

71. Quinn K, Shalowitz MU, Berry CA, Mijanovich T, Wolf RL. Racial and ethnic disparities in diagnosed and possible undiagnosed asthma among public-school children in Chicago. *Am J Public Health*. 2006;96:1599–1603.

72. Ferris TG, Kuhlthau K, Ausiello J, Perrin J, Kahn R. Are minority children the last to benefit from a new technology? Technology diffusion and inhaled corticosteroids for asthma. *Med Care*. 2006;44:81–86.

73. Akinbami LJ, LaFleur BJ, Schoendorf KC. Racial and income disparities in childhood asthma in the United States. *Ambul Pediatr*. 2002;2:382–387.

74. Canino G, Koinis-Mitchell D, Ortega AN, McQuaid EL, Fritz GK, Alegria M. Asthma disparities in the prevalence, morbidity, and treatment of Latino children. *Soc Sci Med*. 2006;63:2926–2937.

75. Federico MJ, Liu AH. Overcoming childhood asthma disparities of the inner-city poor. *Pediatr Clin North Am*. 2003;50:655–675, vii.

76. Gold DR, Wright R. Population disparities in asthma. *Annu Rev Public Health*. 2005;26:89–113.5

77. Sin DD, Svenson LW, Cowie RL, Man SF. Can universal access to health care eliminate health inequities between children of poor and nonpoor families? A case study of childhood asthma in Alberta. *Chest*. 2003;124:51–56.

78. Swartz MK, Banasiak NC, Meadows-Oliver M. Barriers to effective pediatric asthma care. *J Pediatr Health Care*. 2005;19:71–79.
79. Ellickson PL, Bird CE, Orlando M, Klein DJ, McCaffrey DF. Social context and adolescent health behavior: does school-level smoking prevalence affect students' subsequent smoking behavior? *J Health Soc Behav*. 2003;44:525–535.
80. Ellickson PL, Orlando M, Tucker JS, Klein DJ. From adolescence to young adulthood: racial/ethnic disparities in smoking. *Am J Public Health*. 2004;94:293–299.
81. Ellickson PL, Tucker JS, Klein DJ. High-risk behaviors associated with early smoking: results from a 5-year follow-up. *J Adolesc Health*. 2001;28:465–473.
82. Juarez P, Schlundt DG, Goldzweig I, Stinson N Jr. A conceptual framework for reducing risky teen driving behaviors among minority youth. *Inj Prev*. 2006;12(suppl 1):i49–i55.
83. Bachman JG, Wallace JM Jr., O'Malley PM, Johnston LD, Kurth CL, Neighbors HW. Racial/ethnic differences in smoking, drinking, and illicit drug use among American high school seniors, 1976–89. *Am J Public Health*. 1991;81:372–377.
84. Wallace JM Jr., Bachman JG, O'Malley PM, Johnston LD, Schulenberg JE, Cooper SM. Tobacco, alcohol, and illicit drug use: racial and ethnic differences among U.S. high school seniors, 1976–2000. *Public Health Rep*. 2002;117(suppl 1):S67–S75.
85. Browne DC, Clubb PA, Aubrecht AM, Jackson M. Minority health risk behaviors: An introduction to research on sexually transmitted diseases, violence, pregnancy prevention and substance use. *Matern Child Health J*. 2001;5:215–224.
86. Harris KM, Gordon-Larsen P, Chantala K, Udry JR. Longitudinal trends in race/ethnic disparities in leading health indicators from adolescence to young adulthood. *Arch Pediatr Adolesc Med*. 2006;160:74–81.
87. Cuffe SP, Waller JL, Addy CL, et al. A longitudinal study of adolescent mental health service use. *J Behav Health Serv Res*. 2001;28:1–11.
88. Kodjo CM, Auinger P. Predictors for emotionally distressed adolescents to receive mental health care. *J Adolesc Health*. 2004;35:368–373.
89. Padgett DK, Patrick C, Burns BJ, Schlesinger HJ, Cohen J. The effect of insurance benefit changes on use of child and adolescent outpatient mental health services. *Med Care*. 1993;31:96–110.
90. Ringel JS, Sturm R. National estimates of mental health utilization and expenditures for children in 1998. *J Behav Health Serv Res*. 2001;28:319–333.
91. Cossrow N, Falkner B. Race/ethnic issues in obesity and obesity-related comorbidities. *J Clin Endocrinol Metab*. 2004;89:2590–2594.
92. National Center for Health Statistics. *1999–2002 National Health and Nutrition Examination Survey (NHANES)*. Washington, DC: U.S. Government Printing Office; 2005.
93. National Center for Health Statistics. *1999–2003 National Health Interview Survey (NHIS)*. Washington, DC: U.S. Government Printing Office; 2005.
94. Arslanian SA. Metabolic differences between Caucasian and African-American children and the relationship to type 2 diabetes mellitus. *J Pediatr Endocrinol Metab*. 2002;15(suppl 1):509–517.
95. Arslanian SA, Bacha F, Saad R, Gungor N. Family history of type 2 diabetes is associated with decreased insulin sensitivity and an impaired balance between insulin sensitivity and insulin secretion in white youth. *Diabetes Care*. 2005;28:115–119.

96. Dabelea D, Pettitt DJ, Jones KL, Arslanian SA. Type 2 diabetes mellitus in minority children and adolescents. An emerging problem. *Endocrinol Metab Clin North Am*. 1999;28:709–729, viii.

97. Gahagan S, Silverstein J. Prevention and treatment of type 2 diabetes mellitus in children, with special emphasis on American Indian and Alaska Native children. American Academy of Pediatrics Committee on Native American Child Health. *Pediatrics*. 2003;112:e328.

98. Gavin JR III. Insulin resistance syndrome: Implications for the African American population. *Endocr Pract*. 2003;9(suppl 2):28–30.

99. Carnethon MR, Palaniappan LP, Burchfiel CM, Brancati FL, Fortmann SP. Serum insulin, obesity, and the incidence of type 2 diabetes in black and white adults: The atherosclerosis risk in communities study: 1987–1998. *Diabetes Care*. 2002;25:1358–1364.

100. Marshall JA, Hamman RF, Baxter J, et al. Ethnic differences in risk factors associated with the prevalence of non-insulin-dependent diabetes mellitus. The San Luis Valley Diabetes Study. *Am J Epidemiol*. 1993;137:706–718.

101. Robbins JM, Vaccarino V, Zhang H, Kasl SV. Excess type 2 diabetes in African-American women and men aged 40–74 and socioeconomic status: Evidence from the Third National Health and Nutrition Examination Survey. *J Epidemiol Community Health*. 2000;54:839–845.

102. Lee AJ, Hiscock RJ, Wein P, Walker SP, Permezel M. Gestational diabetes mellitus: clinical predictors and long-term risk of developing type 2 diabetes: A retrospective cohort study using survival analysis. *Diabetes Care*. 2007;30:878–883.

103. Barker DJ. Fetal growth and adult disease. *Br J Obstet Gynaecol*. 1992;99:275–276.

104. Barker DJ, Hales CN, Fall CH, Osmond C, Phipps K, Clark PM. Type 2 (non-insulin-dependent) diabetes mellitus, hypertension and hyperlipidaemia (syndrome X): Relation to reduced fetal growth. *Diabetologia*. 1993;36:62–67.

105. Davis JN, Weigensberg MJ, Shaibi GQ, et al. Influence of breastfeeding on obesity and type 2 diabetes risk factors in Latino youth with a family history of type 2 diabetes. *Diabetes Care*. 2007;30:784–789.

106. Melamed S, Shirom A, Toker S, Shapira I. Burnout and risk of type 2 diabetes: A prospective study of apparently healthy employed persons. *Psychosom Med*. 2006;68:863–869.

107. Elmasry A, Lindberg E, Berne C, et al. Sleep-disordered breathing and glucose metabolism in hypertensive men: a population-based study. *J Intern Med*. 2001;249:153–161.

108. Lindberg E, Berne C, Franklin KA, Svensson M, Janson C. Snoring and daytime sleepiness as risk factors for hypertension and diabetes in women—A population-based study. *Respir Med*. 2006;101:1283–1290.

109. Yeh HC, Punjabi NM, Wang NY, Pankow JS, Duncan BB, Brancati FL. Vital capacity as a predictor of incident type 2 diabetes: The Atherosclerosis Risk in Communities study. *Diabetes Care*. 28:1472–1479.

110. Carnethon MR, Jacobs DR Jr., Sidney S, Liu K. Influence of autonomic nervous system dysfunction on the development of type 2 diabetes: The CARDIA study. *Diabetes Care*. 2003;26:3035–3041.

111. Carnethon MR, Kinder LS, Fair JM, Stafford RS, Fortmann SP. Symptoms of depression as a risk factor for incident diabetes: Findings from the National Health and Nutrition Examination Epidemiologic Follow-up Study, 1971–1992. *Am J Epidemiol*. 2003;158:416–423.

112. Abate N, Chandalia M. The impact of ethnicity on type 2 diabetes. *J Diabetes Complications*. 2003;17:39–58.

113. Harris EL, Sherman SH, Georgopoulos A. Black-white differences in risk of developing retinopathy among individuals with type 2 diabetes. *Diabetes Care*. 1999;22:779–783.

114. Heisler M, Smith DM, Hayward RA, Krein SL, Kerr EA. Racial disparities in diabetes care processes, outcomes, and treatment intensity. *Med Care*. 2003;41: 1221–1232.

115. Heisler MB, Rust G, Pattillo R, Dubois AM. Improving health, eliminating disparities: Finding solutions for better health care for all populations. *Ethn Dis*. 2005;15:S1–S4.

116. LeMaster JW, Chanetsa F, Kapp JM, Waterman BM. Racial disparities in diabetes-related preventive care: Results from the Missouri Behavioral Risk Factor Surveillance System. *Prev Chronic Dis*. 2006;3:A86.

117. Schneider EC, Zaslavsky AM, Epstein AM. Racial disparities in the quality of care for enrollees in medicare managed care. *JAMA*. 2002;287:1288–1294.

118. Cowie CC, Port FK, Wolfe RA, Savage PJ, Moll PP, Hawthorne VM. Disparities in incidence of diabetic end-stage renal disease according to race and type of diabetes. *N Engl J Med*. 1989;321:1074–1079.

119. Karter AJ, Ferrara A, Liu JY, Moffet HH, Ackerson LM, Selby JV. Ethnic disparities in diabetic complications in an insured population. *JAMA*. 2002;287: 2519–2527.

120. Kirk JK, D'Agostino RB Jr., Bell RA, et al. Disparities in HbA1c levels between African-American and non-Hispanic white adults with diabetes: A meta-analysis. *Diabetes Care*. 2006;29:2130–2136.

121. Quandt SA, Bell RA, Snively BM, et al. Ethnic disparities in glycemic control among rural older adults with type 2 diabetes. *Ethn Dis*. 2005;15:656–663.

122. National Center for Health Statistics. *Table 77, Health, United States, 2007 with Chartbook on Trends in the Health of Americans*. Hyattsville, MD: Author; 2007.

123. National Center for Health Statistics. *Table 80, Health, United States, 2007 with Chartbook on Trends in the Health of Americans*. Hyattsville, MD: Author; 2007.

124. National Center for Health Statistics. *Table 86, Health, United States, 2005 with Chartbook on Trends in the Health of Americans*. Hyattsville, MD: Author; 2005.

125. Goff DC Jr., Bertoni AG, Kramer H, et al. Dyslipidemia prevalence, treatment, and control in the Multi-Ethnic Study of Atherosclerosis (MESA): Gender, ethnicity, and coronary artery calcium. *Circulation*. 2006;113:647–656.

126. Woodard LD, Kressin NR, Petersen LA. Is lipid-lowering therapy underused by African Americans at high risk of coronary heart disease within the VA health care system? *Am J Public Health*. 2004;94:2112–2117.

127. Ananthakrishnan AN, Schellhase KG, Sparapani RA, Laud PW, Neuner JM. Disparities in colon cancer screening in the Medicare population. *Arch Intern Med*. 2007;167:258–264.

128. Koroukian SM, Xu F, Dor A, Cooper GS. Colorectal cancer screening in the elderly population: Disparities by dual Medicare-Medicaid enrollment status. *Health Serv Res*. 2006;41:2136–2154.

129. Shokar NK, Carlson CA, Weller SC. Prevalence of colorectal cancer testing and screening in a multiethnic primary care population. *J Community Health*. 2007;32:311–323.

130. Chen JY, Diamant A, Pourat N, Kagawa-Singer M. Racial/ethnic disparities in the use of preventive services among the elderly. *Am J Prev Med*. 2005;29:388–395.

131. Influenza vaccination coverage among adults aged ≥ 50 years and pneumococcal vaccination coverage among adults aged ≥ 65 years—United States, 2002. *MMWR*. 2003;52:987.

132. Chen JY, Fox SA, Cantrell CH, Stockdale SE, Kagawa-Singer M. Health disparities and prevention: Racial/ethnic barriers to flu vaccinations. *J Community Health*. 2007;32:5–20.

133. Rangel MC, Shoenbach VJ, Weigle KA, Hogan VK, Strauss RP, Bangdiwala SI. Racial and ethnic disparities in influenza vaccination among elderly adults. *J Gen Intern Med*. 2005;20:426–431.

134. Cromwell J, McCall NT, Burton J, Urato C. Race/ethnic disparities in utilization of lifesaving technologies by Medicare ischemic heart disease beneficiaries. *Med Care*. 2005;43:330–337.

135. Kales HC, Mellow AM. Race and depression: Does race affect the diagnosis and treatment of late-life depression? *Geriatrics*. 2006;61:18–21.

136. Kales HC, Neighbors HW, Blow FC, et al. Race, gender, and psychiatrists' diagnosis and treatment of major depression among elderly patients. *Psychiatr Serv*. 2005;56:721–728.

137. Parker C, Philp I. Screening for cognitive impairment among older people in black and minority ethnic groups. *Age Ageing*. 2004;33:447–452.

138. Chui HC, Gatz M. Cultural diversity in Alzheimer disease: The interface between biology, belief, and behavior. *Alzheimer Dis Assoc Disord*. 2005;19:250–255.

139. Guerrero M Jr., Heller PL. Sociocultural limits in informed consent in dementia research. *Alzheimer Dis Assoc Disord*. 2003;17(suppl 1):S26–30.

140. States RA, Susman WM, Riquelme LF, Godwin EM, Greer E. Community health education: Reaching ethnically diverse elders. *J Allied Health*. 2006;35:215–222.

141. Volker DL. Control and end-of-life care: Does ethnicity matter? *Am J Hospice Palliative Med*. 2005;22:442–446.

142. Newman J, Davidhizar RE, Fordham P. Multi-cultural and multi-ethnic considerations and advanced directives: Developing cultural competency. *J Cultural Diversity*. 2006;13:3.

143. Searight HR, Gafford J. Cultural diversity at the end of life: Issues and guidelines for family physicians. *Am Fam Phys*. 2005;71:515.

144. Levine RS, Foster JE, Fullilove RE, et al. Black-white inequalities in mortality and life expectancy, 1933–1999: Implications for healthy people 2010. *Public Health Rep*. 2001;116:474–483.

145. Feldman RH, Fulwood R. The three leading causes of death in African Americans: Barriers to reducing excess disparity and to improving health behaviors. *J Health Care Poor Underserved*. 1999;10:45–71.

146. Shi L, Macinko J, Starfield B, Politzer R, Xu J. Primary care, race, and mortality in US states. *Soc Sci Med* 61:65–75, 2005

147. Satcher D, Fryer GE Jr., McCann J, Troutman A, Woolf SH, Rust G. What if we were equal? A comparison of the black-white mortality gap in 1960 and 2000. *Health Aff (Millwood)*. 2005;24:459–464.

148. Andrulis DP, Siddiqui NJ, Gantner JL. Preparing racially and ethnically diverse communities for public health emergencies. *Health Aff (Millwood)*. 2007;26:1269–1279.

149. Hsu CE, Mas FS, Jacobson HE, Harris AM, Hunt VI, Nkhoma ET. Public health preparedness of health providers: Meeting the needs of diverse, rural communities. *J Natl Med Assoc.* 2006;98:1784–1791.

150. U.S. Department of Health and Human Services. *Healthy People 2010 Midcourse Review Executive Summary.* Washington, DC: U.S. Government Printing Office; December 2006.

151. U.S. Agency for Healthcare Research and Quality. *National Healthcare Disparities Report, 2005.* Rockville, MD: U.S. Department of Health and Human Services; 2006.

152. Keppel K, Pamuk E, Lynch J, et al. Methodological issues in measuring health disparities. *Vital Health Stat.* 2005;2:1–16.

153. Keppel KG, Pearcy JN. Measuring relative disparities in terms of adverse events. *J Public Health Manag Pract.* 2005;11:479–483.

154. Keppel KG, Pearcy JN, Klein RJ. Measuring progress in Healthy People 2010. *Healthy People 2010 Stat Notes.* 2004;25:1–16.

155. American Association of Medical Colleges. *U.S. Physicians by Race and Ethnicity, 2004.* AAMC Data Warehouse: Minority Physician Database Applicant-Matriculant File, and AMA Physician Masterfile. Washington, DC: Author; 2006.

156. Castillo-Page L, ed. *Minorities in Medical Education: Facts & Figures 2005.* Washington, DC: American Association of Medical Colleges; 2005:24.

157. Kaiser Family Foundation. *Distribution of Medical School Graduates by Race/Ethnicity, 2005.* StateHealthFacts.org. Washington, D.C., Author; 2005.

158. Advisory Committee on Student Financial Assistance. *Access Denied—Restoring the Nation's Commitment to Equal Educational Opportunity.* Washington, DC: U.S. Department of Education; 2001:ix–39.

159. Cohen GL, Steele C. A barrier of mistrust: How negative stereotypes affect cross-race mentoring. In Aronson J, ed. *Improving Academic Achievement: Impact of Psychological Factors on Education.* Boston: Academic Press; 2002:xxvii –395.

160. Perry T, Steele C, Hilliard AG. *Young, Gifted, and Black: Promoting High Achievement Among African-American Students.* Boston: Beacon Press; 2003.

161. Sander R. A systemic analysis of affirmative action in American law schools. *Stanford Law Rev.* 2005;57:367–484.

162. Cohen JJ. The consequences of premature abandonment of affirmative action in medical school admissions. *JAMA.* 2003;289:1143–1149.

163. Morgan RC Jr. Impact of anti-affirmative action on medical school enrollment. *J Natl Med Assoc.* 2001;93:8S–10S.

164. Boulware LE, Cooper LA, Ratner LE, LaVeist TA, Powe NR. Race and trust in the health care system. *Public Health Rep.* 2003;118:358–365.

165. Corbie-Smith G, Thomas SB, St George DM. Distrust, race, and research. *Arch Intern Med.* 2002;162:2458–2463.

166. Adegbembo AO, Tomar SL, Logan HL. Perception of racism explains the difference between Blacks' and Whites' level of healthcare trust. *Ethn Dis.* 2006;16:792–798.

167. Halbert CH, Armstrong K, Gandy OH Jr., Shaker L. Racial differences in trust in health care providers. *Arch Intern Med.* 2006;166:896–901.

168. Stepanikova I, Mollborn S, Cook KS, Thom DH, Kramer RM. Patients' race, ethnicity, language, and trust in a physician. *J Health Soc Behav.* 2006;47:390–405.

169. Arkin EB, National Cancer Institute (U.S.). Office of Cancer Communications. *Making Health Communication Programs Work: A Planner's Guide.* Bethesda, MD: U.S. Department of Health and Human Services; 1989.

170. Institute of Medicine (U.S.). Committee on Communication for Behavior Change in the 21st Century. *Improving the Health of Diverse Populations: Speaking of Health: Assessing Health Communication Strategies for Diverse Populations.* Washington, DC: National Academies Press; 2002.

171. Bertakis KD. The communication of information from physician to patient: a method for increasing patient retention and satisfaction. *J Fam Pract.* 1977;5:217–222.

172. Crane JA. Patient comprehension of doctor-patient communication on discharge from the emergency department. *J Emerg Med.* 1997;15:1–7.

172. Frost MH, Thompson R, Thiemann KB. Importance of format and design in print patient information. *Cancer Pract.* 1999;7:22–27.

173. Schillinger D, Piette J, Grumbach K, et al. Closing the loop: physician communication with diabetic patients who have low health literacy. *Arch Intern Med.* 2003;163:83–90.

174. Doak CC, Doak LG, Root JH. *Teaching patients with low literacy skills.* Philadelphia: J. B. Lippincott; 1996.

175. Ford S, Mai F, Manson A, Rukin N, Dunne F. Diabetes knowledge—Are patients getting the message? *Int J Clin Pract.* 2000;54:535–536.

176. Panja S, Starr B, Colleran KM. Patient knowledge improves glycemic control: Is it time to go back to the classroom? *J Investig Med.* 2005;53:264–266.

177. Povlsen L, Olsen B, Ladelund S. Diabetes in children and adolescents from ethnic minorities: Barriers to education, treatment and good metabolic control. *J Adv Nurs.* 2005;50:576–582.

178. Kreps GL. Disseminating relevant health information to underserved audiences: implications of the Digital Divide Pilot Projects. *J Med Libr Assoc.* 2005;93: S68–73.

179. Kreps GL, Gustafson D, Salovey P, et al. The NCI Digital Divide Pilot Projects: Implications for cancer education. *J Cancer Educ.* 2007;22:S56–60.

180. Lorence D, Park H. Study of education disparities and health information seeking behavior. *Cyberpsychol Behav.* 2007;10:149–151.

181. Lorence DP, Park H, Fox S. Racial disparities in health information access: resilience of the Digital Divide. *J Med Syst.* 2006;30:241–249.

182. Nielsen-Bohlman L, Panzer AM, Kindig DA, Institute of Medicine (U.S.). Committee on Health Literacy. *Health Literacy: A Prescription to End Confusion.* Washington, DC: National Academies Press; 2004.

183. Kutner MA, National Center for Education Statistics. *The Health Literacy of America's Adults: Results from the 2003 National Assessment of Adult Literacy.* Washington, DC: U.S. Department of Education, National Center for Education Statistics; 2006.

184. Rudd RE, Zobel EK, Fanta CH, et al. Asthma: in plain language. *Health Promot Pract.* 2004;5:334–340.

185. Weiss BD, Coyne C. Communicating with patients who cannot read. *N Engl J Med.* 1997;337:272–274.

186. U.S. Census Bureau. Percent of people 5 years and over who speak a language other than English at home. 2005 universe: Population 5 years and over, Table GCT1601. In *2005 American Community Survey.* Washington, DC: U.S. Department of Commerce, Economics and Statistics Administration; 2005.

187. Civil Rights Act of 1964, Title VI. In *Public Law* 88 ed., 1964.
188. Fisher TL, Burnet DL, Huang ES, Chin MH, Cagney KA. Cultural leverage: Interventions using culture to narrow racial disparities in health care. *Med Care Res Rev.* 2007;64:243S–282S.
189. Narayan MC. The national standards for culturally and linguistically appropriate services in health care. *Care Manag J.* 2001;3:77–83.
190. Tocher TM, Larson E. Quality of diabetes care for non-English-speaking patients. A comparative study. *West J Med.* 1998;168:504–511.
191. National Standards for Culturally and Linguistically Appropriate Services in Health Care. *Final Report.* Washington, DC: U.S. Department of Health and Human Services, Office of Minority Health; 2001.
192. Flores G, Laws MB, Mayo SJ, et al. Errors in medical interpretation and their potential clinical consequences in pediatric encounters. *Pediatrics.* 2003;111:6–14.
193. Ngo-Metzger Q, Massagli MP, Clarridge BR, et al. Linguistic and cultural barriers to care. *J Gen Intern Med.* 2003;18:44–52.
194. Hoffmann-Goetz L, Friedman D. Disparities in Coverage of cancer information in ethnic minority and mainstream mass print media. *Ethn Dis.* 2005;15:332–340.
195. Duerksen S, Mikhail A, Torn L, et al. Health disparities and advertising content of women's magazines: A cross sectional study. *BMC Public Health.* 2005;18:85.
196. Albrecht T, Bryant C. Advances in segmentation modeling for health communication and social marketing campaigns. *J Health Commun.* 1996;1:65–80.
197. Freimuth V, Quinn S. The contributions of health communication to eliminating health disparities. *Am J Public Health.* 2004;94:2053–2055.
198. Thackeray R, Neiger B. Using social marketing to develop diabetes self-management education interventions. *Diabetes Educ.* 2002;28:536–540.
199. Renahy E, Chauvin P. Internet uses for health information seeking: A literature review. *Rev Epidemiol Sante Publique.* 2006;54:263–275.
200. Burstin H. Traversing the digital divide. *Health Aff (Millwood).* 2000;19:245–249.
201. Eng TR, Maxfield A, Patrick K, Deering MJ, Ratzan SC, Gustafson DH. Access to health information and support: A public highway or a private road? *JAMA.* 1998;280:1371–1375.
202. Schloman BF. The digital divide: how wide and how deep? *Online J Issues Nurs.* 2004;9:7.
203. Vidyasagar D. Digital divide and digital dividend in the age of information technology. *J Perinatol.* 2006;26:313–315.
204. Whaley KC. America's digital divide: 2000–2003 trends. *J Med Syst* 28:183–195, 2004
205. Urban air pollution and health inequities. A workshop report. *Environ Health Perspect.* 2001;109(suppl 3):357–374.
206. Morello-Frosch R, Lopez R. The riskscape and the color line: Examining the role of segregation in environmental health disparities. *Environ Res.* 2006;102: 181–196.
207. Morello-Frosch R, Jesdale BM. Separate and unequal: residential segregation and estimated cancer risks associated with ambient air toxics in U.S. metropolitan areas. *Environ Health Perspect.* 2006;114:386–393.
208. Cooper LA, Hill MN, Powe NR. Designing and evaluating interventions to eliminate racial and ethnic disparities in health care. *J Gen Intern Med.* 2002; 17:477–486.

209. Farquhar SA, Michael YL, Wiggins N. Building on leadership and social capital to create change in 2 urban communities. *Am J Public Health*. 2005;95:596–601.

210. Jones L, Wells K. Strategies for academic and clinician engagement in community-participatory partnered research. *JAMA*. 2007;297:407–410.

211. Sherer JL. Neighbor to neighbor. Community health workers educate their own. *Hosp Health Netw*. 1994;68:52–56.

212. Mendel P, Meredith LS, Schoenbaum M, Sherbourne CD, Wells KB. Interventions in organizational and community context: A framework for building evidence on dissemination and implementation in health services research. *Adm Policy Ment Health*. 2007;35:21–37.

213. Daniels NA, Juarbe T, Moreno-John G, Perez-Stable EJ. Effectiveness of adult vaccination programs in faith-based organizations. *Ethn Dis*. 2007;17:S15–22.

214. Wolf MS, Gazmararian JA, Baker DW. Health literacy and functional health status among older adults. *Arch Intern Med*. 2005;165:1946–1952.

215. Wolf MS, Gazmararian JA, Baker DW. Health literacy and health risk behaviors among older adults. *Am J Prev Med*. 2006;32:19–24.

216. Shortage of minority dentists threatens dental health of underserved. *Dent Today*. 2001;20:36.

217. Elwood TW. Overview of allied health personnel shortages. *J Allied Health*. 1991;20:47–62.

218. Cohen JJ, Gabriel BA, Terrell C. The case for diversity in the health care workforce. *Health Aff (Millwood)*. 2002;21:90–102.

219. Mitchell DA, Lassiter SL. Addressing health care disparities and increasing workforce diversity: The next step for the dental, medical, and public health professions. *Am J Public Health*. 2006;96:2093–2097.

220. Acosta D, Olsen P. Meeting the needs of regional minority groups: The University of Washington's programs to increase the American Indian and Alaskan native physician workforce. *Acad Med*. 2006;81:863–870.

221. Crowley S, Fuller D, Law W, et al. Improving the climate in research and scientific training environments for members of underrepresented minorities. *Neuroscientist*. 2004;10:26–30.

222. Gates PE, Ganey JH, Brown MD. Building the minority faculty development pipeline. *J Dent Educ*. 2003;67:1034–1038.

223. Thomson WA, Ferry PG, King JE, Martinez-Wedig C, Michael LH. Increasing access to medical education for students from medically underserved communities: One program's success. *Acad Med*. 2003;78:454–459.

224. Potts JT Jr. Recruitment of minority physicians into careers in internal medicine. *Ann Intern Med*. 1992;116:1099–1102.

225. Zayas LE, McGuigan D. Experiences promoting healthcare career interest among high-school students from underserved communities. *J Natl Med Assoc*. 2006;98:1523–1531.

226. Andersen RM, Davidson PL, Atchison KA, et al. Pipeline, profession, and practice program: Evaluating change in dental education. *J Dent Educ*. 2005;69: 239–248.

227. Duncan DT. Health careers for racial/ethnic minorities: Planting the seeds early in the pipeline. *Ethn Dis*. 2006;16:623.

228. Fincher RM, Sykes-Brown W, Allen-Noble R. Health science learning academy: A successful "pipeline" educational program for high school students. *Acad Med*. 2002;77:737–738.

229. Wallen GR, Rivera-Goba MV, Hastings C, Peragallo N, de Leon Siantz ML. Developing the research pipeline: Increasing minority nursing research opportunities. *Nurs Educ Perspect.* 2005;26:29–33.

230. Cooper LA, Roter DL, Johnson RL, Ford DE, Steinwachs DM, Powe NR. Patient-centered communication, ratings of care, and concordance of patient and physician race. *Ann Intern Med.* 2003;139:907–915.

231. Koehn PH. Health-care outcomes in ethnoculturally discordant medical encounters: The role of physician transnational competence in consultations with asylum seekers. *J Immigr Minor Health.* 2006;8:137–147.

232. Koehn PH, Sainola-Rodriguez K. Clinician/patient connections in ethnoculturally nonconcordant encounters with political-asylum seekers: A comparison of physicians and nurses. *J Transcult Nurs.* 2005;16:298–311.

233. van Ryn M, Burke J. The effect of patient race and socio-economic status on physicians' perceptions of patients. *Soc Sci Med.* 2000;50:813–828.

234. Finucane TE, Carrese JA. Racial bias in presentation of cases. *J Gen Intern Med.* 1990;5:120–121.

235. Weiss BD, Blanchard JS, McGee DL, et al. Illiteracy among Medicaid recipients and its relationship to health care costs. *J Health Care Poor Underserved.* 1994;5:99–111.

236. Guidance Memorandum. January 29, 1998. Title VI prohibition against national origin discrimination—Persons with limited-English proficiency. Washington, DC: U.S. Department of Health and Human Services; 1999. Accessed at: http://www.hhs.gov/ocr/lepfinal.htm

237. Tervalon M, Murray-Garcia J. Cultural humility versus cultural competence: A critical distinction in defining physician training outcomes in multicultural education. *J Health Care Poor Underserved.* 1998;9:117–125.

238. Hobgood C, Sawning S, Bowen J, Savage K. Teaching culturally appropriate care: A review of educational models and methods. *Acad Emerg Med.* 2006;13: 1288–1295.

239. Park ER, Betancourt JR, Kim MK, Maina AW, Blumenthal D, Weissman JS. Mixed messages: residents' experiences learning cross-cultural care. *Acad Med.* 2005;80:874–880.

240. Koehn PH, Swick HM. Medical education for a changing world: Moving beyond cultural competence into transnational competence. *Acad Med.* 2006;81:548–556.

241. Farmer P. *Pathologies of Power: Health, Human Rights, and the New War on the Poor: With a New Preface by the Author.* Berkeley: University of California Press; 2005.

Chapter 2

Race/Ethnicity, Trust, and Health Disparities: Trustworthiness, Ethics, and Action

John R. Stone, MD, PhD

Annette Dula, PhD

O ver the past several decades, health professionals, institutions, and programs have paid great attention to the lack of ethnic/minority trust in the U.S. healthcare system.[1] This focus is associated with efforts to eliminate racial or ethnic disparities in health and health care. Also, low participation of minorities in biomedical research (and thus questionable translatability of research results) has provoked investigation into distrust of biomedical research as a cause of nonparticipation. Furthermore, public health literature displays a concern about trust and stresses its importance in work with communities. However, we hold that focus on trust should be a secondary issue—that trustworthiness is the key concern in eliminating health and healthcare disparities. But addressing trustworthiness—what it includes and ethically what we do about it—reasonably should begin with a discussion of trust. So we will illustrate.

In this chapter, we first explain why building such trust helps eliminate these disparities. Then, we argue that even more important is developing **trustworthiness** in health professionals; researchers; and related structures, policies, and programs.[2] We explain that trustworthiness promotes conversion of "rational distrust" into "rational trust." But what should trustworthiness be about? The answer to this question is ultimately an ethical one. What moral reference points should guide health professionals, researchers, and related structures; institutions; and policy formation regarding trustworthiness and the health of racial or ethnic minorities? What actions should follow?

We try to provide substantial initial answers to these questions. We weave threads from the literature into a fabric that we believe is a useful ethical framework for addressing trustworthiness. We then recommend a set of guiding ethical principles. Finally, we recommend a set of action guides that are consistent with the framework. However, the best way to understand trustworthiness and related ethical responsibilities is first to get a fix on trust.

Trust and Trustworthiness: Meanings, Distinctions, and Relevance

Trust

Trust is essential for positive patient–provider relationships, recruiting and retaining research participants, and effective partnering with communities.[3–6] However, significant evidence document that racial and ethnic minorities often significantly distrust professionals and/or systems, organizations, and other entities that engage in health care, research, and public health.[4,7] Tragedies involving the care and support of minorities after Hurricane Katrina were poignant reminders of why these groups should distrust public health and governmental actions. Responses suggested that officials put greatest priority on rescuing whites.[8] But what do **trust** and **distrust** mean?

Those Who Trust

Consider those who trust: (1) Trustors are vulnerable; they are susceptible to the trusted's beneficial or harmful intent. (2) Trustors expect that the trusted will act in the trustor's best interests.[9] For example, a trusting patient expects that healthcare professionals will act caringly, communicate clearly, and diagnose competently. (3) Trustors have positive emotional attitudes that can enhance healing and promote collaboration.[3,4]

Kinds of Trust

Several approaches help us get a handle on trust. One classification relates to objects of trust. "Personal trust" targets discrete individuals and relies on personal experience. "Social trust" concerns groups and depends on secondary information.[3,4] Thus, someone may trust her own doctor and yet *dis*trust doctors generally. Another approach employs the relationship of trust to reasons. "Blind trust" exists when trust persists despite good reasons to the contrary (presuming a competent reasoner). Solomon and Flores contrast such irrational trust with "authentic trust" that rests on a *conscious decision* that there are good reasons to trust.[10] Their "authentic trust" includes what we and others term "rational trust."[9,11]

As a working definition, **rational trust** is trust that a reasonable person would hold after assessing the grounds for that trust. Adequately defining the elements of something like rational trust is notoriously difficult, including questions about what reasonable people would conclude. However, we propose that key among these elements are that (1) the trustor has and exercises capacities for making sound judgments; (2) to the trustor, there appear to be sufficient reasons to trust; and (3) the trustor understands these reasons and concludes that they are sufficient for (warrant or justify) trust. A corollary is that (4) lacking are reasons that the trustor understands would justify distrust or suspension of judgment. This is what philosophers call a fallibist account. The trustor could be mistaken. For example, what the trustor thinks are sufficient reasons might actually be false or contrary reasons that might have been overlooked.

This working definition of trust allows degrees or strengths of rational trust. For example, someone could reasonably say that based on the evidence (say, from personal observation and testimony from acquaintances), she somewhat or highly trusts that a researcher or physician will serve the trustor's best interests. Many healthcare choices require that people proceed without full trust. An example is the need to make quick decisions when serious threats to health require urgent responses. Then we often consent to treatment on the judgment that those who propose to help us are *trustworthy enough*. We conclude that our odds look better if we go with them, although we would ideally prefer that we have a higher level of trust before consenting. Also, the related emotional attitudes of reasonable trustors should track their degree of trust.

Dimensions of Trust

Another way to decipher trust and discern good reasons for trusting involves the use of domains or "dimensions" as a way to analyze characteristics and practices of professionals and institutions or structures. For example, Hall and colleagues suggest that the dimensions of honesty, competence, loyalty or fidelity, and confidentiality are elements of general trust in physicians and relate to serving patients' best interests. "Global trust" is another dimension in their model, a synthesis more or less of the other dimensions that serves as a kind of pervasive element.[3,12]

Such dimensions of trust in physicians can be used both analytically and normatively. In the first instance, investigators can empirically determine whether proposed dimensions are grounds for people's trust. Hall and co-investigators found that those they assessed did not dissect out bases for trust along these dimensional lines. However, we think provisionally that such dimensions have normative implications—that when manifested they should be among grounds for trusting physicians. We will shortly note a caveat, but first we consider how the dimensions concept could be fruitfully employed in other areas.

Wallerstein and Duran stress the importance of power, privilege, integrity, and cultural humility in community-based participatory research.[6] Thus, normative dimensions of trust here might include (1) shared power, (2) unpacked and mitigated privilege, (3) integrity, and (4) cultural humility and sensitivity. Other possibilities are (5) full sharing of relevant information and results with communities (transparency), (6) culturally sensitive and equitable forums that promote questions and provide clear answers about the research, (7) emphasis on do-no-harm and nondeceptive research policies, and (8) strict avoidance of treatment without appropriate consent.[5] Further promising dimensions regarding research are (9) community benefit, and (10) sustained community-researcher relationships that are reciprocal. Our general point is that the dimensions concept is a valuable method for discerning what should be bases for rational trust. Also, we will later show that dimensions are important ways to analyze what should be the grounds of trustworthiness.

Although the concept of dimensions is an attractive way to understand and set normative standards for rational trust, there are pitfalls. Dimensions can include hidden and unwanted biases or assumptions. "Fidelity" is a good example. Stress on fidelity might involve a one-way orientation about how professionals should advance patients', participants', or community members' interests. Without a counterbalancing dimension, this orientation can sustain professional power over patients because the emphasis is on a "looking after." Thus, "checking" or counterbalancing dimensions such as mutuality and empowerment may be very important as grounds for rational trust. The overarching point is that a proposed dimension should be critically reviewed for features that may promote morally unacceptable arrangements. Such critical review should include **perspectival humility**—that our (always) limited viewpoints mean that diverse parties should provide scrutiny. Given this caveat, we conclude that the dimensions concept is a useful way to discern what should be the bases for rational trust.

Why Trust Matters

Now that we have some explanation of trust, we are better positioned to consider in more detail why it matters. In health care, trust promotes communication, timely care, healing, patient loyalty to physicians, less litigation, and adherence to treatment recommendations.[3,4,11] In public health and community-based participatory research, trust fosters and sustains collaborations with communities.[6,8,13] Trust also promotes participation in biomedical research, better research outcomes, and improved communication between participant and researcher.[14] Further, there is growing awareness that successful intersectoral efforts of disciplines, other entities, and communities are essential for eliminating health disparities.[15,16] Trust is crucial for success in these endeavors.

Rational Distrust

Distrust matters because trust matters. Comparable to the prior discussion, distrust is rational if a distrustor with appropriate capacities judges that there are sufficient reasons for distrust and the distrustor understand those reasons.[11] Comparably, this is also a fallibist account in that rational distrust can be mistaken.

In addressing trust issues, health professionals and institutions must understand that good historical and contemporary reasons justify racial and ethnic minorities' rational distrust of health care, public health, and biomedical research. Such distrust is a logical outcome of "historical trauma" and "intergenerational wounding" imposed on African Americans, Latino Americans, American Indians, Asian Americans, and others.[4,6,17,18] This traumatic past, continued negative experiences, and extensive documentation of unequal treatment warrant ethnic minority judgments *that health professionals, institutions, and policies often cannot be trusted to act as equitably and respectfully with them as with whites.*[18–21]

Granted, there may be many cases in which the distrust is not justified. Nevertheless, rational or *irrational* distrust can have an anti-healing effect.[4,22] Whatever the cause, distrust increases demands for specialist referrals even if unnecessary, decreases adherence to treatment plans, and reduces organ donations.[11] Rational or irrational distrust lowers participation in clinical trials and impairs community collaboration with public health programs and academic institutions.[4,5,8] Reducing health gaps and healthcare inequalities will require addressing both kinds of distrust. What it takes to reverse irrational distrust will incompletely overlap with strategies aimed at eliminating rational distrust. But the reasons for rational distrust are foundational—*the lack of trustworthiness* at societal, institutional/structural, and professional levels.[4,20,21,23]

Trustworthiness

In providing a working definition of trustworthiness, the focus moves to the object of trust. People and institutions or structures (including programs, practices, organizations, systems, universities, and policies) are trustworthy if there are sufficient reasons to trust them.

Our health care is untrustworthy. Extensive evidence documents that inferior health care for racial/ethnic minorities is common.[20,21,24] The main causes are unclear, but patients' preferences are not the primary explanation. The later point is quite important because a primary focus on preferences places the main moral responsibility in minorities—a blame-the-victim orientation—and ignores how other societal disparities like education and income affect the health of populations. Also, even when a patient elects inferior or inadequate treatment, suspicion regarding physician motives may explain why the patient chose that treatment.[25] Comparable explanations for preferences might be obtained in research and public health; that is, suspicion regarding researchers' or public health officials' motives may explain why people elect not to participate in research or follow advice about health habits or early disease detection and treatment. Thus, operating in the background may be a rational distrust that flows from prior untrustworthiness.

Research has been untrustworthy. Biomedical and public health researchers promulgated egregious abuses upon racial or ethnic minorities. The U.S. Public Health Service (USPHS) Syphilis Study in Tuskegee, Alabama, is the classic example, but it is only one among many.[17,18,26] Also, significant exclusions of minorities have reduced the probability that research outcomes translate to them, as we noted earlier. Further, given the disparities in access to quality health care, African American and other underserved populations fear that benefits derived from research will not be equitably bestowed to them.

As Annette Baier observes, trust is slowly built and fragile, but evidence of untrustworthiness quickly destroys it.[9(p.131)] She writes, "Once the stronger have abused the trust of the weaker, the burden of truth is on them [the stronger] to patiently demonstrate their goodwill, to attempt to show new trustworthiness, should they thereafter want to recover anyone's trust."[9(p.149)] Thus, building trustworthiness and subsequent rational trust can be very difficult.

Guiding Development of Trustworthiness

As we suggested, the concept of dimensions is useful in determining how to develop trustworthiness. Consider the dimensions we noted earlier regarding trust in physicians. For example, patients ought to place themselves in a surgeon's hands only if they have good reason to judge that the surgeon is technically competent (competence dimension), or they should discuss personal matters with a psychiatrist only if the latter will honor confidentiality (confidentiality dimension). Similarly, people should agree to become research participants only if they conclude that the process of informed consent honestly conveys methods and risks (dimension of honesty in informed consent), among other things. Communities should collaborate with institutions in community-based participatory research only if they perceive that there are sufficient reasons to believe the latter will honor their commitments (faithfulness dimension). These are merely examples. Considerable work must be done in developing the appropriate dimensions. In developing and in deciding how to assess them, all major stakeholders should be informed and should participate in decisions, especially served communities. One attractive model for community involvement employs collaborative enterprises that draw on concepts of community-based participatory research.[6] Ethically, what should guide such efforts? We next offer an answer.

Addressing Trustworthiness: From Theory to Principles to Action Guides

Background Moral Theory

We ground our ethical framework particularly in a theory of social justice that Madison Powers and Ruth Faden recently proposed for public health and health policy.[15] They argue that societies should ensure social conditions such that everyone can have a "sufficient" level of basic elements necessary for well-being, those elements being health, respect, personal security, reasoning, attachment, and self-determination.[27] Their theory is "nonideal" in that when working to advance well-being by providing sufficient levels of these elements, practicalities such as natural disasters, geography, available resources, societal infrastructure, lifestyles, and the like can influence what ought to be done. Although the ideal may be unachievable because of practical constraints, this is not to assert that the status quo is to be accepted or that the context is unalterable. The theory calls for continued effort to eliminate negative influences on health. It establishes the general importance of improving health to a sufficient level for well-being within a conception of justice—a key basis for the ethical framework and practical guidelines that we now offer.

Powers and Faden explain that providing a sufficient level of health and well-being for everyone requires broad analyses and solutions that show how different social influences interact.[28] Examples are inequalities in health care, wealth, housing, education, and lifestyle. A caveat is that many investigators and research funding priorities ignore that unjust and adverse social inequalities promote unhealthy and anti-well-being lifestyles.[29] We can only highlight a few key elements of Powers and Faden's important theory.

Ethical Framework for Addressing Trust and Trustworthiness

Our framework of ethical principles draws from three elements in Powers and Faden's theory: (1) their general conception of justice, (2) people's equal and significant moral worth, and (3) respect as a dimension of well-being. That everyone has equal and significant moral worth is a crucial precept for establishing that everyone should be provided equitable and adequate means for sufficient health as an element of well-being. Also, Powers and Faden note that John Rawls and other moral philosophers stress the importance of *respect* in human flourishing. With illustrative narratives, Sarah Lawrence-Lightfoot portrays the importance of respect in the work of healthcare professionals.[30] Our framework describes how moral worth flows into a *principle* of respect that supports respect as a dimension of well-being.

These four principles comprise our basic framework: (1) equal and substantial respect, (2) justice, (3) care, and (4) community. They give more guidance than a theory, but they are still quite general. The principles apply to professionals in public health, health care, and health/biomedical research; their respective institutions, agencies, or systems; and related policies. What the principles imply can vary with context.[31] Our general idea is to provide moral anchors or benchmarks for assessment of trustworthiness and trust issues, and what to do about them.

Principle of Equal and Substantial Respect

The core principle of **respect** holds that all should be treated with equivalent and significant recognition and regard. This principle is the key moral guideline for developing and sustaining trustworthiness in health institutions and building corresponding trust in communities of color and other racial or ethnic minorities. Implications of the principle of equal and substantial respect tie to the ethical idea that everyone's dignity should be promoted, honored, preserved, or restored—related to the Kantian view that people should be treated as ends.[32,33] As we stated earlier, the key underlying concept is that everyone has equal and significant moral worth.[15,32–37] When systems and professionals provide unequal services and sustain inequalities that maintain health disparities, and when societies could eliminate those inequalities but do not, then these actions fundamentally violate equal and substantial respect *and* justify rational distrust.

Although related, the principle of equal and substantial respect is distinct from the action of showing respect. The principle gives general guidance. To show respect is to do what the principle implies and is ultimately what matters. As Powers and Faden argue, *showing* respect and *having* self-respect are important elements of well-being.[38] Also relevant in eliminating health disparities are historical and continued inequalities and mistreatment that make racial and ethnic minorities very sensitive in general to respect and disrespect. Perception that a health professional, program, or institution respects them will dispel rational distrust and build trust because showing respect is a good reason to think that professionals or institutions are trustworthy—that they will advance the interests of racial and ethnic minorities as much as they will whites.

Other important aspects of the principle of equal and substantial respect include the following:

1. People should be "treated" (how they are generally approached or considered) equivalently regardless of irrelevancies such as race/ethnicity per se.

2. Equivalent treatment does not imply color blindness. Experience and identity related to race or ethnicity can influence what are best approaches to many issues related to health; people should be recognized for who they are. The "recognition" element of equal and substantial respect focuses on everyone as discrete individuals and fosters their agency when reasonably possible—enabling and building individual capacities.[30,32] Recognition includes how people's supposed "race," ethnicity, gender, and comparable aspects may influence efforts to enhance or sustain their health. For example, a doctor might diplomatically inquire whether a member of an ethnic or racial minority is significantly distrustful and adjust his or her efforts accordingly.

3. Showing respect includes advocating for or protecting people when needed. (Here we target health-related endeavors.)

4. Such respect applies to *individuals and communities*, but the latter is often neglected. This omission motivated the separate principle of community that is discussed later.

5. We should treat everyone *well*.[37]

6. Such respect includes the subsidiary and familiar principle in health care: "respect for autonomy."[31]

The principle of equal and substantial respect incorporates several dimensions (reasons to trust) of trustworthiness: offering particularized health care; fostering the agency of patients and research participants; promoting collaborative public health endeavors; honoring people's rights to voice opinions and their freedom to be heard at all levels of health and healthcare institutions; and preserving dignity through culturally sensitive transactions, including provision of adequate cover during physical examinations.

A common error in applying ethical principles is to focus moral scrutiny too narrowly. Professionals may treat patients or clients respectfully but ignore broader adverse influences on health that professionals' systems and institutions promulgate. We mentioned this caveat earlier. Avoiding such errors requires a culture of continuing *critical reflection* and *review* of:

1. Institutional *structures* (programs, policies, personnel composition and roles, etc.) that sustain and influence practices.
2. *Relationships* of structures and professionals with served individuals and communities, including present and past.
3. *Outcomes* of health professionals' practices.

Critical reflection here requires (1) careful thinking about what the principle of equal and substantial respect actually implies for institutions, practices, and policies and (2) adopting the critical stance that good intentions can still lead to disrespect. *Review* builds on critical reflection and stresses outcome assessments (evidence) that determine (1) if racial/ethnic minorities are indeed treated equally for equivalent medical or public health needs compared with majority populations and (2) if truly individualized, culturally appropriate, context-appropriate, and competent services are provided.[39] Another focus of review is whether people with greater health needs have greater presumptive priority for services—invoking the principle of justice.

Principle of Justice

Our principle of **justice** stresses fairness aspects of justice *that flow from the principle of equal and substantial respect.*[40,41] This principle of justice implies the following elements of fairness *that in turn comprise dimensions of trustworthiness*. There should be:

1. Equal consideration or treatment for equivalent problems or needs. Thus, it is unfair that ethnic minorities receive less pain control intervention for long bone fractures and treatments to open blocked coronary arteries in acute myocardial infarction are administered less quickly.[24,42]

2. Unequal responses proportional to nonequivalent conditions, with greater provisional priority to those with worse health or greater threats to health. For example, someone with severe diabetic ketoacidosis should get care before a person with a closed fracture without evidence of compromised vasculature or another impending catastrophe. Or, in public health, given limited resources, remediation efforts should first be directed at the population with the "worse" health even if they can be helped somewhat less than a group significantly better off.[15]

3. Efficient use of resources. Given limited resources and qualified by priority to the worse off, resources should be used to benefit as many people as possible. (Although often considered a utilitarian or consequentialist approach, justice actually requires efficient use of resources. However, efficiency is not the primary focus of justice. On this point, also see the following discussion about Powers and Faden's account of justice in public health.)

4. Significant involvement of served communities in decisions about addressing health inequalities.[43]

5. Compensation for past unequal treatment. This relatively unexplored area needs considerable attention. Suppose an institution historically has deliberatively avoided allocating sufficient resources to a community despite knowledge that the community had major needs. Such unequal treatment would be grounds for employing extra resources to assist that community at a later time. Served communities should have a major voice in such discussions. The principle of community addresses some of these issues.

In promoting trustworthiness, outcome assessments and causal analyses should be conducted in light of the preceding elements. Results should ground revisions of policies, systems, and practices. Thus, the ultimate focus of justice is on positive change to eliminate unequal treatment.[44]

Regarding whether to give priority to the worse off, Powers and Faden observe that the basic ethical approach in public health has been utilitarian or consequentialist, constrained by justice. That is, the greatest aggregate net health gain has been the primary goal, often cashed out as helping the greatest number of people. This approach gives no priority to health improvement among the most disadvantaged or worse off unless they will have greater health gains than the better off. Here, justice acts as a side constraint to what consequentialist moral reasoning may indicate. Instead, Powers and Faden argue that justice, *as a theory*, should direct public health efforts with efficiency as a modifier. We agree and employ the same considerations in our principle of justice. Thus, being more disadvantaged means, by default, greater priority for measures to improve health. Efficiency is then a subsidiary principle that calls for maximizing health outcomes for as many people as justice allows. (Maximizing aggregate net benefit does not always imply helping the greatest number of people, given that benefit amount matters.) Our fairness dimensions of justice retain this secondary role for efficiency. However, even when anchored in equal and substantial respect, a principle of justice can be rather sterile or nonhumanistic. One way to enrich justice is through care.

Principle of Care

The principle of **care** emphasizes that whatever the health-improving effort, pervasive and humanistic caring is the goal for each individual. Caring includes trustworthiness dimensions of empathy, supportiveness, kindness, honesty, and thoughtfulness.[36] Such caring is often associated with clinical work, but it should also play a prominent role in public health and research. Further, the work of feminist scholars Carol Gilligan and Nell Noddings suggests that the ethic of caring should play a central role in developing social practices and policies that benefit the worse off.[45,46] The principle of care we envision is consistent with their broader view of care. That is, attunement to the principle should involve especially a concern for the needs of the worst off. This implication of caring is partly an extension or specification of equal and substantial respect. Such caring expresses regard, recognition, or support for people's dignity and suffering. Also, the principle of justice supports these implications of caring.

Although the primary outcome of applying such a care principle is greater trustworthiness, implementing it will enhance trust through its positive effect on relationships between health professionals or institutions and their target populations.[47] A perception of genuine caring promotes judgments that professionals and institutions are respectful.

In assessing care trustworthiness, evaluation instruments addressing the preceding dimensions would obviously need development and validation. Tackling those issues is beyond the present scope. Finally, the principle of caring guides relationships with both individuals and communities. However, a specific principle of community is also helpful.

Principle of Community

Our principle of **community** also flows from the core principle of equal and substantial respect for persons and connects with the principles of care and justice. This principle requires that affected communities have major roles in determining and evaluating practices and policies that affect them—the community-agency dimension that is commensurate with requirements of the respect principle.[36] Strong community input helps ensure that its interests are served. Additionally, considerations of justice as fairness imply that those who will bear burdens and benefits should have a significant voice about interventions or research that will produce those outcomes. Moreover, those affected will have knowledge, perspectives, and traditions that bear on what the community deems to be burdens and benefits. Blumenthal describes a set of principles that one community–academic collaboration employs.[48] These principles could be rich sources for developing a set of dimensions for such partnering. Also, McQuiston and colleagues provide useful comments regarding agency building.[49]

Another key dimension of the community principle is the pursuit and practice of **cultural humility**. Our concept of cultural humility is based on the work of Tervalon and Murray-Garcia, and one of us (JRS) has which is elaborated elsewhere.[36,37,39] Readers might also consider literature on the culture and paradigms of biomedicine.[50,51] For us, cultural humility requires health professionals and institutions to appreciate that:

1. Their perspectives are influenced by their embeddedness in biomedical, public health, and research goals, values, and conceptual models.
2. Their policies and practices often maintain dominance and superior power, typically aligned with whiteness and male gender.
3. Their attitudes and beliefs often unconsciously include biases, prejudices, and stereotypes toward other cultures.[20,39,52]
4. Their cultural understandings are often incomplete.

Our concept of cultural humility is partly an attitude and a perspective about cross-cultural efforts to eliminate health inequalities among racial and ethnic minorities. But cultural humility also implies *action* that includes personal and collective efforts to understand and to eliminate biased, disrespectful, and prejudiced attitudes, beliefs, behaviors, policies, and practices. Thus, cultural humility involves *transformation* of individuals and institutions through self-knowledge and action—a *journey*.[53]

Caveats About the Framework

We have introduced an ethical framework that can help guide efforts to build and sustain trustworthiness as an important step toward eliminating health disparities involving racial and ethnic minorities. We suggested that the principles could yield a number of useful dimensions for analyzing trustworthiness and ultimately for determining what should be changed or sustained. However, the framework has limitations:

1. We may have omitted other core principles. For example, one of us (JRS) and a colleague elaborated a separate principle of critical trustworthiness in another venue to stress the need for critical review.[36] However, here we judged that our discussion sufficiently highlighted this need.

2. Useful sub-principles could be delineated regarding various disciplines and situations. An example is how to show respect. Also, when things do not go well, there may be a need for elaborating obligations of apology, regret, and amends.[54] Fiester argues that articulating such obligations avoids tendencies to employ general principles merely as topical lists that promote superficial and incomplete applications. We agree.

3. A complete moral framework would include virtues or positive character traits. For example, to be respectful, fair, and caring as guided by the respective principles requires that health professionals are certain kinds of persons with certain dispositions and attitudes. Education and training programs should identify, inculcate, and enhance such traits.

4. A complete account should draw on Critical Race Theory (as well as on feminist and other critical literature that targets power and gender issues) and analyses of racial and ethnic identity, including whiteness.

5. We briefly review justifications, explanations, and objections.

6. We touch on how our framework should flow into decision processes, an issue that connects with an expanding literature on fair and deliberative democratic decision processes.[55–57]

What Health Professionals and Institutions Should Do

The principles we have discussed are fine, readers may be thinking, but they are vague or indeterminate. We agree. The general ethical principles in the framework need specification and particularization. That is, their generality should flow into more fine-tuned guides for action about trustworthiness. This is the specification move. Then, what those action guides imply for a given context—how to implement and prioritize implementation of those guides—will depend significantly on local factors: the particularization. In other words, context will determine further specification or fine-tuning of the action guides. Experience with implementation recursively leads to even more reflection on the principles and action guides, sometimes leading to modification. Such review may in turn lead to changes in a particular implementation. This is the well-known strategy of striving for a reflective equilibrium. Crucially, those reflections should always be in light of the ultimate goal of insuring trustworthiness that will help eliminate racial and ethnic health inequalities.

We now provide a fairly detailed specification of action guides for promoting trustworthiness that can help eliminate health disparities. As with the principles, the list may need additions and changes. Given these cautions, Whitehead's four categories of actions are a useful beginning:[58]

1. Strengthen individuals (focus on those with a "deficit").
2. Strengthen communities (another "deficit" focus).
3. Improve living and working conditions.
4. Promote healthy macro-policies.

We add the following:

1. Diversify workforces fairly, including health professionals and other institutional and program personnel.[43,59]
2. Promote so-called intersectoral work among diverse disciplines, groups, and communities in order to address the intersecting causes of health inequalities.[15,16]
3. Ensure fair allocation of resources.
4. Ensure equal, high-quality, and humanistic care, dealings, or treatment.
5. Promote and sustain fair partnerships with communities, including major community input and mutually respectful relationships in which all strive for cultural proficiency.
6. Develop transparent and amendable processes and policies with community partners and other disciplines that help ensure fair decisions, balance of power, openness to grievances and accountability, and welcoming of diverse modes of expression and conducting business (including cultural humility).[4,9(pp.161–162),43]
7. Promote continuing outcome assessments of whether policies, practices, and programs are trustworthy regarding the elimination of health inequalities.
8. Develop programs and practices based on analyses of trustworthiness that enhance patient, client, and community trust and dispel rational distrust.

9. Ensure accountability.

10. Act on the assumption that practices, policies, and workforce composition promote racial or ethnic health *inequalities* until proven otherwise.[60]

11. Learn and promote effective strategies for change.[61]

12. Individual professionals should reflect critically and constructively on how their racial, ethnic, cultural, and professional identities, concepts, beliefs, and attitudes should be transformed.[53]

Any serious effort to build and sustain trustworthiness must promote these action guides or something comparable in order to eliminate health and healthcare disparities related to race and ethnicity. We have omitted justifications for these action guides. We invite readers to reflect on whether they are consistent with the ethical framework and background moral theory that this chapter delineates.

Note that particularizing these action guides will include at least three steps: (1) reflection and possible modification in light of the area of work (e.g., health care, research, and public health), (2) further possible modification in light of local issues, and (3) additional changes based on community input. Also, implementing such action guides to promote trustworthiness is very challenging. In addressing healthcare inequalities related to race and ethnicity, for example, we previously described some major challenges and obstacles for healthcare institutions.[62]

SUMMARY

This chapter argues that trust issues are very important in addressing health inequalities related to race and ethnicity but that fostering trustworthiness is the fundamental need. Our scope included health care, research, and public health. We examined trust, rational distrust, and trustworthiness, including the importance of each. We showed that the concept of dimensions is a useful way to analyze trustworthiness and understand how to promote it. We next sketched a background moral theory that supports the chapter's core: an ethical framework for addressing trustworthiness issues in health disparities. Our framework consists of these four ethical principles: (1) equal and substantial respect, (2) justice, (3) care, and (4) community. We elaborated on these principles, showed their interconnectedness, and noted some caveats. The final section provided action guides for addressing trustworthiness in order to eliminate racial and ethnic health disparities. We noted that the action guides require additional steps of specification and particularization that depend on discipline, context, and community input. We stressed the importance of partnering and collaboration with affected communities and among various disciplines.

REFERENCES

1. Some writers use scare quotes around *race* or *racial* to denote that race is a social construction rather than an intrinsic biological or genetic category. Ethnicity is already widely recognized as socially constructed.

2. Crawley LM. African-American participation in clinical trials: Situating trust and trustworthiness. *J Natl Med Assoc.* 2001;93(suppl 12):14S17S.

3. Hall MA, Dugan E, Zeng B, Mishra AK. Trust in physicians and medical institutions: What is it, can it be measured, and does it matter? *Milbank Q.* 2001;79(4):613–639.

4. Gamble VN. Trust, medical care, and racial and ethnic minorities. In Satcher D, Pamies RJ, eds. *Multicultural Medicine and Health Disparities.* New York: McGraw-Hill; 2006:437–448.

5. Corbie-Smith G, Thomas SB, St. George DMM. Distrust, race, and research. *Arch Intern Med.* 2002;162(21):2458–2463.

6. Wallerstein NB, Duran B. Using community-based participatory research to address health disparities. *Health Promot Pract.* 2006;7(3):312–323.

7. Dula A. African American suspicion of the healthcare system is justified: What do we do about it? *Camb Q Healthc Ethics.* 1994;3:347–357.

8. Cordasco KM, Eisenman DP, Glik DC, Golden JF, Asch SM. "They blew the levee": Distrust of authorities among hurricane Katrina evacuees. *J Health Care Poor Underserved.* 2007;18:277–282.

9. Baier AC. *Moral Prejudices: Essays on Ethics.* Cambridge, MA: Harvard University Press; 1995.

10. Solomon RC, Flores F. *Building Trust in Business, Politics, Relationships, and Life.* New York: Oxford University Press; 2001.

11. DeVille K, Kopelman LM. Diversity, trust, and patient care: Affirmative action 25 years after Bakke. *J Med Phil.* 2003;28(4):489–516.

12. Although Hall and colleagues' "global trust" could be descriptively correct, we do not further discuss it because we fail to see that it should have the normative role that the following text suggests.

13. Inviting public participation in clinical research: Building trust through partnerships. October 26–27, 2004. Public Trust Workshop Work Group. Gonzalez-Amezcua R, Browne R. (co-chairs). http://copr.nih.gov/reports/October_2004 _COPR_WORKSHOP_Proceedings.pdf. Accessed March 17, 2007.

14. Corbie-Smith G, Moody-Ayers S, Thrasher AD. Closing the circle between minority inclusion in research and health disparities. *Arch Intern Med.* 2004;164(13): 1362–1364.

15. Powers M, Faden R. *Social Justice: The Moral Foundations of Public Health and Health Policy.* New York: Oxford University Press; 2006.

16. Mullings L, Schulz AJ. Intersectionality and health: An introduction. In Schulz AJ, Mullings L, eds. *Gender, Race, Class, & Health: Intersectional Approaches.* San Francisco: Jossey-Bass; 2006:3–17.

17. Gamble VN. Under the shadow of Tuskegee: African Americans and health care. *Am J Public Health.* 1997;87(11):1773–1778.

18. Brandon DT, Isaac LA, LaVeist TA. The legacy of Tuskegee and trust in medical care: Is Tuskegee responsible for race differences in mistrust of medical care? *J Natl Med Assoc.* 2005;97(7):951–956.

19. Cose E. *The Rage of a Privileged Class.* New York: HarperCollins; 1993.

20. Smedley BD, Stith AY, Nelson AR, eds. *Unequal Treatment: Confronting Racial and Ethnic Disparities in Healthcare.* Washington, DC: National Academies Press, Institute of Medicine; 2003.

21. Agency for Healthcare Research and Quality (2005). National Health Disparities Report (NHDR). (AHRQ Publication No. 06-0017) http://www.ahrq.gov/qual/nhdr05/nhdr05.pdf. Accessed July 1, 2007.

22. Thom DH, Campbell B. Patient-physician trust: An exploratory study. *J Fam Pract.* 1997;44(2):169–176.

23. Atrash HK, Hunter MD. Health disparities in the United States: A continuing challenge. In Satcher D, Pamies RJ, eds. *Multicultural Medicine and Health Disparities.* New York: McGraw-Hill; 2006:3–31.

24. Bradley EH, Herrin J, Wang Y, et al. Racial and ethnic differences in time to acute reperfusion therapy for patients hospitalized with myocardial infarction. *JAMA.* 2004;292:1563–1572.

25. Armstrong K, Hughes-Halbert C, Asch DA. Patient preferences can be misleading as explanations for racial disparities in health care. *Arch Intern Med.* 2006;166(9):950–954.

26. Byrd WM, Clayton LA. Racial and ethnic disparities in health care: A background and history. In Smedley BD, Stith AY, Nelson AR, eds. *Unequal Treatment: Confronting Racial and Ethnic Disparities in Healthcare.* Washington, DC: National Academies Press, Institute of Medicine; 2003:455–527.

27. Powers and Faden's account draws on prior work of John Rawls, Amartya Sen, Martha Nussbaum, Amartya Sen, and Norman Daniels, among others.

28. Schulz AJ, Mullings L, eds. *Gender, Race, Class, & Health: Intersectional Approaches.* San Francisco: Jossey-Bass; 2006.

29. Geiger HJ. Health disparities. What do we know? What do we need to know? What should we do? In Schulz AJ, Mullings L, eds. *Gender, Race, Class, & Health: Intersectional Approaches.* San Francisco: Jossey-Bass; 2006:261–288.

30. Lawrence-Lightfoot S. *Respect: An Exploration.* Cambridge, MA: Perseus; 2000.

31. Beauchamp TL, Childress JF. *Principles of Biomedical Ethics.* New York: Oxford University Press; 2001.

32. Hill TE. *Respect, Pluralism, and Justice: Kantian Perspectives.* New York: Oxford University Press; 2000.

33. Nussbaum, MC. *Women and Human Development: The Capabilities Approach.* New York: Cambridge University Press; 2000.

34. Buchanan, A. Justice, *Legitimacy, and Self-determination: Moral Foundations for International Law.* New York: Oxford University Press; 2004.

35. Stone J. Importance of community input—A moral framework for disaster planning. *Practical Bioethics.* 2007;2(4) & 3(1–2):9–11.

36. Stone J, Parham G. An ethical framework for community health workers and related institutions. *Fam Community Health.* 2007;30(4):351–363.

37. Stone J. Healthcare inequality, cross-cultural training, and bioethics: Principles and applications. *Camb Q Health Ethics.* 2008;17(2):216–226.

38. In light of people's equal moral worth, others have prominently framed the importance of showing respect within considerations of upholding human dignity, treating

people as ends, and promoting human flourishing through the promotion and preservation of core "capabilities." The most prominent here are Amartya Sen and Martha Nussbaum. Powers and Faden explain how their account fits with Sen's and Nussbaum's work, as well as John Rawls's.

39. Tervalon M, Murray-García J. Cultural humility versus cultural competence: A critical distinction in defining physician training outcomes in multicultural education. *J Health Care Poor Underserved*. 1998;9(2):117–125.

40. For readers familiar with John Rawls's theory of justice, we are not employing his technical sense of "justice as fairness." See Beauchamp and Childress's account for a nuanced discussion of a principle of justice.

41. Rawls J. *A Theory of Justice*. Cambridge, MA: Harvard University Press; 1971.

42. Green CR. Assessing and managing pain. In Satcher D, Pamies RJ, eds. *Multicultural Medicine and Health Disparities*. New York: McGraw-Hill; 2006:343–359.

43. Stone JR. Race and healthcare disparities: Overcoming vulnerablity. *Theor Med Bioeth*. 2002;23:499–518.

44. Lurie N. Health disparities—Less talk, more action. *N Engl J Med*. 2005;353(7): 727–729.

45. Gilligan C. *In a Different Voice: Psychological Theory and Women's Development*. Cambridge, MA: Harvard University Press; 1982.

46. Noddings N. *Starting at Home: Caring and Social Policy*. Berkeley: University of California Press; 2002.

47. Collins TC, Clark JA, Petersen LA, Kressin NR. Racial differences in how patients perceive physician communication regarding cardiac testing. *Med Care*. 2002;40(suppl 1):I27–I34.

48. Blumenthal DS. A community coalition board creates a set of values for community-based research. *Prev Chronic Dis*. 2006;3(1):A16. Epub December 15, 2005.

49. McQuiston C. Choi-Hevel S, Clawson M. Protegiendo nuestra comunidad: Empowerment participatory education for HIV prevention. *J Transcult Nurs*. 2001;12(4):275–283.

50. Weber L. Reconstructing the landscape of health disparities research: Promoting dialogue and collaboration between feminist intersectional and biomedical paradigms. In Schulz AJ, Mullings L, eds. *Gender, Race, Class, & Health: Intersectional Approaches*. San Francisco: Jossey-Bass; 2006:21–59.

51. Fox RC, Swazey JP. Examining American bioethics: its problems and prospects. *Camb Q Healthc Ethics*. 2005 Fall;14(4):361–373.

52. Núñez A, Robertson C. Cultural Competency. In Satcher D, Pamies RJ, eds. *Multicultural Medicine and Health Disparities*. New York: McGraw-Hill; 2006:371–388.

53. Murray-García JL, Harrell JA, García EG, Gizzi E, Simms-Mackay P. Self-reflection in multicultural training: Be careful what you ask for. *Acad Med*. 2005;80: 694–701.

54. Fiester A. Viewpoint: Why the clinical ethics we teach fails patients. *Acad Med*. 2007;82(7):684–689.

55. Gutmann A, Thompson D. Deliberating about bioethics. *Hastings Cent Rep*. 1997; 27(3):38–41.

56. Daniels N. Justice, health, and healthcare. *Am J Bioeth*. 2001;1(2):2–15.

57. Fleck L. Healthcare justice and rational deliberation. *Am J Bioeth*. 2001; 1(2):20–21.

58. Whitehead, M. A typology of actions to tackle social inequalities in health. *J Epidemiol Community Health*. 2007;61:473–478.

59. Pamies RJ, Hill GC, Watkins Jr. L, McNamee MJ, Colburn L. Diversity and the health-care workforce. In Satcher D, Pamies RJ, eds. *Multicultural Medicine and Health Disparities*. New York: McGraw-Hill; 2006:405–426.

60. Bostick N, Morin K, Benjamin R, Higginson D. Physicians' ethical responsibilities in addressing racial and ethnic healthcare disparities. *J Natl Med Assoc.* 2006;98(8):1329–1334.

61. Farmer P. *Pathologies of Power: Health, Human Rights, and The New War on the Poor*. Berkeley: University of California Press; 2003.

62. Dula A, Stone JR. Wake-up call. Health care and racism. *Hastings Cent Rep.* 2002;32(4):48.

Chapter 3

Justness, Health Care, and Health Disparities

Judith Lee Kissell, PhD

The modern, postindustrial world has begun, fairly recently (if belatedly), to pay attention to issues of justness as related to health care. I use the term **justness** to avoid the connotations that *justice* suffers in the discussion of distribution of healthcare resources. Too often the justice discussion is reduced to impotence by introducing arguments that validate the notion of health care as a commodity and the supremacy of the market system. Recognition in the United States by national agencies to a series of crises has all contributed to our willingness finally to "listen up." These crises include the presence of health disparities within our population: 46 million people who lack health insurance; the underinsured; and the differences in coverage for mental illness, whether by private insurance or publicly funded programs.

Various approaches have been taken to address the "justness in healthcare" problems as a question of ethics and moral responsibility. The most influential way of thinking about healthcare ethics in latter part of the 20th century addressed *justice* as one of four major principles. More recent efforts of all the healthcare professions and their organizations have striven to make this issue part of their vision of "professionalism." University admissions offices have made service, or volunteering among the underserved, a serious consideration for admission to their professional schools of health sciences. Once again we are being serious, hopefully more serious, about universal coverage.

In one sense, the idea that healthcare professionals *must* make unfairness in access to health care a part of their personal and professional agenda appears to be *urged* on a more or less ready-to-listen constituency.

When any crises (such as the ones mentioned earlier) are discussed, the feeling surfaces that there is also the afterthought, "and besides, it's an *ethical* issue."

And herein lies the problem—that the problems of justness and health disparities are often considered to be mere add-ons, mere appendages, to caring for the ill and the healthcare professions. In this chapter, I argue not that it is *appropriate* that there be a chapter in a book on health disparities to address *also* the ethics of this problem, but that we ought to consider justness by its nature to be *intrinsically related* to heath disparities. To make this argument, I must argue (1) that health care be integrally connected to what it means to be human and (2) that justness be a part of enhancing the capability to live more and to be more. Finally, I must show that however justice or justness are considered in relation to health care, they transcend personal obligations that are part of the clinician–patient relationship and also belong to the realm of ethics that is societal.

Here I must also mention my use of "justness" as opposed to "justice"—a term that is hotly debated, often with negative results for those who are underserved and underprivileged in our society. I will propose a particular way of thinking about the meaning of health care as a social good and how it ought to be distributed and why. By using "justness," I signal my unwillingness to enter into the fray of "which" justice we are talking about, a discussion that has traditionally weighed down the topic in the past.

It is difficult to discuss any ethical concerns without paying at least a nod to the principles approach first introduced in 1979 by Tom L. Beauchamp and James F. Childress in their *Principles of Biomedical Ethics*.[1] That book, now in its fifth edition, marked a beginning for medical ethics in the developed world that put the spotlight on the primacy of the relationship between the clinician and the patient that has persisted ever since. While this book has been an extremely important contribution to the understanding of the ethics of health care, it will be important in this chapter to carefully investigate how a misinterpretation of the fourth principle they espouse—justice, as simply another part of the relationship between clinicians and patients—has led us to where we are today. That the book recognized the importance of this principle is a plus, but its legacy has been the contest among different theories that has ensued.

Few theoreticians of justice throw a light as helpful to us as Michael Walzer, in his *Spheres of Justice*.[2] Walzer's insights provide a helpful lens through which to look at how health care as a social good belongs to everyone. Another important contributor to how we think about this matter is Amartya Sen, Nobel Prize–winning laureate in economics, who has had the audacity to write about economics from the viewpoint of the poor.[3] Sen contributes an essential element of thinking about justness, human flourishing, and health care with his development of the concept of *capabilities*, a concept that has become part of the lexicon of justice issues for philosophers and ethicists. Standing on the shoulders of these giants, I make my case about the intrinsic nature of justness in health care.

The Idea of Health Disparities

The concept of **health disparities** as it is commonly used by the National Center on Minority Health and Health Disparities (NCMHHD) is of fairly recent origin. The NCMHHD itself dates from 1990, and the first strategic plan, established by the National Institutes of Health, was first published in 2003.[4] What healthcare professionals probably think of when they hear this term is the data showing that the treatment women and minorities receive differs markedly from that given to white men. These cases of disparity, according to the research, have little to do with socioeconomic status. Certain groups of people in the United States receive substandard treatment for identical illnesses and/or conditions regardless of their insurance status, despite their financial situation, irrespective of their social status. Documentation of these disparities points at the least to prejudice, stereotyping, and lack of care of these minority groups. The concept of disparities in health care is not exhausted by this relatively narrow idea.

More recent analysis on the part of healthcare agencies such as National Institutes of Health (NIH) and the Centers for Disease Control (CDC) points to lack of access of minorities and the poor for any kind of health care at all. Such analysis focuses on the socioeconomic roots of the medically underserved and the need for us as a nation to ensure that all persons receive the health care they need.[5] This broader perspective on what health disparities are and how they occur points to the realities of the social strata of American life. The U.S. Department of Health and Human Services has set goals for the nation to eliminate such diversity in health conditions of different populations. Their second goal for the *Healthy People 2010* project reads: "The second goal of *Healthy People 2010* stems from the observation that there are substantial disparities among populations in specific measures of health, life expectancy, and quality of life. The second goal is to eliminate health disparities that occur by race and ethnicity, gender, education, income, geographic location, disability status, or sexual orientation."[6]

Clearly the poor and the marginalized suffer from differences in access and differences in care. Most marginalization eventually boils down to socioeconomic status—if not originally, then certainly when large amounts of a person's resources have been spent on health care; certainly when lack of adequate care has meant the loss of a person's job; certainly when the loss of job means the loss of health insurance; certainly when a person's shelter security has disappeared; certainly when a person's food security has vanished; certainly when healthcare costs have resulted in personal bankruptcy; certainly when a person must choose between food and medication.

In a broad sense, marginalization of patients from the more standard sources of health care can be a result of how much money a person has or what job he or she works at, but it can also result from the nature of that person's condition, such as AIDS or mental illness; his or her unfamiliarity with the English language; his or her age, such as occurs with the very young and the very old; or where a peson lives, such as those who live in greatly underserved rural and urban areas. Health disparities come about as the consequences of all these factors.

However we view health disparities—whether as disparate treatment of women and minorities or as the differences in health that result from conditions of marginalization—they are clearly matters of justness. We often require a certain amount of mental gymnastics, though, to make us see that the move from disparities to justness to ethics is not more than an artificial move: "We have this matter of health disparities, and oh yes! There are also ethics matters involved."

How Justness and Health Disparities Might Be Considered an Ethics Afterthought

Justice and the "Georgetown Mantra"

Questions of justice have been part and parcel of bioethics since the current version emerged during the latter quarter of the 20th century. Principlism is perhaps the most popular of the theoretical approaches to bioethics and was explicated by Beauchamp and Childress in their *Principles of Biomedical Ethics*; it is sometimes referred to as the "Georgetown Mantra" because of the university affiliation of its authors. Principlism held center stage for a long time in this field and remains important. Most who "speak" bioethics are familiar with the four principles: autonomy, beneficence, nonmalfeasance, and justice. Some of the procedures that flow from these principles, such as informed consent, have found their way into the law and into the standards of healthcare practice.

Principlism is largely an enlightenment approach to healthcare ethics, with a deep and thorough emphasis on pluralism and its implications for society that the enlightenment brought about and of which we are so fond in the United States. While beneficence and nonmalfeasance are important parts of this system of ethics, the principle that has come to be stressed is **autonomy**, or the right for each of us to act according to our own preferences, even in matters of more socially relevant ethical concerns.

Thus, discussion about principlism has much more to do with patient autonomy and self-determination than with physician beneficence or justice. Often, in earlier years, problems of access were raised about whether given therapies were putting an undue burden on the resources of the system or the community or even the patient's family. But the usual response in ethics education was something of the order, "This is a discussion about ethics (meaning principles) and not about economics. And while the principle of justice may be closely related to economics, what we're really concerned with is the clinician–patient relationship."

Early editions of the Beauchamp and Childress book raised justice mainly as a principle for dealing with a society that found itself with limited resources, growing healthcare technologies, and a growing older population with increased healthcare needs. The issues covered had to do with such matters as theories of justice, rationing, whether there is a right to health care, how healthcare resources should be allocated, and so forth. Many questions revolved around economic concerns, theories of just distribution, and the property rights of individuals rather than with justness as integral ethical concern. Justice indeed appeared as a question of ethics, but one that was peripheral just because the attitude of principlism has been that we have before us a veritable buffet of theories of justice, of which we are free to choose. Principlism is basically inimical toward, if not at war with, the idea that health care is a fundamentally moral enterprise. My decision to use the term "justness" arises from the antagonistic nature of the discussions that take place about justice within principlism.

Discussions on rights to health care inevitably have met the wall of "Rights entail duties: you may have a right to health care, but you'll have a hard time proving that I have a duty to provide it"; or "Who is my neighbor?"; or the libertarian version of the right, ". . . to act in accordance with his own choices, unless those actions infringe on the equal liberty of other human beings to act in accordance with their choices."[7]

Rationing became a big part of the discussion early on, but it met with and was defeated by some of the arguments mentioned earlier. The discussion about rationing at least has had the advantage of bringing to light the realization that whether or not we do it formally and explicitly, we certainly ration health care by default. We may not have an official version such as the infamous Oregon plan, but one way or another, because resources are limited, only certain people have access to certain kinds of treatment.[8]

On the whole, while the principles approach to bioethics at least acknowledges that justice questions exist, it spends considerable energy determining which, if any, theory of justice warrants a more fair distribution of health care. It spends much of its drive highlighting issues that want for good theoretical bases for rights, for rationing, and for the just allocation of resources. But the justice principle has an even more particular problem that it shares with justness in health care.

One of the effects of the popularity of the principles approach has been the emphasis in ethics on how clinicians and patients are to relate, thus stressing the obligations of the clinician and the rights of the patient. Justice or justness, however else it is conceived, is not primarily about the relationship, although there are aspects of health disparities in which this relationship may predominate. In general, however, justice and justness have to do with societal values and how we as a society appraise who we are and for what and whom we are responsible. Many of the problems in health care that seem intractable when approached from the principles approach come about from reasons that transcend the individual. While the personal is one legitimate "realm of ethics," the institutional and societal are the sources of some of our most challenging problems, including justness and health disparities in its widest sense.[9]

The Turn Toward "Professionalism"

More recently, justness in health care has come to be discussed in terms of **professionalism**. Some examples of how this concept affects physicians, for instance, can be found in the literature of the American Medical Association (AMA) in its *Declaration of Professional Responsibility: Medicine's Social Contract with Humanity*, Code of Ethics, and Strategies for Teaching and Evaluating Professionalism (STEP) program; the American Board of Internal Medicine (ABIM); the American College of Physicians; the American Society of Internal Medicine; and the European Foundation of Internal Medicine in its *Physician's Charter*. These organizations have all made admirable efforts to promote responsibilities of the physician for service to the poor and underserved both in their own members and among medical schools.

The AMA's *Principles of Medical Ethics* states: "A physician shall support access to medical care for all people."[10] Their *Declaration of Professional*

Responsibility states that its members will "[a]dvocate for social, economic, educational and political changes that ameliorate suffering and contribute to human well-being."[11] The STEP program is designed to promote the teaching of professionalism in medical schools. The *Physician's Charter* says, "The medical profession must promote justice in the health-care system, including the fair distribution of health-care resources. Physicians should work actively to eliminate discrimination in health care, whether based on race, gender, socioeconomic status, ethnicity, religion, or any other social category."[12]

The professionalism approach has been a worthy effort to confront the growing problems of access. But there are two major problems with this effort as it envisions justness. The first has to do with the degree to which statements about professionalism and justness assume the principle of justice to be simply the fourth element of the relationship between clinicians and patients after respect for autonomy, beneficence, and nonmalfeasance. Professionalism makes an invalid, if valiant attempt to deal with the problems of justness as though they belong primarily at the level of individual, personal ethics.

Professionalism statements attempt to lay the responsibility for justness at the door of the individual by, for example, articulating the responsibilities of caregivers in terms of nondiscrimination; being knowledgeable about how to get free or inexpensive drugs for patients who cannot afford them; advocacy for reform; and, as is sometimes implied, pro bono service. And, in fact, to stress these responsibilities among clinicians is reasonable and necessary because they understand the issues better than do others. But to treat the demands of justness as the same kind of principle as respect for patient autonomy or beneficence is a category mistake. To do so is to fail to recognize that most of our really serious bioethics problems, and especially the justness ones, are institutional and societal. The real issue in health disparities is universal coverage, and this is of course a problem for the much wider society. (The British studies and New York's Health Insurance Program have demonstrated that even with health insurance there are still health disparities.)

Being nondiscriminatory toward the patient certainly lies at the feet of the clinician as a personal responsibility. In fact, nondiscrimination is an excellent example of how basic social values also exist as personal obligations. Thus, for example, respect for the dignity of the individual and belief, at least in theory, that all [humans] are created equal—which we read about in the Constitution—demands that all of us treat one another with fairness and impartiality and that we promote procedural justice in our areas of public responsibility. This same nondiscrimination is also a prime example of how a societal value belongs to all of us as a people, as well as to each of us as individuals.

The second major problem with the professionalism approach has to do with the idea of the **social contract**. It is sometimes difficult to grasp how ethically problematic is the philosophical context in which the idea of "contract" is couched. This justification of professionalism fails to recognize how justness is integral to health care itself, and not simply an add-on and an afterthought. While some statements from professional organizations are more closely related than others to the ideals of justness, they are all at least broadly based on the idea that there is a contract among society's members that binds them together. Almost all professions use this terminology to explain their responsibilities toward society. In principle, professionalism is linked to obligations that arise because of the many prerogatives, including access to people's private lives, education, and social status that accrue to members of the health professions. The idea is that these clinicians owe something back to the society because of the privileges that the society accords them.[13]

While this concept may sound good to those of us steeped in the enlightenment tradition of political freedoms and individual rights, the tradition has several serious problems, many of which reflect my concern with principlism. The most serious problem is that a social contract theory is not essentially an ethical theory, but rather a political one. Not that political theory is not or should not be ethical—but rather, and more importantly, that it isn't *health care*–ethical. It has no *essential* relationship to health care. Moreover, the concept has been adopted by organizations in part because it is fully compatible with the market approach that is the source of many of the justness problems that lead to health disparities in the first place.

One of the worst threats presented by the notion of the social contract is precisely that it is socially constructed, and that the society that constructs it may change its mind.[14]

When society alters its values and priorities, including the ones related to health care, its commitments and contracts may change with it. While this concern may sound like too much philosophy, we would do well to remember that we have indeed changed our attitudes toward our healthcare responsibilities as the fashions have changed. We were, after all, once a nation in serious search of *genetic* health, that is, eugenics (the aim being, not to *care for* its citizens with serious healthcare problems, but rather to use forced sterilizations to *prevent* these citizens ever being born in the first place). Some claim we are still looking in that direction.

The notion of the contract is firmly based on the idea that a contract must be freely entered into, and if freely entered into, freely departed from. The *Declaration of Professional Responsibility*, for instance, claims that "The *Declaration* is enforced *solely* [emphasis added] by the honor of its signatories and their respect for the profession. . . ." and "The *Declaration* is a powerful symbolic statement calling all physicians to uphold and celebrate medicine's historical covenant with society." The *Declaration* clearly states its historical limitations, claiming that it has been careful in its use of language lest some more universal language "turn off" the dedication of some physicians.

Other problems with the social contract approach to defining professionalism are more directly related to the responsibility of healthcare professionals toward the poor and underserved. One of the most significant problems is that traditionally, only a select few ever get to be signatories. While this argument was very obvious when the idea was first introduced in the 17th century (clearly women and slaves didn't get to sign up) the same argument appears to hold today, when the poor, children, the undocumented, ethnic minorities, the mentally ill, and the hungry get little consideration in social arrangements.

It would indeed be difficult to articulate in what manner these marginalized persons find themselves bound to those of us who are more privileged and more affluent. Do we imagine ourselves bound to them at all? Think, for instance, of the criteria for admission into medical schools where performance in examinations, more easily coped with by those who attend well-funded public schools or private schools, are thought to be the major, if not the *only*, gauge for providing medical care to a public comprised of such a wide variety of ethnic, racial, economic, language, and cultural groups—many of whom would prefer to be cared for by someone like themselves.

The turn toward professionalism as a way to address the needs of the poor and underserved is a worthwhile and admirable effort. However, the idea that justice constitutes the fourth principle of the clinician–patient relationship as a purely personal ethical obligation and that the emphasis should be on the social contract idea of professionalism has serious flaws.

Justness from a New View

One of the effects of the **marketplace vision** of health care is that it blinds us to the view of how caring and healing relate to the basic meaning of being embodied, embedded human beings. Instead it places the focus of justness on distribution of a commodity. When we think of health care in this way—and we are encouraged to do so in many ways, ranging from health insurance plans to cost-effectiveness reports of therapies to the percentage of the gross domestic product that is spent on health care—justness becomes the best way to distribute the goods that money can buy. But health and health care are more than that.

Early enlightenment discussions on health care focused on the goods of society, their scarcity, how they might be allocated, and what gives people a right to the goods they can claim. The emphasis on goods, how they are distributed, and the historical association with private property and economics made it seem as if there must be a single principle that would explain how distribution should be justified. And indeed, most theories of justice have sought to find this single principle.

Moreover, many theories assume that all goods are at least metaphorically commodities and can therefore be distributed, and, if distributed, they can also be given a common value. That is, values of all things are somehow commensurable. They can be measured with a common measuring stick. Given the importance of the market, it seemed that there could also be one currency by which all goods that could be distributed could also be valued. Increasingly in the developed world, that measure has come to mean money.

It is the temptation of the philosopher, including the justice philosopher, to find the grand unified theory that will first identify and categorize the "goods of society." This same theory should then be capable of explaining the criteria according to which these goods should be distributed. Philosophers also like to assume that their theories can be universally applied, that is they lend themselves equally and in the same way in all time and all places. Michael Walzer, in his *Spheres of Justice*, suggests that life is more complicated than that, and he offers a different view of justice that not only challenges this philosophical conceit, but will help us see justness as integral to the ethics of health care.[2]

Walzer points out that to argue for an exhaustive list of social goods, or a single principle by which to distribute them, is to misapprehend what distributive justice is all about. Within our societies, we distribute entities or goods as diverse as ritual eminence, membership, power, honors, and offices and more specific entities such as shelter, clothing, jewelry, art, and books. Note that all goods are "social goods" in that they belong to and find their meaning as part of a social process. Not only do societies have a wide variety of goods and meanings of these goods, but they then develop varied criteria by which they are justly meted out. Some of these criteria that exist in our society are what is earned, such as when assigning grades; qualifications, such as when awarding offices; friendship and love, which have no need of explanation; and free exchange, such as in the marketplace.

Philosophers of justice often proceed as if the goods come first in the order of priority, and then decisions are made about more or less fair or just ways of distributing them. But in fact, the order is most likely just the other way around. Rather than a theory of distribution predominating in the determination of justness, what is helpful is first to arrive at a theory of the goods that are then distributed in accord with the meaning and significance of those goods. Inevitably and invariably, goods have meanings that anyone in a particular society understands before they ever come into possession of them. Moreover, despite what theories of private property might have us believe, goods are not things that relate merely on a one-to-one basis to their owners. All goods have meanings that are, and can only be, social. Because meanings are socially constructed, they change with time and place. Thus, for instance, a purple cloak held a special significance in the middle ages that meant that it could be distributed only by a special criteria that probably had something to do with blood (royal) and rank (also royal). Today you and I can buy purple clothing if we have the money.

In other words, the meaning has to come before the criteria for distribution are established. We have to know the importance of the purple cloak before we can decide who can have it, why they can have it, and how they can get hold of it. To understand how each entity is to be distributed, we must understand its *meaning* in the time and place in which we are considering.

Like the cloak, property was not always a matter of the market because not everyone was entitled to own property; historically, women were not so entitled and, in some places, still are not. During some phases of Western history, private property did not exist and, in some cultures, still does not. Or property may have more properly been allotted by reason of blood or a person's position in the family. Offices were often inherited, and the right to vote depended once again on gender and blood.

It becomes more apparent that for each good, or each kind of good, there is a proper and improper, a just and unjust, manner of distribution. The propriety or justness of the distribution is intrinsically tied to the social meaning of the good. Injustice—unjustness—arises when the allotment of the entity occurs in an inappropriate manner. Thus, we have unjustness when honors and public offices are purchased, grades are given because of friendship, and love is given as a reward. There should begin to arise in our mind questions about the nature of health care as a social good. But first we have one more element of Walzer's theory to consider.

Walzer recognizes in most cultures that one means of distribution comes to dominate the system—termed the "dominant" means.[2] It is dominant by reason of its being able to come into possession of more and more goods. We easily recognize how money and market exchange have come to dominate in our society as the means of exchange for almost every good we can think of. Domination itself can be seen as unjustness as increasing numbers of good in our society come to be influenced by money—just think of access to a good education, lobbying efforts to influence legislative process, and campaign spending to determine who wins an office.

There is probably no better example than health care, though, to show how a method of distribution can become dominant and then enter inappropriately into areas in which its presence is ethically unacceptable. Even in the past several decades, health care was thought to belong to the realm of compassion and mercy for the sick and suffering. As drugs, appliances, and interventions became more sophisticated, capitalism became more invested in the field. Both private insurance and government programs ensured payment of clinicians and hospitals, further promoting moneyed interests in all fields of health care.

The domination of money in this field has changed how we regard health and health care as a social good. Rather than being seen as a basic means to secure physical survival and to promote the individual's ability to seek the good things in life, it has become, in the most destructive sense, a commodity. And the same domination has altered the way we think about the just means for distributing health care. Rather than being seen as a good distributed in response to need, health care has increasingly become big business and access to it much the same as access to an expensive car, a big house, or a special piece of jewelry.

The dominance of money in health matters seems to have considerably crippled our common sense. We, as a nation, are faced with many severe illnesses: heart disease, respiratory illness, diabetes, and obesity, to name a few. We can begin to deal with these problems with low-tech solutions. Yet we make little investment, either monetary or politically, in trying to educate the public about the dangers of bad diet and smoking. Government subsidies pour into the production of corn and corn sweeteners, but little goes into the production of fruits and vegetables. While other countries are sensitive to the effects of promoting products full of sweeteners to children and so restrict them, it is carte blanche for advertising to American children. Our officials worry more about loss of lobbying dollars than they do about the devastating effects of diabetes, obesity, and dental caries. Cities vote to remove fluoride from their water. Government plans put only limited funds into home health visits and services such as hospice. Industries trade or sell pollution limits so that total pollution is not reduced, and we lower pollution standards so that we can grow yet more corn for yet more purposes. We ignore less costly ways of insuring health because health protections are sold or compromised in the marketplace of lobbying.

The kinds of health care that get promoted are new drugs, organ transplants, new dental appliances, and ways to whiten teeth—because these investments in our health make money. Health care as a social good has evolved in our society. Of more historical immediacy, we can see how health care has become big business so that almost any other view of it has been eclipsed.

And most discouraging—and disgraceful—of all, we are the only developed country in the world without universal healthcare coverage for our citizens. We spend more, get less.

On the other side, the very fact that we may be paying more attention to our responsibilities to deliver health care give us hope. For example, think of the attention given to professionalism among healthcare disciplines, health disparities, the numbers of uninsured or underinsured, coverage for pharmaceuticals in social programs (however poorly designed they are from the patient's point of view), and the social determinants of health.

The idea that we are embodied persons for whom health and health care are the foundations for all else that we value and for all other social goods is a start. The revelations given to us by studies about the social determinants of health and careful thought given to public health help us to see that without certain social goods basic to how we flourish in our physicality, there is little use in talking about life, liberty, and the pursuit of happiness—and the celebrated equality into which we are all supposedly born.

Amartya Sen, 1998 Nobel Laureate in economics, tells us that the true measurement of economic development takes its most important meaning from how it expands peoples' capabilities, and "emancipation from the enforced necessity to 'live or be less,'" and services, he reminds us, echoing Walzer, are not valuable in themselves.[3] They are of value only because of how they benefit people and expand their capabilities. Freedom to pursue happiness, much less to achieve it, he reminds us "is a question of the command that people have over their lives" thus reiterating the primary observation of the architects of the social determinants of health.[15]

Those of us who are privileged take for granted access to clean air and water, control over our careers and our lives, and freedom from food and shelter insecurity. But these structural elements of our culture, which we may think exist for all of us, are absent in the lives of many, even in our own country, as a result of environmental racism, poor educational facilities, and salaries that make food and shelter iffy propositions.

The idea that we are embodied persons reinforces the idea that the goods we have in our society are social goods and that they receive their meaning from us. We cannot speak blithely of the values we think so importantly define us:—equality; the right to life, liberty, and the pursuit of happiness—without a more careful awareness of what they mean to those less fortunate than we. We must heed Sen's warning about the importance of recognizing how we may be failing to give our fellow citizens the chance to develop their capabilities. People who can't afford their medications; or whose only access to health care is the emergency room; or who sit in a classroom with a serious, persistent toothache are necessarily forced to "live and be less."

SUMMARY

Justness and health care are, by their very nature related. Although in the early days of contemporary medical ethics, the issues of access were given short shrift, we are increasingly coming to realize that the lack of access to health care and the resulting health disparities are the most important and pressing ethical issues in health care.

Various attempts have been made to place emphasis on this problem and to bring a sense of urgency to remedying it. Our strongest tradition of healthcare ethics is principlism, which has its roots in the enlightenment. In that tradition, individual rights, including property rights, predominate. A closer look at the philosophical basis of that tradition causes us to doubt whether enlightenment thinking draws a portrait of ourselves that we recognize.

We experience ourselves as embodied beings embedded in a family, a society, a language group, a narrative. Given that new picture of ourselves, health and health care can be seen as the bedrock upon which our lives and our search for happiness are founded. As a social good, health care cannot be a commodity, but rather something necessary to all of us if we are to live more and to be more.

We should fit our methods of distribution to the meanings of the goods we have in a society to distribute. A good such as health care that is so intimately tied up to what it means to be human should be available to all—a necessity that can best be arrived at by instituting in the United States a system of universal health coverage.

REFERENCES

1. Beauchamp TL, Childress JF. *Principles of Biomedical Ethics*. New York: Oxford University Press; 1979.
2. Walzer M. *Spheres of Justice*. New York: Blackwell Publishers; 1984.
3. Sen A. *Goods and People, Resources, Values, and Development*, Cambridge, MA: Harvard University Press; 1984.
4. National Institutes of Health, *The NIH Almanac*. Available at: http://www.nih.gov/about/almanac/organization/NCMHD.htm. Accessed April 2, 2007.
5. Centers for Disease Control. *Eliminating Racial & Ethnic Health Disparities*. Available at: http://www.cdc.gov/omh/AboutUs/disparities.htm. Accessed April 2, 2007.
6. U.S. Department of Health and Human Services, *Healthy People 2010: Midcourse Review, Executive Summary*. Available at: http://www.healthypeople.gov/data/midcourse/html/introduction.htm. Accessed April 3, 2007.

7. Hospers J. The Libertarian manifesto. In James P. Sterba, ed. *Justice: Alternative Political Perspectives*, Belmont, CA: Wadsworth Publishing; 1999:24–25.
8. Fleck LM. Just caring: Oregon, health care rationing, and informed Democratic deliberation. *J Med Philosophy.*, 1994;19:367–388.
9. Glaser JW. The institutional side of healthcare ethics. *Focus.* Fall 2000:3.
10. American Medical Association. *Principles of Medical Ethics.* Chicago, IL: American Medical Association; 2001:1.
11. American Medical Association. *Declaration of Professional Responsibility.* Chicago, IL: American Medical Association; 2008:1.
12. Medword. *Physician's Charter.* 2008. Available at: http://www.medword.com/PhysiciansCharter.html. Accessed May 28, 2008.
13. Cruess SR, Johnston S, Cruess RL. Professionalism for medicine: Opportunities and obligations. *Med J Australia.* 2002;4:208–211.
14. Pellegrino ED. The internal morality of clinical medicine: A paradigm for the ethics of the helping healing professions. *J Med Philosophy.* 2001;26:559–789.
15. Marmot M, Wilkinson R., eds. *Social Determinants of Health.* London: Oxford University Press; 2005.

Chapter 4

The Role of Academic Medical Centers in the Elimination of Racial and Ethnic Health Disparities

M. Roy Wilson, MD, MS

Vanessa Gamble, MD, PhD

In October 1985, the *Report of the Secretary's Task Force on Black and Minority Health*—also known as the Heckler Report in recognition of then Secretary of Health and Human Services, Margaret Heckler—was released.[1] This landmark report extensively documented disparities between the health status of blacks, Native Americans, Hispanics, and Asian/Pacific Islanders compared with whites. It found that 60,000 excess deaths occurred each year in minority populations—deaths that probably would not have occurred had the persons been white. The task force identified six causes of death—cancer, cardiovascular disease and stroke, cirrhosis, diabetes, homicide and accidents, and infant mortality—that together accounted for more than 80% of the excess deaths observed in minority populations.

The Heckler Report placed racial and ethnic disparities in health onto the national research and health policy stage. Indeed as Senator Edward Kennedy put it, "the issue of health disparities did not seriously capture national attention until 1985, when Margaret Heckler . . . released the *Report of the Secretary's Task Force on Black and Minority Health*, which detailed the many stark differences in health between blacks and whites."[2(p. 453)] The task force's recommendations to Secretary Heckler included more research and data collection on minority health, increased educational outreach to minority communities, improved healthcare access for minority populations, and increased coordination between federal agencies on minority health issues. In response to the report, in January 1986 the U.S. Department of Health and Human Services (DHHS) established the Office of Minority Health (OMH) to develop strategies to improve minority health in the future. The Heckler Report served as the impetus for the formation of an infrastructure on minority health at both the national and state levels. In 1990, the National Institutes of Health (NIH) created the Office of Research on Minority Health to coordinate the development of NIH policies, goals, and objectives related to minority research and research training programs. By 2004, 35 states and territories had established some kind of office, commission, council, or advisory panel on minority health. Of note, task force recommendations focused on actions to be taken by federal and state governments and not by external entities such as medical and other health professions schools.

Yet, as long as health disparities exist among different segments of our society, academic medical centers and the issue of health disparities are inexorably linked. Academic medical centers provide clinical care to a disproportionate share of our nation's health disparity populations, they train the vast majority of the healthcare workforce of the future, they generate new knowledge about disease pathogenesis and processes, and they translate that knowledge into new treatments and cures. Academic medical centers thus have enormous potential to affect the elimination of health disparities within our population. Indeed, academic medical centers are uniquely positioned to do so.

When Secretary Heckler created the Task Force on Black and Minority Health, she charged it to examine what she called a "national paradox—*a continuing disparity in the burden of death and illness experienced by blacks and other minority Americans as compared with our nation's population as a whole*" (Heckler's emphasis). She noted that although there had been steady gains in the health status of minority Americans, "the stubborn disparity remained an affront both to our ideals and to the ongoing genius of American medicine."[1] More than 20 years later, this "national paradox" or, more appropriately this national disgrace, remains an affront to the ideals of the health professions.

Health professions (education and medical education specifically) have historically been considered a public good. All segments of our society pay their share of taxes, and it is a reasonable expectation that the product of these public dollars inure to the good of the commonwealth. The existence of health disparities challenges the egalitarian principle that forms the core of the notion of public good. To the extent that academic medical centers benefit from the support of public dollars—albeit some more directly than others—there exists a moral obligation for academic medical centers to be leaders in the elimination of health disparities.

The Institute of Medicine (IOM) report, *Unequal Treatment: Confronting Racial and Ethnic Disparities in Health Care*, had a tremendous impact on focusing attention on disparities as a national dilemma and on the need for various stakeholders, including academic medicine, to take leadership roles in tackling this problem.[3] Dr. Risa Lavizzo-Mourey, president of the Robert Wood Johnson Foundation and co–vice chair of the IOM committee that issued the report, astutely commented that the report was "incredibly powerful because it put in one place, with the power of the IOM behind it, data that were compelling to people who had not been previously compelled to believe that this was an important issue."[4] The report found that a large body of research existed that documented significant variation in the rates of medical procedures by race, even when insurance status, income, age, and severity of disease were taken into account. It identified several potential sources for these disparities, including health systems–level factors (financing, structure of care, cultural and linguistic barriers), patient-level factors (patient preferences, poor adherence, biological factors), and clinical-level factors (physician bias, lack of cultural competence). The report concluded that comprehensive and multilevel approaches were needed to eliminate racial and ethnic disparities. Indeed, several of the report's final recommendations focus on areas that are clearly under the purview of academic medical centers: (1) increasing the proportion of underrepresented racial and ethnic minorities in the health profession, (2) integration of cross-cultural education into the training of health professionals, and (3) further research to identify the sources of racial and ethnic disparities and to develop intervention strategies. An additional role that academic medical centers can assume is that of advocate for programs and policies that increase diversity in health professions education and that support funding for diversity and disparities research.

Recruiting for Diversity

The past several decades have witnessed a profound demographic change, and the rate of change is currently accelerating. In August 2007, the Census Bureau announced that "minorities" now make up the majority in almost 30% of the most populous counties in the United States and 10% in all counties.[5] These demographic changes will continue, and it is anticipated that within 40 years, the majority of the U.S. citizenry will be comprised of groups currently classified as "minority."[6] Yet, the composition of the healthcare workforce remains not only unrepresentative of the general population, but the diversity gap between the health professions and the general population is widening. Eliminating this diversity gap can contribute greatly to reducing health disparities.

Research that shows how minority healthcare professionals are more likely to practice in minority communities underscores the link between a diverse healthcare workforce and health disparities. Keith and colleagues examined data collected from the class of 1975 medical school graduates by the Association of American Medical Colleges to ascertain the choices of practice location, specialty, specialty board certification, and patient population served.[7] The results of this study showed that almost twice the proportion of minority graduates as compared with nonminorities were practicing in federally designated, manpower shortage areas. In addition, significantly more underrepresented minority physicians chose primary care specialties as compared with white physicians, and family and general practitioners were the most likely to serve manpower shortage areas.

Two studies in California assessed the impact of race on practice patterns, and both yielded similar results. Davidson and Montoya examined data collected using a survey of 1974 and 1975 graduates of seven of California's eight medical schools.[8] The study revealed that minority physicians were more likely than white physicians to be practicing in or adjacent to areas designated as having a healthcare personnel shortage (53% vs. 26%). A more recent study by Komaromy and colleagues used data from the AMA Masterfile and from the U.S. Census Bureau to explore the geographic distribution of California physicians and the characteristics of the communities they served.[9] Similar to the studies by Keith and colleagues and by Davidson and Montoya, this study showed that black and Hispanic physicians were more likely to practice in the areas with fewer primary care physicians per capita and in poorer areas as compared with white physicians. Overall, physicians tended to practice in areas with relatively high proportions of residents of their own race/ethnicity.

The link between a racially and ethnically diverse healthcare workforce and clinical practice among the health disparity population is thus well established. With regard to academic medical centers, one of the most important determinants of success in achieving a racially and ethnically diverse student body—who make up the healthcare workforce of the future—is leadership at the top. Most leaders of academic medical centers value diversity, and many have deeply held convictions about educational opportunities for disadvantaged and underprivileged minorities. Although essential, such personal beliefs are not sufficient; the difficult work is in incorporating those personal values into the organizational culture.

Academic medical centers can take a number of steps toward better achieving diversity:

- The achievement of diversity must be incorporated into the strategic plan of the institution, and leaders at all levels of the institution must be held responsible and accountable for implementation of the plan.
- The institutional officer with overall responsibility for diversity must be placed high in the organizational hierarchy, and this person must have the title and qualifications commensurate with other institutional leaders at this level.
- Implementing and maintaining diversity programs can be costly, and they do not generate revenue for the most part. Institutional support to sustain and expand these programs must be assured.
- Affirmative action is under attack. Rather than retrenching and "playing it safe," academic medical centers must take full advantage of the flexibility afforded by state and federal laws for the achievement of racial and ethnic diversity.

Cultural Competency Training

Dr. Joseph Betancourt, director of the Massachusetts General Hospital's Disparities Solution Center, reminds us that, "Cultural competence is not a panacea that will single-handedly improve health outcomes and eliminate disparities, but a necessary set of skills for physicians who wish to deliver high-quality care to all patients."[10] Prompted by the growing recognition of the impact of racial and ethnic disparities, by the increasing diversity of the nation's population, and by accreditation and legislative mandates, many academic medical centers have developed educational programs in cultural competence. Yet the teaching of cultural competence has encountered several challenges in academic medical centers, including the following:

- Variability in the definition of cultural competence.
- A range in expectations of what should be learned.
- Marginalization in the curriculum.
- Risk of oversimplification and stereotyping.
- Inadequate integration of material throughout the curriculum.
- A scarcity of effective evaluation methods.
- Inadequately prepared faculty.
- Lack of institutional support.

In response to these challenges and with funding from the Commonwealth Fund, the Association of American Medical Colleges (AAMC) released the Tool for Assessing Cultural Competence Training (TACCT) in 2005.[11] This curriculum evaluation tool identifies five domains of cultural competence education:

- Cultural competence—rationale, context, and definition.
- Key aspects of cultural competence.
- Understanding the impact of stereotyping on medical decision making.
- Health disparities and factors influencing health.
- Cross-cultural clinical skills.

Challenges remain, and academic medical centers must work to solidly institutionalize cultural competence at all levels of training. The TACCT warns, "A cultural competence curriculum cannot be an add-on to the present medical school curriculum. If issues such as culture, professionalism, and ethics are presented separately from other content areas, they risk becoming deemphasized as fringe elements or of marginal importance." Despite the acceptance of the importance of cultural competence in the training of medical professionals and the growth of educational programs on the topic, residents report that they are inadequately prepared to treat patients from diverse cultures.[12,13]

In Domain III, "Understanding the Impact of Stereotyping on Medical-Decision-Making," the TACCT did not shy away from tackling the controversial issue of the role of physician bias, stereotyping, and prejudice as contributing factors in the perpetuation of racial and ethnic disparities in health status. Research has clearly identified these as factors. In 1990, the Council on Ethical and Judicial Affairs of the American Medical Association responded to the growing research on racial and ethnic disparities in treatment. It contended that patient characteristics such as income, education, and cultural beliefs contributed to these disparities. However, it acknowledged that physicians' attitudes toward minority patients were also operational. The Council wrote, "Disparities in treatment decisions may reflect subconscious bias. . . . The health care system like all of society has eradicated this [racial] prejudice."[14(p. 2346)] Since the release of this report, additional research has provided further evidence of the role of subconscious bias on treatment decisions and possibly on treatment outcomes. Van Ryn and Burke used survey data to examine whether patients' race and socioeconomic status affected physicians' perceptions of patients.[15] They found that physicians were more likely to have negative perceptions of black patients than white patients and believed that black patients were more likely to be noncompliant with medical advice, less intelligent, and more likely to abuse drugs and alcohol. Schulman and colleagues assessed physicians' recommendations for management of chest pain after they viewed vignettes of "patients" (actually actors) who complained of symptoms of coronary artery disease.[16] The "patients" were divided by race (black or white), sex, age (55 or 70 years), level of coronary risk, and the results of an exercise stress test. The authors found that physicians were less likely to recommend cardiac catheterization procedures for women and blacks than for men and whites. In a similar study, Rathore and colleagues analyzed the influence of race and sex on medical students' perceptions of patients' symptoms.[17] They found that the students were more likely to provide a diagnosis of definite angina for a white male "patient" (also an actor portraying a patient) than for a black female "patient" even though the "patients" had identical symptoms of angina. More recently, Green and colleagues conducted a study to ascertain whether residents exhibited subconscious bias and whether the magnitude of such bias affected thrombolysis recommendations for black and white male patients with acute coronary syndromes.[18] They found that residents held more negative attitudes toward the black patients than they did toward the white patients. More troubling is that these attitudes influenced their clinical decision making. Residents who held the most negative attitudes toward black patients were less likely to prescribe the recommended therapy to the black patients. Despite the large body of research that has demonstrated the role of physician behavior in contributing to health disparities, there is less understanding about the interventions to change these behaviors. As such, it is critical that academic medical centers develop and evaluate educational interventions to address physician and medical student bias.[19]

Mandates developed by accreditation bodies for undergraduate and graduate medical education have underscored the urgency of cultural competence education for medical students and residents. In February 2000 the Liaison Committee on Medical Education (LCME), a joint body of the American Medical Association (AMA) and the AAMC that is responsible for accreditation of medical schools in the United States and Canada, adopted cultural competence accreditation standards. These standards read:

> The faculty and students must demonstrate an understanding of the manner in which people of diverse cultures and belief systems perceive health and illness and respond to various symptoms, diseases, and treatments.
>
> Medical students must learn to recognize and appropriately address gender and cultural biases in themselves and others, and in the process of healthcare delivery.[20]

The Accreditation Council for Graduate Medical Education (ACGME), which is responsible for the accreditation of postgraduate medical training programs in the United States, has also established accreditation policies that focus on cultural competence. The ACGME has identified six general competencies for residency education. Two of them—professionalism and interpersonal and communication skills—include expectations regarding cultural competence. Residents are expected to "communicate effectively with patients, families, and the public, as appropriate, across a broad range of socioeconomic and cultural backgrounds" and to "demonstrate sensitivity and responsiveness to a diverse patient population, including but not limited to diversity in gender, age, culture, race, religion, disabilities."[21]

Legislation has also been introduced at the state level to require that medical schools teach cultural competence. In an unprecedented move, New Jersey enacted legislation in March 2005 that requires that all medical school students in New Jersey receive cultural competency training and makes cultural competency training a condition of licensure for physicians. Washington State has also passed legislation requiring that all health professional schools integrate multicultural health into their curricula by July 2008. Other states, including Ohio, New York, and Illinois, are considering similar legislation.[22] The message is clear: if academic medical centers do not create voluntary cultural competence programs and communicate their effectiveness to lawmakers, the move toward mandatory action will increase.

Health Disparities Research

One of the distinguishing features of academic medical centers is the volume and quality of basic and health-related research that they conduct. Almost by definition, research is part of the mission of all academic medical centers. Regardless of the size of the research enterprise, funding opportunities exist for individual academic medical centers to further expand upon their research, particularly as it relates to health disparities.

As the name might imply, the Minority Health and Health Disparities Research and Education Act of 2000 (Public Law 106-525) highlighted the importance of research and health professions education in the campaign against health disparities. One of its major provisions was the elevation of the NIH Office of Minority Health to the National Center for Minority Health and Health Disparities (NCMHD). The new Center's objectives included coordinating NIH disparities research efforts, funding research programs on health disparities and minority health, supporting health disparity training programs, and providing education loan relief for health professionals who conduct health disparities research. Another provision of the bill directed the Agency for Healthcare Research and Quality (AHRQ) to conduct and support research on health disparities and to issue a health disparities report. Finally, the act authorized the Health Resources and Services Administration (HRSA) to support research and demonstration projects to train healthcare professionals to reduce healthcare disparities.

Although the areas of focus for AHRQ and HRSA are broad, both offer a vast array of research and training programs that directly and indirectly affect health disparities. Examples include AHRQ's Excellence Centers to Eliminate Racial and Ethnic Health Disparities (EXCEED) programs and HRSA's Centers of Excellence (COE) and Health Careers Opportunity Programs (HCOP). EXCEED fosters the building of capacity for health services research that seeks to reduce racial/ethnic health disparities. The programs focus on augmenting the research skills and abilities of ethnically diverse researchers and institutions and on developing sustainable and meaningful research relationships with communities and community organizations. The COE program is intended to improve health professions training for diverse populations. Designated health professions schools are eligible to apply for this grant if they meet required general conditions regarding: (1) certain historically black colleges and universities, (2) Hispanic individuals, (3) Native American individuals, and (3) enrollment of underrepresented minorities above the national average for such enrollments of health professions schools. The HCOP provides grants to eligible accredited schools and health educational entities. The goal of the HCOP is to increase the number of individuals from disadvantaged backgrounds entering and graduating from health and allied health professions programs in order to increase diversity in the health professions workforce. HCOP focuses on intervening at the earliest level and throughout the educational pipeline to develop a sufficient applicant pool of academically prepared and competitive students to enter and graduate from such programs.

The NCMHD continues the legacy of the former NIH Office of Research on Minority Health in partnering with the NIH Institutes and Centers to support programs of health disparities research. However, with the designation of "Center" status, NCMIID now awards grants and contracts independently. NCMHD's focus is exclusively on health disparities. It achieves its goals with a wide breadth of programs that facilitate (1) the development of health disparities research infrastructure and capacity building; (2) funding of meritorious basic, clinical, and population-based health disparity research; and (3) training of health disparity research professionals.

Advocacy

The Association of Academic Health Centers, Association of American Medical Schools, Association of Schools of Public Health, American Dental Education Association, American Association of Colleges of Nursing, American Association of Colleges of Pharmacy, and many other national organizations involved with health care and health professions education have been strong and effective advocates for programs that increase diversity in the healthcare workforce and that support diversity and disparities research. Individual academic medical centers, through their leadership, must join these national organizations in these advocacy efforts. Academic medical centers are invariably enormously important to the state in which they are located. Thus, leaders of academic medical centers typically enjoy substantial influence with state and federal legislators. Due to this reality, they can play an important role in influencing legislation that affects many of the contributors to health disparities.

A review of the recent funding history of Title VII and VIII programs would suggest that such advocacy is needed now more than ever. Titles VII and VIII of the Public Health Service Act authorize a variety of initiatives for training programs to improve the geographic distribution, quality, and racial and ethnic diversity of the healthcare workforce. Administered through HRSA, Title VII programs support physician, dentist, and health professions training, with most of the funding dedicated to training in primary care medicine, dentistry, and health professions students diversity. Title VIII programs fund advanced and basic nurse education and nursing workforce diversity.

The fiscal year (FY) 2008 budget submitted by President George W. Bush cut funding for Titles VII and VIII to $10 million. In stark contrast, the FY2007 budget for Title VII was $184,746,000, and for Title VIII it was $149,679,000. Congress approved a 1.6% (House Labor-HHS Committee) to 23.6% (Senate Labor-HHS Committee) increase from FY2007 for Title VII and 10.7% (House Labor-HHS Committee) to 13.4% (Senate Labor-HHS Committee) for Title VIII. The entire increase contemplated by Congress went unfunded, however, as final budget negotiations forced a 1.76 % recision in budgets across the board. The recision, plus the impact of earlier budget cuts meant the FY2008 funding for both programs would be substantially less than what was funded just 3 years previously (FY2005 for both programs was $450,213,000 versus FY2007 of $334,425,000).[23] At the time of this writing (April 2008), President Bush has submitted a 2009 budget that completely eliminates funding for Title VII programs and cuts $46 million, or about 26%, from Title VIII programs.

Further, between 2005 and 2006, funding for Title VII was cut by about 52%—from \$291,017,471 to \$144,668,633. Every state in the nation, including the District of Columbia and Puerto Rico, suffered huge decreases in funding—with the exception of Indiana, which had an increase of 0.021%. While the largest states had the largest cuts (California, \$15,479,514; New York, \$10,510,741; Texas, \$9,592,326), one state, Wyoming, lost all funding for the program.[24]

During the same period, HRSA Centers of Excellence funding was cut by \$21.8 million or 65%. HRSA used the remaining portion, about \$12 million, to maintain funding for four historically black colleges and universities. The additional 30 Centers of Excellence were no longer funded. Funding for the HCOP was cut by \$32 million or about 89%. HRSA used the remaining \$4 million for the historically black colleges and universities; the other 80 HCOP programs lost their funding.[25]

As a group, academic medical centers are currently facing unprecedented fiscal challenges in relation to their clinical care and research missions. In addition, many state-supported academic medical centers have experienced dramatic cuts in recent years in state funds designated to support education and capital construction. As committed to the cause of eliminating health disparities as they may be, the financial reality is that the vast majority of academic medical centers cannot make up the federal funding cuts of programs—such as those discussed earlier—through their institutional budgets. Continued and even enhanced funding is essential for the nation to fully benefit from the enormous contributions that academic medical centers can make in the campaign to eliminate health disparities. Academic medical centers, in partnership with national organizations that represent the various health professions, must assume a greater leadership role in advocacy.

SUMMARY

Racial and ethnic minorities in the United States receive a lower quality of health care than nonminorities. Michael Byrd and Linda Clayton, in their prodigiously researched, two-volume book, *An American Health Dilemma*,[26,27] have documented that the roots of American racial and ethnic health and healthcare disparities are more than 2,000 years old. Whether the medical and scientific communities have been directly responsible, or only complicit, in this sordid history is debatable. However, it is clear that the causes of the present-day persistence of health disparities are complex and that academic medical centers have influence over many of these. Notwithstanding its historical role, academic medical centers must now assume leadership in eliminating racial and ethnic health disparities.

REFERENCES

1. U.S. Department of Health and Human Services. *Report of the Secretary's Task Force on Black and Minority Health*, vol. 1, Executive Summary. Washington, DC: U.S. Government Printing Office; 1986.
2. Kennedy EM. The role of the federal government in eliminating health disparities. *Health Affairs*. 2005;24:452–458.
3. Smedley BD, Stith AY, Nelson AR. *Unequal Treatment: Confronting Racial and Ethnic Disparities in Health Care*. Committee on Understanding and Eliminating Racial and Ethnic Disparities in Health Care, Institute of Medicine. Washington, DC: National Academies Press; 2003.
4. Institute of Medicine. "Unequal Treatment, One Year Later." Webcast, March 19, 2003. Available at www.kaisernetwork.org/healthcare/iom/19mar2003.
5. Roberts S. Minorities now form majority in one-third of most-populous counties. *New York Times*, August 9, 2007. Online version accessed August 29, 2007.
6. U.S. Census Bureau. *Statistical Abstract of the United States: 2001*. Washington, DC: Author; 2001:17, Table 15.
7. Keith SN, Bell RN, Swanson AG, Williams AP. Effects of affirmative action in medical schools: A study of the class of 1975. *N Engl J Med*. 1985;313:1519–1525.
8. Davidson RL, Montoya R. The distribution of medical services to the underserved: A comparison of majority and minority medical graduates in California. *Western J Med*. 1996;334:1305–1310.
9. Komaromy M, Grumback K, Drake M, et al. The role of black and Hispanic physicians in providing healthcare for underserved population. *N Engl J Med*. 1996;334:1305–1310.
10. Betancourt JR. Cultural competence—Marginal or mainstream movement. *N Engl J Med*. 2004;351:953–955.
11. Association of American Medical Colleges. Tool for Assessing Cultural Competent Training: TACCT. Available at: http://aamc.org/meded/tacct/start.htm. Accessed August 27, 2007.
12. Weissman JS, Betancourt JR, Campbell EG, et al. Residents' physicians' preparedness to provide cross-cultural care. *JAMA*. 2005;284:1058–1067.
13. Park ER, Betancourt JR, Kim MK, et. al. Mixed messages: residents' experiences learning cross-cultural care. *Acad Med* 2005;80:874–880.
14. Council on Ethical and Judicial Affairs. Black-white disparities in health care. *JAMA*. 1990;263:2344–2346.
15. van Ryn M, Burke J. The effect of patient race and socio-economic status on physicians' perception of patients. *Soc Sci Med* 2000;50:813–828.
16. Schulman KA, Berlin JA, Harless W, et al. The effect of race and sex on physicians' recommendation for cardiac catheterization. *N Engl J Med*. 1999;340:618–626.
17. Rathore SS, Lenert LA, Weinfurt KP, et al. The effects of patient sex and race on medical students' ratings of quality of life. *Am J Med*. 2000;108(7):561–566.
18. Green AR, Carney DR, Pallin DJ, et al. Implicit bias among physicians and its prediction of thrombolysis decisions for black and white patients. *J Gen Int Med*. 2007;22:1231–1238.
19. Burgess DJ, Fu SS, van Ryn M. Why do providers contribute to disparities and what can be done about it? *J Gen Int Med*. 2004;19:1154–1159.
20. Liaison Committee on Medical Education. *Accreditation Standards*. Available at: www.lcme.org. Accessed August 27, 2007.

21. Accreditation Council for Graduate Medical Education. *General Competencies.* Available at: http://www.acgme.org/outcome/comp/compFull.asp. Accessed August 27, 2007.

22. National Consortium for Multicultural Education for Health Professionals. *Medical Cultural Competence Legislation and Regulation.* Available at: http://cultural meded.stanford.edu/news/laws.html. Accessed August 27, 2007.

23. Website of the Association of American Medical Colleges. Available at: http://www .aamc.org/advocacy/hpnec. Accessed March 14, 2008.

24. Website of the Association of American Medical Colleges. "Health Professions Funding." http://www.aamc.org. Accessed December 8, 2008.

25. Website of the U.S. Department of Health and Human Services Health Resources and Services Administration. Available at: http://bhpr.hrsa.gov. December 8, 2008.

26. Byrd WM, Clayton LA. *An American Health Dilemma. Volume 1. A Medical History of African Americans and the Problem of Race: Beginnings to 1900.* New York: Routledge; 2000.

27. Byrd WM, Clayton LA. *An American Health Dilemma. Volume 2. Race, Medicine, and Health Care in the United States: 1900–2000.* New York: Routledge; 2002.

Chapter 5

Nursing Perspectives in Addressing Health Disparities

Valda Ford, RN, MPH, MS

"We just want to be treated like everybody else."

I was invited to meet with 20 Somali women, recent immigrants living in Omaha, Nebraska, to discuss some of their concerns about health and new realities in America. I had never addressed a group of recent African immigrants before and was a little intimidated about the encounter. In seeking advice from a local "expert" on immigrant issues, I was told to "not worry about coming on time, take a casual approach to the encounter, and everything would just be fine." She could not have been more wrong. I intentionally arrived two minutes late—rationalizing that I was not "early" and assuming this would be culturally appropriate. To my shock, every single Somali woman was already present and they had been waiting for me almost three hours! These women considered my visit of high importance to them and their community. I was completely embarrassed. The clincher was when I asked the ladies what they wanted me to do for them. They said that ever since their arrival in America they had been treated like slaves and less than intelligent human beings. They wanted me to educate them on how "to be treated like everybody else" and "as real people."

My four-hour encounter with these women revealed my own deep ignorance about what is really taking place outside of the United States and started me on a journey of new discoveries. Those Somali women were proud, nurturing, and protective of their families and community, yet they simply wanted someone to show them how to "receive better treatment as human beings." I considered myself an international traveler and lecturer on health and cultural competency, and yet I had walked into that meeting clueless. I was determined to never let that happen again.

"Water, water everywhere, but who's stopping to drink?"

I was invited to speak to a group of white women at a luncheon meeting in a small town in suburban Nebraska. The topic of my discussion was about improving the general state of their health, maintaining a proper diet, drinking plenty of water, and exercising in a safe place. This was a group of educated, middle-class women, so it was quite a surprise when someone asked me, "Why do we need to drink so much water and why don't coffee, tea, and soft drinks fill the same needs?" I had come prepared to talk about general health and give an overview of fluid and electrolytes, but the general murmur in the room quickly showed me that these women, despite being educated and middle to upper class, really didn't understand the biological importance of water. I decided not to give a suboptimal presentation, but to do a "Basic Water 101" overview for these women. The response from the group was positive. That day I learned that there was a difference in "dumbing down" and adjusting the content of a presentation to fit the needs of the audience. My stereotyping almost kept me from giving a good, effective, and group-specific presentation. Yes, stereotyping does get in the way—regardless of the group!

"Never trust anybody over 30? Why, they're talking about me!"

I was asked to speak to a class of ethnically mixed students at one of Omaha's largest alternative schools. These students had dropped out or otherwise been removed from the mainstream public school system. Most were ethnic minorities, and many were from single-parent, low-income households or the products of substandard school experiences. I was to give one of those "pull yourself up by your boot straps; you can do it" kind of presentations with a big dose of health education on the side. The students questioned why I would have anything to say that could be relevant to their daily existence.

They were tough on me—merciless even. I could easily have finished my presentation, walked out of that classroom, wiped the sweat off my face, and never returned. But, I was determined to return and get it right.

It took about six visits with those students before I understood how to connect and communicate with them; I learned through my perseverance. They were so jaded by the "helicopter" approach of well-meaning adults (drop down, drop off supplies/wisdom, drop out of sight, and never be seen again), that the most important thing they needed to see from me was that I cared enough to keep coming back and that I was not there only as part of a "research project" or "graduate paper requirement." Once I gained their trust, I introduced a wide array of health-related subject matter. These young people were extraordinarily attentive and demonstrated attitudinal changes that would improve their overall health and well-being.

"Oh, come on, Valda. You're being much too sensitive!"

Every time I move to a new city, one of the first concerns I have is to develop a relationship with a new personal healthcare provider. Several years ago, I was referred to one particular physician by at least 20 nurses in my new hometown—high praise, indeed! I went to her office for my first appointment. The front office staff was very friendly and accommodating. I was introduced to the doctor while I was still fully clothed (something that allows me to feel more like an equal in the relationship), and we spoke in-depth about my health history before I was requested to undress. Then she gave me one of the most thorough physical examinations I had ever had. I felt, wow, I have really found an excellent health provider. Near the end of the exam she told me with great sincerity how much she really enjoyed talking to me because I was "so educated." My ears perked, but I remained silent. After all, I had switched to the passive mode of a patient. Moments later, she said she wondered who I had to talk to because she knew that I was a recent arrival to town. When I told her that I was a part of a large organization with lots of women and that I had many people available to talk to, she stated that she was talking about personal and confidential conversations. I told her I had plenty of long-time friends and a few relatives in the area and that I saw them all very frequently. Then the doctor said, "No, I mean someone to talk to on your level; someone as intellectual as you are." When I reiterated that I had plenty of intellectually capable colleagues and relatives, she responded in a way that convinced me that she did not, or chose not, to hear my protestations. As if this was not bad enough, she continued to talk about "we" and "they" while I mentally shrank away from her. Before long she was lamenting the poor work ethic of African Americans and using other disturbing and demeaning stereotypes.

Somehow, as she repeated her delight and surprise at the fact that I was "educated," she seemed to be considering me a confidant and a near-equal and therefore felt it appropriate to talk to me like the most rare and anomalous occurrence—a "good" minority. This doctor, in terms of her clinical skill set, was one of the best physicians I had ever encountered, and I would refer anyone to her for her dedication and professionalism. Additionally, she was well known for her mission to make her practice available to people who are vulnerable or who may not have health insurance. But, disappointingly, even *she* had come to expect that people who look like me would be relatively unintelligent, inarticulate, and crude. If she represents the best in potential professionalism and service to minorities and the underserved, what else is out here? Worse yet, when colleagues asked about my interaction with the doctor and I related this story, their responses were all too often, "Oh Valda—you're just being too sensitive."

The preceding anecdotes occur thousands of times a day throughout the American healthcare system. Nurses have the unenviable task, but the extraordinary vantage point, of reflecting upon how to understand and manage more effectively the wide-ranging differences in health outcomes for the nation's citizens. The role of the nurse in the improvement of the public's health is essential, especially as it relates to health disparities and the cultural competency needed to provide optimum health care from bedside to community.

In every example given, the healthcare professional (myself included) was well meaning. However, good intentions are not enough to avoid creating the very circumstances professionals should strive to avoid—a lack of cultural proficiency, which results in a lack of trust.

The Role of Nurses in Promoting Cultural Competency

Nurses have been perceived as the most ethical and honest of U.S. professionals.[1] The public's confidence in nurses provides a major opportunity to decrease disparities if we assume that the perception of honesty directly relates to the kind of trusting relationships needed to effect change. According to Madeleine Leininger, an essential aspect of relationship building for nurses is moving from stranger to trusted friend.[2] In today's healthcare environment, where interactions are determined on a time versus quality indicator, nurses bridge the gap created by a continually shortened clinic visit. According to the American Nurses Association's Code for Nurses, "The nurse, in all professional relationships, practices with compassion and respect for the inherent dignity, worth, and uniqueness of every individual, unrestricted by considerations of social or economic status, personal attributes, or the nature of health problems."[3] All nurses should strive to create environments that encourage quality healthcare practices because all patients deserve quality care. Health care that is insensitive to differences in that socially mandated condition called *race*, specifically health practices and needs of different groups, can be harmful.

While the Code for Nurses is commendable, research to date has shown that healthcare providers' diagnostic and treatment decisions, as well as their attitudes about patients, are influenced by patients' race and/or ethnicity and stereotypes.[4] Nurses have an even greater opportunity to counter inappropriate or biased treatment decisions by developing relationships with people who are generally perceived as disadvantaged. With the clinical and inpatient expectations of insurance companies being shorter provider visits, the nurse must be the liaison between medical provider and patient in order to promote good health and eliminate health disparities.

Demographic Challenges to Contemporary Nurses

There are about 56 million Americans who do not live where they can find a primary care provider. Nearly one out of every five Americans "are medically disenfranchised, meaning they have inadequate or no access to primary care physicians . . ." and more than 47 million are uninsured.[5] "While more than half of the uninsured have no regular source of health care, most people living in medically disenfranchised areas *have* health insurance."[5] Why is this important? Nurses must be aware that having health insurance does not automatically mean that a person has access to care.

Barriers to care go beyond lack of physicians, health insurance, transportation, income, and language skills.[5] As such, it is critically important that nurses make every effort to educate patients as well as accommodate their travel needs when making patient appointments.

"In underserved areas, there is a current need for 16,000 additional physicians and 9,000 additional dentists. It is estimated that by 2010, 1,000,000 nurses must be added to alleviate the nursing shortage."[6] The shortage in each health profession averages between 20% and 25%.[7] In July 1999, half of all people living in the United States were aged 36 or older, almost 3 years older than the median age in April 1990.[6] The aging of the baby boom generation is partially responsible for this increase. As they moved into their middle years, "the population aged 45 to 49 grew 41 percent and the group aged 50 to 54 swelled 45 percent. However, the oldest age category also experienced substantial gain during this period. Between April 1, 1990, and July 1, 1999, the population aged 85 and older passed 4 million, a 38-percent gain over the 9-year period. Age differences were evident by race and ethnicity."[6] The two youngest groups were the Hispanic population and American Indian/Alaskan Native population. About half of the people in both these groups were aged 27 or younger. The median age for blacks was 30, and for the Asian/Pacific Islander, it was 32; the non-Hispanic white population was the oldest group with a median age of 38.[6]

Nurses Bridging the Gaps

If nurses are to bridge the gaps created by shortened clinic visits and hospital stays, lack of interpreters, and dramatic shifts in cultural and linguistic needs, then it is reasonable to conclude that there need to be more nurses. Health disparities exist throughout the United States, and the nursing shortage is experienced by all areas of the country. While methods vary, "many strategies are being designed to alleviate the problem."[8] "Congress reacted to the pervasive nursing shortage . . . by passing legislation in 2002 designed to stimulate the growth of the nursing profession and to enhance the attractiveness of nursing as a profession. The Nurse Reinvestment Act (NRA), Public Law 107-205, was signed August 1, 2002."[9]

According to a recent study, there are nearly 500,000 registered nurses (RNs) who are licensed but choose not to work in the field of nursing.[10,11] The reasons for this problem include but are not limited to "declining interest in and satisfaction with nursing . . . aging of the RN workforce, increased employer demand, and the need for more intensive nursing care by sicker patients."[8] Other reasons based on the author's observation include suggested frustration at the inability to communicate with patients due to linguistic and cultural differences and the failure of healthcare organizations to take the need for interpreters, translators, and cultural guides (diverse staff representative of the community demographics) seriously when hiring or developing strategic plans.

Gordon Lafer asserts, "there is no shortage of nurses in the United States."[12] According to private and federal sources, "the number of licensed registered nurses in the country who are choosing not to work in the hospital industry due to stagnant wages and deteriorating working conditions is larger than the entire size of the imagined 'shortage.' Thus, there is no shortage of qualified personnel—there is simply a shortage of nurses willing to work under the current conditions."[12] Those "current conditions" include surprise and dismay at the number of people moving into areas not typically viewed as refugee and immigrant catchment areas, and, therefore, not equipped with adequate resources.[13]

"Conflicting expectations of nurses . . . and lack of opportunity to provide comprehensive care emerged as the most important issues for experienced nurses today."[11] Nurses work with patients with higher acuity ratings in hospitals and with greater needs as outpatients. The healthcare industry needs to implement improved staffing levels to provide quality care.[12,14] Nurses should have the opportunity to work in systems in which culturally competent care is considered the norm and should have access to training and technical assistance on the culturally and linguistically appropriate services (CLAS) standards.[5,9,13]

Regardless of the actual or perceived nursing shortage, the present healthcare system is not equipped to allow for culturally competent care without the likelihood of "compassion fatigue."[15] Many organizations have turned to foreign-educated nurses as the answer.[9,12,14] There are advantages and disadvantages to recruiting and hiring foreign-educated nurses. Advantages include reduced costs (compared with the use of temporary nursing staffers) and the ability to keep beds open. The disadvantages are usually lack of English-language proficiency, religious and cultural differences, and real or perceived resentment of special treatment (i.e., special diversity classes, prolonged extra training, and racial/ethnic discrimination by a formerly homogeneous staff).[8,9,11,16]

Recent interviews with nursing executives revealed that hiring foreign nurses "increased the ability of hospitals to respond to the needs of a diverse patient community . . . U.S. nurses consistently recognized that having some extra 'hands on deck' made their lives better. It is, after all, nurses themselves who suffer most when there is a critical shortage."[14,17] *Nurse executives may fail to understand the nuances of problems created when more staff is added without accounting for a lack of cultural competency embedded in the present hospital culture and exacerbated by the introduction of new, different, and still culturally incompetent staff.*

Reasons for health disparities are numerous but in general are due to lack of primary care, health insurance, education, and overall financial instability[4] as well as the perception that minorities are unwilling to participate in clinical research, which could help eliminate health disparities. "Classic public health doctrine holds that the major determinants of the health of every population group lie in the social order: the physical, biological, social, economic, and political environments in which its members, in the main, live."[18]

To equip themselves with appropriate skills to provide culturally competent care and eliminate barriers to improved health outcomes, nurses and public health professionals must first understand the role of culture—"the learned and shared beliefs, values and life ways of a designated or particular group . . ."[2] While knowing about cultures is important, it is not sufficient to be simply culturally aware.

It is the responsibility of healthcare organizations and schools to provide students and employees with the education and training necessary to provide culturally competent care. Additionally, any healthcare organization receiving federal financial assistance is *required* to employ the CLAS standards as a part of standard operating procedure.[19] Implementation of the CLAS standards should reduce inequities in the delivery of health care services.[19] The standards were developed in 2000 in accordance with Title IV of the Civil Rights Act of 1964.[20] Title IV says that "no person in the United States shall, on the ground of race, color, or national origin, be excluded from participation in, be denied the benefits of, or be subjected to discrimination under any program or activity receiving Federal financial assistance."[20]

It is not within the scope of this chapter to fully address the CLAS standards; however, the 14 standards are listed here for information only and are self-explanatory.

Culturally Competent Care

1. Healthcare organizations should ensure that patients/consumers receive from all staff members effective, understandable, and respectful care that is provided in a manner compatible with their cultural health beliefs and practices and preferred language.

2. Healthcare organizations should implement strategies to recruit, retain, and promote at all levels of the organization a diverse staff and leadership that are representative of the demographic characteristics of the service area.

3. Healthcare organizations should ensure that staff at all levels and across all disciplines receive ongoing education and training in culturally and linguistically appropriate service delivery.

Language Access Services

4. Healthcare organizations must offer and provide language assistance services, including bilingual staff and interpreter services, at no cost

to each patient/consumer with limited English proficiency at all points of contact, in a timely manner during all hours of operation.

5. Healthcare organizations must provide to patients/consumers in their preferred language both verbal offers and written notices informing them of their right to receive language assistance services.

6. Healthcare organizations must assure the competence of language assistance provided to limited English proficient patients/consumers by interpreters and bilingual staff. Family and friends should not be used to provide interpretation services (except on request by the patient/consumer).

7. Healthcare organizations must make available easily understood patient-related materials and post signage in the languages of the commonly encountered groups and/or groups represented in the service area.

Organizational Supports

8. Healthcare organizations should develop, implement, and promote a written strategic plan that outlines clear goals, policies, operational plans, and management accountability/oversight mechanisms to provide culturally and linguistically appropriate services.

9. Healthcare organizations should conduct initial and ongoing organizational self-assessments of CLAS-related activities and are encouraged to integrate cultural and linguistic competence-related measures into their internal audits, performance improvement programs, patient satisfaction assessments, and outcomes-based evaluations.

10. Healthcare organizations should ensure that data on the individual patient's/consumer's race, ethnicity, and spoken and written language are collected in health records, integrated in the organization's management information systems, and periodically updated.

11. Healthcare organizations should maintain a current demographic, cultural, and epidemiological profile of the community as well as needs assessment to accurately plan for and implement services that respond to the cultural and linguistic characteristics of the service area.

12. Healthcare organizations should develop participatory, collaborative partnerships with communities and utilize a variety of formal and informal mechanisms to facilitate community and patient/consumer involvement in designing and implementing CLAS-related activities.

13. Healthcare organizations should ensure that conflict and grievance resolution processes are culturally and linguistically sensitive and capable of identifying, preventing, and resolving cross-cultural conflicts or complaints by patients/consumers.

14. Healthcare organizations are encouraged to regularly make available to the public information about their progress and successful innovations in implementing the CLAS standards and to provide public notice in their communities about the availability of this information.[21]

With the acknowledgement of health disparities, health professionals and regulatory agencies recognized the need for clear guidelines for a beleaguered healthcare delivery system.[4,7] The CLAS standards were developed to offer some specificity and "are intended to be inclusive of all cultures and not limited to any particular group or subgroup. However, they are especially designed to address the needs of racial, ethnic, and linguistic populations that experience unequal access to health services."[19] Ultimately, the aim of the standards is to contribute to the elimination of racial and ethnic health disparities and to improve the health of all Americans via culturally competent care.

Adding Insult to Injury

A patient walked into the emergency room after driving 40 miles from the site of a workplace accident. His face was wrapped in his shirt, and his shirt was soaked with blood. The patient was immediately taken into an exam room where his face was examined. Beneath the bloody shirt was a deep wound running from forehead to chin. While disfiguring and obviously painful, the patient had escaped life-threatening injury. A team of people worked to help the man and, though he was unable to speak English, they were able to determine that he had been injured while doing his work as a migrant worker. A friend of the patient, who had arrived with him, explained in halting English the details of the accident, interpreted basic social and medical information, and assisted in giving discharge instructions. During the course of treatment, the nurse went for a suture tray and extra suture material. The doctor, expressing disgust that there was another one of "them" using up his taxpayer dollars, refused the suture material offered by the nurse and told the nurse to get larger suture material. The nurse explained that she had the appropriate size of suture for a facial injury—the type that would leave the least visible scars in the future. While the team was obviously uncomfortable with the doctor's insistence on using suture that would leave very ugly scars, the nurse and other team members felt helpless to change the patient's fate.

The fact that this behavior noted is unethical is obvious. The fact that the patient received less than the optimal care is obvious. The fact that the nurse and the rest of the team felt helpless for fear of reprisals from the doctor and/or hospital administration may not be so obvious. And, what may not come immediately to mind is the knowledge that the patient and the ad hoc interpreter were denied respect, ethical treatment, and culturally competent care. Whatever outreach progress may have been achieved in that community was essentially wiped out with a single act; the physician provided medically adequate care (minimally) but not culturally competent care.

The Many Faces of Patient Vulnerability

A study by Lehman and colleagues shows that African American men are "less likely to receive a diagnosis of a mood disorder and more likely to receive a diagnosis of schizophrenia" than their white counterparts and are "less likely to receive a diagnosis of a co-morbid affective or anxiety disorder."[21] Evidence continues to grow that clinician bias and lack of cultural competency are "likely causing race-linked biases in diagnosis and therefore in treatment."[21] Additionally, clinicians create opportunities for disparity when they fail to use balanced research samples or unbiased tools to assess pathology, and are unaware of or unwilling to "control for socioeconomic status, education, and urbanicity."[21] "These remarkably consistent findings suggest that clinicians should be mindful of the extent to which cultural factors influence their diagnostic approach."[21] Nurses are, again, in a position to make note of variations in medication administration, adverse effects, and outcomes and to assist in clinical decision making or offer other avenues to ameliorate biased treatment and outcomes. Nurses must also ensure that they are aware of long-standing stereotypes (e.g., African Americans have greater pathology, and are in need of more medications, than their white counterparts).

Disparities exist for many reasons, not the least of which are provider perceptions, biases, lack of knowledge, and embarrassment or resentment.[4] Friedman and Borum note that in a "review of 258 medical records 80% of African American patients and 25% of white patients had hypertension. Of the African American patients with hypertension, 58% were prescribed medication to lower hypertension and 42% were never prescribed blood pressure medication. Of the white patients, 86% were prescribed blood pressure meds and 14% were never prescribed meds to lower blood pressure."[22] Simply looking at the differences in percentages of blacks and whites who had meds prescribed in this study along with the evidence of similar diagnostic and treatment regimens in other studies confirms the fact that the disparities in medical management are substantial.[4,22] While there may be many variables to explain variations in health outcomes, there should be no attempt to ignore the obvious: that there is, in fact, "unequal treatment."[4,21,22]

The Ground Meat Parable, or "If I really listen I will understand."

After working in two refugee camps in Ghana and up to 20 different camps in Sri Lanka, I was heading for my final project of 2005—a camp for Liberian refugees in Sierra Leone. I was working with two amazing young women, both undergraduates from Ivy League schools in the United States, and I felt it my responsibility to improve the possibilities for open and honest communication between those of us from the United States and those who were representing the refugees. Not surprisingly, the representatives from the nongovernmental organization were nearly as young as the students—all under age 30. After experiencing some major communication breakdowns and other problems related to the concepts of respect and overfamiliarity, I took the opportunity to have a sit-down meeting before the work began. I asked the spokesperson of the group to feel free to correct us if we made mistakes in what we said or the methods we used to approach our patients and others in the refugee community. I went on to explain that after many months of work with varying volunteers, I felt badly that sometimes, in trying to help, we actually were extremely offensive or insensitive. I requested that they act as our cultural guides and act quickly to correct our faux pas. One of the young men spoke up and said, "I would like to respond to you by telling you the parable of the ground meat." When we agreed, he told a story of a man who was drowning. As the man struggled and struggled to get to the shore, ever afraid of the white water in the rushing river, he pulled at reed after reed—with no success. As the roar of the waterfall became evident and he became more and more tired, he began to give up hope. Just as he was about to give himself up to the river and accept his fate, he saw the glint of something metallic on the shore. He reached deep into himself one more time and fought to get to the shore. As he reached the shore he saw that the metallic object was a sword—sharp on both sides. Undaunted, he reached for the sword and attempted to pull himself from the churning waters. His hands were sliced by the sharp blade but he fought past the pain, past the blood, and past the probability of permanent injury in order to save himself from certain death. After repeated cuts he was able to pull himself out of the water and save his life.

At the end of the story he said, "I hope that you can see why, based on this parable, we will never tell you when you hurt us. Our needs are great and overwhelming, like the river. Our source of salvation may be more like the blade—sharp, cutting, painful—but in the end, still salvation." He thanked us and ended the meeting.

As we walked away from the meeting, I was overcome with grief about the man's statements. He had come to believe that regardless of the inappropriateness of the comments or the brutality and pomposity of the service delivery, ultimately services were delivered. Speaking up or correcting the holder of the services might lead to a temporary or permanent cessation of services. The services might not be as good overall, but they were services nonetheless. My reflection on his story was interrupted by one of the student volunteers who said, "What did what you asked and what he said have to do with 'ground meat'?" After a moment I realized what had happened. The student had heard "ground meat" rather than "drowning man" and, as we talked about the moral of the story, we laughed at how the failure to get a clarification early on had created a situation in which the rest of the message was lost. As we continued toward our meager rooms, we discussed the issues of power and privilege and the devastating understanding that we, as women, nurses, and students, were still in the "privileged" class. We came to understand that our role is to assess for vulnerability and take personal responsibility for doing what we can, with the most information available, to help some of the most vulnerable people—regardless of the way they look, pray, or approach the world.

We came to call this story the Parable of the Ground Meat to point out each person's responsibility in facilitating effective communication. This story is a telling commentary on the urgent need for culturally competent care delivery in our very diverse world.

REFERENCES

1. The Gallup Poll. Honesty/ethics in professionals; December 2006. Available at: http://www.galluppoll.com/content/?ci=1654&pg=1. Accessed August 31, 2007.
2. Leininger M. *Transcultural Nursing: Concepts, Theories, Research and Practices*, 2nd ed. New York: McGraw-Hill; 1995.
3. American Nurses Association, Code of ethics with interpretive statements; 2001. Available at: http://nursingworld.org/ethics/code/protected_nwcoe813.htm. Accessed August 31, 2007.

4. Institute of Medicine. Committee on Understanding and Eliminating Racial and Ethnic Disparities in Health Care. *Unequal Treatment*. Washington, DC: National Academy of Sciences; 2002.

5. National Association of Community Health Centers & The Robert Graham Center. *Access Denied: A Look at America's Disenfranchised*. Washington, DC: National Association of Community Health Centers; 2007.

6. U.S. Census Bureau. *Population Profile: America at the Close of the Twenty-first Century. U.S. Census Population Statistics* [online]. March 2001. Available at: http://www.census.gov. Accessed August 31, 2007.

7. Swartz K, Artiga S. *Kaiser Commission on Medicaid and the Uninsured: Health Insurance Coverage and Access to Care for Low-income Non-Citizen Adults*. Washington, DC: Kaiser Family Foundation; 2007.

8. Skillman SM, Palazzo L, Keepnews D, Hart LG. Characteristics of registered nurses in rural versus urban areas: Implications for strategies to alleviate nursing shortages within the United States. University of Washington Center for Health Workforce Studies; 2005. Available at: http://depts.washington.edu/uwrhrc/uploads/CHWSWP91.pdf. Accessed August 31, 2007.

9. National Advisory Council on Nurse Education and Practice. *Third Report to the Secretary of Health and Human Services and the Congress*. U.S. Department of Health and Human Services, Health Resources and Services Administration; November 2003. Available at: http://bhpr.hrsa.gov/nursing/NACNEP/reports/third/2.htm. Accessed August 31, 2007.

10. National Center for Health Workforce Analysis. *Projected Supply, Demand, and Shortages of Registered Nurses 2000–2020*. U.S. Department of Health and Human Services Bureau of Health Professions; 2002. Available at: http://www.ahca.org/research/rnsupply_demand.pdf. Accessed August 31, 2007.

11. Forsyth S, McKenzie H. *A Comparative Analysis of Contemporary Nurses' Discontents. Journal of Advanced Nursing*; 2006. Available at: http://www.blackwell-synergy.com/doi/abs/10.1111/j.1365-2648.2006.03999.x. Accessed August 31, 2007.

12. Lafer G. Hospital speedups and the fiction of a nursing shortage. *Labor Studies J.* 2005;30:27–46.

13. Boyd-Ford V. *The Role of Cultural Competence in Clinical Competence*. Philadelphia, PA: American Nurses Association Biennial Conference; 2002.

14. Levine RE. Testimony of Ruth E. Levine, senior health economist, World Bank, for hearing on rural and urban health care needs; 2001. Available at: http://judiciary.senate.gov/oldsite/te052201si-levine.htm. Accessed August 31, 2007.

15. Mulligan L. Overcoming compassion fatigue; 2004. FindArticles.com. Accessed August 31, 2007. Available at: http://findarticles.com/p/articles/mi_qa3940/is_200408/ai_n9438202. Accessed April 4, 2008.

16. Davis CR, Kritek, PB. *Healthy Work Environments: Foreign Nurse Recruitment Best Practices*. Association of Nurse Executives; 2005. Available at: http://www.aone.org/aone/pdf/ForeignNurseRecruitmentBestPracticesOctober2005.pdf. Accessed August 31, 2007.

17. World H. The recruits: Despite the red tape and expense, U.S. facilities find it worthwhile to recruit nurses from overseas to alleviate the shortage. *Nurse Week*; 2004. Available at: http://www.nurseweek.com/news/features/04-06/recruits_print.html. Accessed August 31, 2007.

18. Byrd WM, Clayton LA. *An American Health Dilemma: A Medical History of African Americans and the Problem of Race*. New York: Routledge; 2000.

19. U.S. Department of Health and Human Services. *National Standards on Culturally and Linguistically Appropriate Services*. The Office of Minority Health; 2001. Available at: http://www.omhrc.gov/templates/browse.aspx?lvl=2&lvlID=15. Accessed August 31, 2007.

20. 88th Congress, H. R. 7152. Civil Rights Act of 1964. U.S. Information; 1964. Available at: http://www.usdoj.gov/crt/cor/coord/titlevistat.htm. Accessed August 31, 2007.

21. Lehman A, et al. *Practice Guideline for the Treatment of Patients with Schizophrenia*, 2nd ed. Washington, DC: American Psychiatric Association; 2004.

22. Friedman M, Borum ML. Colon cancer screening consultations may identify racial disparity in hypertension diagnosis and management. *J Natl Med Assoc.* 2007; 99:525–526.

Chapter 6

Full Circle: The Qualified Medical Interpreter in the Culturally Competent Healthcare System

Janet E. Bonet, BA

The purpose of this chapter is to explore medical interpreting as an element of organizational cultural competence. It discusses interpreters' bilingual proficiency and considers standards of practice that include cultural competence as an essential component of qualified professional interpreters' skill set. This exploration is organized on three basic premises that are well documented in existing literature on healthcare disparities and language access: (1) many people in need of health care in the United States are of limited English proficiency (LEP), requiring an interpreter to achieve meaningful access to health care services[1]; (2) healthcare providers realize language access is a significant factor in serving LEP populations and want to communicate effectively with patients and their families[2]; and (3) healthcare providers and patients prefer to work with *qualified* interpreters.[3,4]

Since the 2000 U.S. Census, many scholarly and popular publications have described the major demographic shifts reflected in the United States's metamorphosis as increasing numbers of refugees and immigrants join American communities. According to the U.S. Census Bureau's 2006 American Community Survey, nearly 60,000,000 people in the United States speak a language other than English in their home.[5] Satellite television, the Internet, and wireless communications shrink the world, bringing remote cultures into our personal spaces. The same technology that makes geopolitical boundaries disappear in the minds of new generations alters traditional assimilation patterns by keeping immigrants in regular contact, albeit virtual, with their ethnic origins. In the pre-digital age, geographic distance isolated immigrants and engendered social and linguistic assimilation; today, diverse cultural identities of immigrants are reinforced daily. The world becomes seemingly borderless, yet the volume of immigration and information flow makes everyone more conscious of how diverse the world is and how difficult it is to overcome language barriers. But these barriers must be overcome for many reasons, including healthcare needs and public health. The swelling tide of immigration raises healthcare challenges to a level in which regulatory requirements and market demands must compel healthcare systems to provide culturally competent services. Community medical clinics become multicultural, multilingual worlds within single neighborhoods—the human frontline of culture clash and the organizational finish line for judging a health system's cultural competence.

Cultural competence on an organizational scale refers to the larger concept of having the necessary structure and policy around which departments design procedures in the form of standard practices utilized by individual members of the organization. Each individual must become personally culturally competent in his or her occupation, proactively putting cultural competence into practice. In other words, no matter how many policy and procedure manuals might be written, an organization will not become culturally competent until the individuals within it are culturally competent.

The Why and How of Language Access in Health Care

On August 11, 2000, President Bill Clinton signed Executive Order 13166: *Improving Access to Services for Persons with Limited English Proficiency*, requiring ". . . the Federal agencies work to ensure that recipients of Federal financial assistance provide meaningful access to their LEP applicants and beneficiaries."[1] Language is part of culture and part of national origin, and discriminatory treatment based on language is against the law. Making the connection between language access and civil rights was an important step, bringing national attention to something that had been hidden in plain sight. Healthcare systems, state and local agencies, and individual service providers initially considered it just another unfunded federal mandate. Human resources and compliance officers saw it as a huge new headache for employee training and risk management. Patients, public health organizations, and community advocates were given hope of healthcare services becoming more culturally appropriate through improved linguistic access. Of particular significance in Executive Order 13166 is the phrase, "meaningful access." It refers to the quality of service being such that the LEP patient will understand as much via the interpreter as the *non*-LEP patient would understand directly from the healthcare provider. As Holly Mikkelson, a professional in the forefront of interpreter training, puts it, "The goal of interpreted communications is to eliminate linguistic and cultural barriers and allow the participants to carry out their business as if there were no interpreter present."[6] Equality of care is the objective of culturally and linguistically competent health care.

Putting language access requirements into practice is challenging. The U.S. Department of Health and Human Services (DHHS), in accordance with the Executive Order 13166, issued a directive to all federal agencies, *LEP Guidance*, in 2000; but it was not until 2004 that the Revised U.S. DHHS *LEP Guidance*[7] became available to assist healthcare systems and providers understand how to comply. The 4 years needed to complete the guidance is testament to the complexity of providing language access in health care. The National Standards for Culturally and Linguistically Appropriate Health Care Services (known as CLAS) were published by the U.S. Office on Minority Health in 2001.[8] The standards provide the conceptual framework, practical methods, and organizational resources required to achieve legal compliance. The CLAS handbook states, "These standards for culturally and linguistically appropriate services (CLAS) are proposed as a means to correct inequities that currently exist in the provision of health services and to make these services more responsive to the individual needs of all patients/consumers."[8]

Cultural competence in medicine is no more complicated yet no less ingenious than simple, adaptive innovation. Although often discussed as if it were a recently coined concept and somehow unique to the United States, its timeless nature and global context is illustrated in "The Story of Avicenna," as recently told on Spain's National Public Radio.[9] Abú Alí ibn Sina, known as Avicenna, was a 1st century physician whose cultural sensitivity influenced his approach to treating female patients. Knowing that cultural taboos prevented women from allowing him to touch them, it occurred to Avicenna to make a listening tube of rolled paper in order to hear a woman's heartbeat without touching her directly. We could say the stethoscope was invented as a result of cultural competence. Avicenna and his patients lived with a set of inhibiting cultural norms, as does anyone in any time or place; but he was perhaps unique for his time. Healthcare providers in today's multicultural communities must all be aware that cultural norms, their own as well as their patients', may affect health outcomes. In medical encounters with LEP patients needing an interpreter, this third participant's cultural norms are added to the mix. Some healthcare providers are frustrated by expectations that they must be ethnographers as well as medical professionals when treating an ethnically diverse patient base. A well-trained medical interpreter can be a significant culture-specific resource for healthcare providers in cross-cultural multilingual encounters.

Since publication of the CLAS and U.S. DHHS *LEP Guidance*, professional and academic organizations such as the American Medical Association (AMA) and the University of Northern Iowa have created guides for providers. The AMA, in collaboration with the National Medical Association, formed the Commission to End Health Care Disparities[10] in 2004 and published an *Office Guide to Communicating with Limited English Proficient Patients*,[11] similar to *Bridging the Language Divide: A Pocket Guide to Working Effectively with Interpreters in Health Care Settings*, published by the University of Iowa's Center for Immigrant Leadership and Integration.[12] Other guides and tool-kit publications (such as the *Language Services Action Kit*[13] of the National Health Law Program, and the Access Project) have been created to help immigrant advocate and community service organizations work with healthcare providers to fulfill CLAS standards.

The Professional Interpreter: Beyond Bilingualism

It would be unreasonable, however, to assume "bilingual" to be synonymous with "walking ethnographic encyclopedia." Knowing a language does not necessarily make someone an expert in the related culture. There are thousands of languages around the world, and most of them are spoken somewhere in the United States. There is no Star-Trekian earpiece to make all languages intelligible to all persons, and it takes years to attain fluency in a second language. In the meantime, we remain dependent on human interpreters. Medical interpreting is a specialty in high demand as healthcare systems strive to improve language access. Healthcare systems, from megahospitals to neighborhood clinics, develop language access plans to comply with governmental regulations, attain facility certification, increase patient satisfaction, and improve public heath. Plans include how and where to find language services including volunteers, bilingual staff, independent contractor interpreters, and telephonic language bureaus. Where there is sufficient demand in a particular language, staff interpreters are hired. In contrast to bilingual employees who are used as interpreters in addition to their regular duties, staff medical interpreters consider themselves professional interpreters.

Over the past four decades, medical interpreting has gone through developmental stages to achieve professional status. In the United States during the 1970s, most people thought of interpreting as a generalized concept that started with Malinche or Pocahontas. It came to public attention in the 20th century during the Nuremburg War Trials after World War II. It included *anyone* who interpreted, from United Nations' elite conference interpreters to a child helping mom understand a grocery clerk. By the 1980s, beginning in the coastal states because of their large concentrations of LEP populations, distinctions were made among conference, judiciary, and community interpreting as specialties. In the 1990s, medical interpreting grew out of community interpreting, and medical interpreting training curricula became available. In 1998, the National Council on Interpreting in Health Care (NCIHC) was founded with the primary goal of "establishing a framework that promotes culturally competent health care interpreting, including standards for the provision of interpreter services in health care settings and a code of ethics for interpreters in health care."[14] By 2000, the year Executive Order 13166 was signed by President Clinton, medical interpreting degree and certificate programs had been established in universities and colleges. Professional development associations formed to facilitate training and raise public awareness about the profession.

Specialized dictionaries, glossaries, and more ambitious training curricula are improving continually in response to progress toward professionalization of medical interpreting. There are professional regulatory mechanisms, such as the nationally recognized Code of Ethics[15] and Standards of Practice[16] for medical interpreters by NCIHC, which is currently working to develop and institute a national certification process similar to that of judiciary interpreters. The professional status of medical interpreting is gaining credence at corporate and state agency levels. To qualify as a medical interpreter, liability-conscious facilities and agencies require formal training before anyone, including bilingual staff members, is allowed to interpret. Human resources and healthcare staffs are now trained to select and work with qualified interpreters.

Confronted for the first time with language barriers, healthcare providers may misconstrue ethnic heritage as automatically endowing a person with bilingual ability. Some may assume that an employee's high school Spanish or a patient's friend's basic English is "good enough." **Bilingualism,** absolutely essential for interpreting, is not innate; a person named Lindstrom may not speak Swedish and not everyone named Garcia speaks Spanish. Nor is it reasonable to assume that a person is fully bilingual just because the patient introduces him as his "interpreter" from the job site. Nor is bilingualism the only skill needed to become a qualified interpreter; like any skill, relative levels of ability exist. A person fluent in everyday casual conversation may be inept at the level of comprehension and expression needed in medical settings.

Questions of professional **protocol** arise as well. Will a volunteer from the community center have the full range of language fluency and interpreter skills needed? Can a conscripted family member maintain the doctor/patient confidentiality? Hospital social workers may have the best intentions of Good Samaritans when called to interpret, but are they fully prepared to be impartial in the emergency room treatment of a pedophile? Can a pastor from the local ethnic church stay impartial; that is, can she suspend her personal morality while interpreting and allow a patient to make an independent decision on whether or not to use birth control? Will the patient's uncle give a complete rendition, that is, interpret everything the patient says, even if he thinks it will make another relative look guilty of a crime? A trained interpreter will remain impartial and respect confidentiality; will not delete, embellish, or filter a rendition; and will not allow personal beliefs or conflicts of interest to influence or affect the session.

Beyond protocols and bilingualism is another essential characteristic of a qualified interpreter: **cultural competence**. When they are not members of the same ethnic subgroup as LEP patients for whom they will be interpreting, interpreters must look beyond the requisites of language skills, completeness of rendition, and impartiality to their cultural knowledge and, when in doubt, be willing to unselfishly utilize available resources, including glossaries, documents, and LEP patients or family members. Part of cultural competence is knowing how to ask for information that will help clarify communication. For instance, **regionalisms**, terms used in one geographic region where a language is spoken but not in another, can be stumbling blocks. An example is the Spanish word commonly used in Mexico to mean "bug." The same word is used in some parts of the Caribbean to informally mean "penis." Body parts and bodily functions are almost universally given colorful or funny names because people are embarrassed by talking about them and cultural taboos prohibit it. The open-minded and culturally cued-in, sensitive person will gather this kind of knowledge over time; it becomes a very valuable asset to an interpreter.

Bilingual individuals who have attained superior language proficiency, studied medical vocabulary, trained in interpreting techniques, *and* gained cultural expertise are the most qualified as medical interpreters and therefore are the most valuable in healthcare encounters. Optimal clarity in communicating symptoms is a patient's best way to help healthcare providers determine a correct diagnosis efficiently. Optimal clarity in communicating that diagnosis and course of treatment is the provider's best way to help patients achieve successful health outcomes. The life-and-death scenarios in health care make accurate, timely, and culturally appropriate language services essential and medical interpreting a particularly demanding profession. Examples of the very real costs of not using a qualified medical interpreter are given in personal accounts collected by organizations like NHelp.[13]

Examples as Food for Thought

Consider this reality-based, but fictionalized, example of inappropriate language access services. A patient who recently had her gall bladder removed complains of pain in her abdomen to the clinic doctor's new assistant. The assistant's high school Spanish, aided by the patient's daughter's grade school vocabulary learned in ESL class, interprets the patient's gall bladder pain complaint as bladder discomfort. The doctor listens to the assistant's narrative of the symptoms and rather than bother with the time-consuming effort of finding an interpreter, he is satisfied with the assistant's interpretation and prescribes acetaminophen and cranberry juice. In this case, if there had been no language barrier, the doctor might have discovered the real problem was an untreated postoperative infection that eventually turned deadly. An interpreter is not needed at an autopsy but will be at the court proceedings.

Where does the responsibility fall for a communication failure such as that described? Is it a systemic failure of the hospital for not having a functional policy for LEP patient services? Was it a matter of discriminatory treatment because of national origin, or are all patients treated with equally lax communication practices? Was it an overly confident assistant who considered himself bilingual, even though he was not yet past the "where's the bathroom" level? Or was it the child's fault for not knowing the difference between bladder and gall bladder in her second language? Was the doctor at fault because he found it convenient to trust that the assistant really was bilingual? (After all, the assistant's name sounded like he should be, so what is a doctor to do?) Could it be the deceased patient's fault for trusting her 10-year-old daughter to interpret? (After all, the sign on the door did say "bring your own interpreter.")

Horror stories like this one abound, taking on the character of urban legends. They are used by trainers to frighten novice interpreters and medical providers into realizing that language proficiency and cultural competence are serious business. Dedicated healthcare professionals know that open, clear, and knowledgeable communication makes all phases of health care more efficient and all outcomes more successful. The qualified interpreter, as an integral member of the culturally competent team, can help providers and patients reach successful outcomes less stressfully and more accurately, making the process more time efficient and cost effective.

It is naïve to assume that bilingualism and cultural competency are necessarily mutually inclusive. Just as not all bilingual persons are capable as interpreters, not all linguistically qualified interpreters are culturally competent. In evaluating candidates for interpreter work, providers often make the same mistakes as when they evaluate a patient's need for language services. Nationality is confused with race, which is confused with ethnicity, which is confused with language group. Look at the chain of misconceptions illustrated by this single realistic, but fictional, description. There is an interpreter from Africa who is a Sudanese national. He is a member of the Nuer tribe and speaks Nuer, English, and Arabic. An uninformed person might assume that because he is African he will be culturally competent with all Africans, including African American patients. It might also be assumed that because he speaks Arabic, he will be culturally competent with all Arabic patients. It might also be assumed that he will surely be culturally competent with all Sudanese patients, especially those who speak Nuer. And of course, presumably, because he speaks English, he will be culturally competent with the English-speaking administrators, doctors, and nurses for whom he interprets.

In reality, this Sudanese interpreter's cultural competencies may be much more limited. He does not consider himself part of the African American culture because he is a new immigrant. He defines himself as a Sudanese American and does not like being called black which he does not spell with a capital B. Nor does he consider himself simply African because he considers Africa to be a geographic place, an entire continent in fact, and he knows there are many different groups of peoples there. He may dislike speaking Arabic, of which there are several forms, because his tribe was oppressed by Arabic-speaking tyrants. Within his own Sudanese community, there are distinctions between the northern and southern tribes, and tensions exist between them. He may not want to interpret for Nuer women because it could be considered improper. He speaks English, but his cultural knowledge of American life is very basic, and his misconceptions about how the health system functions could lead to erroneous choices in vocabulary, especially as Nuer is a tribal language that does not have words for all the complex concepts and terminology American medical services require. This means heavy mental lifting for the interpreter to search for analogous, descriptive phrases to communicate those ideas and words that do not exist in his indigenous language. Both the interpreter and the provider must be trained in thinking about cultural concepts and how they apply to all three participants in bilingual healthcare encounters.

Due to limited life experiences, an interpreter may be less sensitive to culture-specific cues than the monolingual healthcare providers and LEP patients themselves. Consider two Spanish/English bilingual women with different life experiences. Betty Jo is a 35-year-old native Iowan of German heritage who learned Spanish as a second language and lived in Guatemala for 5 years while studying for her master's degree. Betty Jo's first and dominant language is English, but she is fluent in both scholarly and everyday Spanish because she studied it formally in high school and college life in Guatemala immersed her in it. Her life there was filled with onsite daily contact with Guatemalans and their culture. Silvia is a 35-year-old first-generation immigrant, born in Guatemala, who moved to the United States with her parents when she was 7 years old and learned English by necessity, eventually earning her nursing degree at a local college in Iowa. Although Silvia's first language is Spanish, she has spoken English in all facets of her daily life except in her parental home and among some friends for the last 28 years, thus her dominant language is English. Spanish is Silvia's heritage language because it was her first language and is the language of her parents. Her formal coursework in Spanish ended when she moved to the United States as a child, and she has not studied since. Her exposure to Guatemalan culture was limited to her family life because in her youth there were so few Guatemalans in Iowa. We can assume equivalent English language skills because both women are college educated in the United States but not so for Spanish. Betty Jo has the greater linguist exposure, vocabulary, and grammatical skills as a result of her life in Guatemala. Her accent in Spanish is flawless. By comparison, Silvia speaks Spanish mostly in family settings and sometimes at the clinic, using a mix of Spanish and English to express complex ideas. Due to minimal formal education in standard Spanish, her Spanish lexicon is filled with false cognates and composite or invented words that blend pronunciation and form between the two languages into "Spanglish." She has a definite American accent because of 28 years living in the United States. Silvia calls herself Guatemalan American and is dedicated to her community in both the ethnic and larger American senses.

Who would be more skilled at interpreting in medical settings? Which of these two women would be more able to respond to the cultural cues from Guatemalan patients and serve as a culture broker? Silvia would be more prepared in English medical vocabulary and concepts than Betty Jo; however, Betty Jo would be more up-to-date on the culture of modern urban Guatemalans because she recently spent many years there in a city. Silvia would probably be more in touch with the special conditions of Guatemalan immigrants working in the packing house due to her community activism and her family history. Each woman has her strengths and weaknesses. Both will probably be used as medical interpreters in the town clinic. What is the moral of this comparison? The easy, commonsense assumptions of ethnicity, bilingualism, and specialty training used to generalize about and select interpreters are often nonsensical and erroneous. Both women should be trained in interpreter skills and cultural competence as it relates to medical interpreting, and each should be given every opportunity to share her special skills and knowledge with the other during that training.

There are many areas of the United States in which the pool of potential interpreters is comprised of individuals like Betty Jo and Silvia, available bilinguals with a wide range of fluency, education, interpreter skills training, and cultural knowledge but not trained in medical interpreting. This is where the full circle of organizational cultural competency comes about, where corporate planning and policy design come together with human resource cultivation. As medical interpreter candidates are recruited, the healthcare system uses its corporate human resources in partnership with postsecondary educational resources to coordinate interpreter training programs designed to strengthen interpreter candidates' skill sets to bring them to a level of professional medical interpreter, solidifying culturally and linguistically appropriate service delivery in health care.

SUMMARY

We began this chapter with three premises: (1) there is a demographic need for language access, (2) healthcare providers want to communicate with their patients, and (3) both patients and providers want qualified interpreters. The law requires language access in health care, responsible organizations support the development of culturally and linguistically appropriate services, and professionalization of medical interpreting offers qualified human resources. A qualified healthcare interpreter has three basic skill sets: (1) high bilingual proficiency—advanced levels of comprehension and expression in both languages; (2) health care knowledge—medical concepts, terminology, and health care; and (3) professional preparation and conduct—trained in and abiding by the professional code of ethics and standards of practice for medical interpreting. But within a healthcare organizations in which cultural competence is given priority, medical interpreters will be considered fully qualified only when a fourth skill set, cultural competency, is included.

The U.S. DHHS *LEP Guidance* for compliance with Title VI sets some parameters for designing language access plans; the CLAS, NHelp, AMA, and NCIHC publications (among others) provide resources for preparing and instituting those plans. Language access solutions include using family and friends, volunteers, bilingual staff when necessary, contract and freelance interpreters when available, and, optimally, full-time staff interpreters. The recent literature generated by government agencies, healthcare systems, academia, and nonprofit groups regarding language access provides three overarching recommendations: (1) the use of minor children should be avoided if at all possible, (2) relatives and friends should be used only in cases when no other interpreter is available, and (3) anyone who is to interpret or use an interpreter should be properly trained in the professional code of ethics and standards of practice for medical interpreters. In addition, it is highly recommended that any healthcare provider who will be using an interpreter also be trained in how to best manage an interpreted encounter and best utilize an interpreter to optimize patient outcomes. Providers and interpreters who have undergone specific diversity training are more comfortable and more capable of addressing the health care of a diverse patient base. Conversely, LEP patients who are given an opportunity to become informed on how an interpreted session is handled are more likely to be proactive participants in the encounter.

When assuming the challenge of attaining cultural competency and evaluating resource allocation, healthcare systems must ask the following questions. What is it worth to be able to communicate with the growing LEP patient base? What portion of the market is LEP? What will it cost for a healthcare system to become culturally and linguistically competent to serve the LEP population?

Oh, what a tangled web the financial gurus weave with their bottom lines when they look at the cost of interpreter services as an isolated number on the budget sheet! Of course it is not that simple. What are the direct and hidden costs of inept communication? Who pays the cost of LEP patients' medical services resulting from incorrect diagnoses because of language barriers? To help providers appreciate the potential for medical errors resulting from poor cross-cultural communication, NHelp and other advocacy groups have collected real-life stories of LEP patients' suffering as a consequence of inadequate or total lack of language services and other scenarios such as those presented in this chapter. Deciding to upgrade to the most modern imaging equipment or creating a language access plan that includes upgrading cultural competency policies for medical interpreters are both matters of good planning. When healthcare systems invest in creating a full-circle approach to culturally and linguistically appropriate service provision, they build stronger organizations. Organizational cultural competency is fortified by a highly qualified pool of culturally competent medical interpreters integrated into the healthcare team. What is good for public health—providers using qualified medical interpreters—is good for the healthcare system's risk management, cost efficiency, and the bottom line.

REFERENCES

1. Executive Order 13166. *Improving Access to Services for Persons with Limited English Proficiency*. August 11, 2000. Available at: http://www.lep.gov/13166/eolep .htm. Accessed April 4, 2008.

2. American Medical Association. *Physicians are becoming engaged in addressing disparities*. April 2005. Available at: http://www.ama-assn.org/ama/pub/category/ 14969.html. Accessed December 12, 2007.

3. Ginsburg J. *Language Services for Patients with Limited English Proficiency: Results of a National Survey of Internal Medicine Physicians*. A White Paper of the American College of Physicians. April 2007;8.

4. Kuo DZ, O'Connor KG, Flores G, Minkovitz CS. Pediatricians' use of language services for families with limited English proficiency. *Pediatrics*. 2007;119:e920e927. Originally published online March 19, 2007. Available at: http://www .pediatrics.org/cgi/content/full/119/4/e920. Accessed April 4, 2008.

5. U.S. Census Bureau. *2006 American Community Survey*. Available at: http://fact finder.census.gov/servlet/STTable?_bm=y&-geo_id=01000US&-qr_name=ACS_ 2006_EST_G00_S1603&-ds_name=ACS_2006_EST_G00_. Accessed December 18, 2007.

6. Mikkelson H. *The Art of Working with Interpreters: A Manual for Health Care Professionals*. 2006. Available at: http://www.acebo.com/papers/artintrp.htm. Accessed December 18, 2007.

7. U.S. Department of Health and Human Services, *Guidance to Federal Financial Assistance Recipients Regarding Title VI Prohibition Against National Origin Discrimination Affecting Limited English Proficient Persons*, 2004. (U.S. DHHS Revised *LEP Guidance*). Available at: http://www.usdoj.gov/crt/cor/lep/hhsrevised lepguidance.html.

8. U.S. Department of Health and Human Services, Office of Minority Health. *National Standards for Culturally and Linguistically Appropriate Services in Health Care, FINAL REPORT*. Rockville MD: IQ Solutions; March 2001:3. Available at: http://www.omhrc.gov/templates/browse.aspx?lvl=2&lvlID=15. Accessed December 12, 2007.

9. National Public Radio of Spain, Radio Televisión Española. *El cuento de Avicena*. May 20, 2007 (c) EL SUEÑO DE ARQUÍMEDES, Angel Rodríguez Lozano. Available at: http://www.ciencia.rne.es. Accessed May 28, 2007.

10. Mission and Vision Statements of the Commission to End Health Care Disparities (see #2). Available at: http://www.ama-assn.org/ama/pub/category/12809.html.

11. *Office Guide to Communicating with Limited English Proficient Patients*, 2nd ed. Available at: http://www.ama-assn.org/go/healthdisparities. Accessed December 18, 2007.

12. Grey MA, Yehieli M, Rodriguez-Kurtovic N. *Bridging the Language Divide: A Pocket Guide to Working Effectively With Interpreters in Health Care Settings*. Cedar Falls, IA: University of Northern Iowa, Iowa Center for Immigrant Leadership and Integration; December 2006. Available at: www.bcs.uni.edu/icili/PDFDocument/hires_handbook.pdf. Accessed December 18, 2007.

13. National Health Law Program (NHelp) and The Access Project. *Language Services Action Kit: Interpreter Services in Health Care Settings*. Revised 2004. Available at: http://www.healthlaw.org/library/item.70355.

14. *Mission and Goals of the National Council on Interpreting in Health Care*. Available at: http://www.ncihc.org/mission.htm. Accessed December 18, 2007.

15. National Council on Interpreting in Health Care. *National Code of Ethics for Interpreters in Health Care*. July 2004. Available at: http://www.ncihc.org/NCIHC_PDF/NCIHC_COE_962005.pdf.

16. National Council on Interpreting in Health Care. *National Standard of Practice for Interpreters in Health Care*. September 2005. Available at: http://www.ncihc.org/NCIHC_PDF/National_Standards_of_Practice_for_Interpreters in Health Care.pdf.

Chapter 7

Cultural Proficiency: Challenges for Health Professionals

Richard L. O'Brien, MD, FACP

Practicing a health profession in a culturally diverse society presents significant challenges. Even defining culture meaningfully in the context of health care is challenging. "Culture has been defined in a number of ways, but most simply, as the learned and shared behavior of a community of interacting human beings."[1] Cultural traits—habits of mind, language, values, beliefs, practices, family and social relationships, behavior—are associated with race, ethnicity, socioeconomic status, educational attainment, occupation or profession, workplace, residential locale, generation, gender, and other circumstances that define a group of persons with common sets of learned behavior. Most individuals belong to more than one culture and find themselves conforming to culturally determined behavior that fits the circumstances in which they find themselves at any given time.

Even the health professions differ in culture. Although all are expected to share commitment to the well-being of those they serve, nurses, pharmacists, physicians, and others use different language and have different expectations, knowledge sets, and habits of mind. The challenge of working together on behalf of others requires understanding different professional cultures, languages, and expectations. Further, professionals bring their own culturally diverse backgrounds into the professions, and this diversity can influence the effectiveness of communication and collaboration on behalf of patients.

But these inter- and intraprofessional cultural differences, although sometimes challenging and demanding intercultural sensitivity and knowledge to ensure the best of care delivered by professionals,[2] are not the primary focus of this chapter. Rather, it addresses those cultural differences arising from different values, beliefs, and traditions affecting understanding of health and disease that determine practices affecting the likelihood of contracting disease, how individuals and groups respond to illness and approaches to treatment, and how professionals approach and deal with patients of cultures significantly different from their own. The cultural differences that are most challenging in professional practice are associated with race, ethnicity, language, socioeconomic status, and gender.

For health professionals to deliver effective care, they must ensure accurate communication; understand and appreciate culturally determined values, beliefs, and practices; and engender trust. Achieving these three goals—communication, cultural understanding, and trust—is usually interrelated in interactions with patients and clients. And it is professionals, not patients, who are responsible for ensuring adequate understanding and communication and developing trusting relationships.

Communication

Different languages are the most obvious barriers to effective communication and create frustrations for patients and professionals. Professionals encounter problems of timely accessibility to translation and are frequently concerned about the accuracy of translation, proficiency of interpreters with medical subjects, and linguistic parallels: are there terms in the patient's language or dialect that accurately reflect the medical term and context?

Federal law requires that hospitals and practices provide interpreters' services as needed.[3] Most hospitals and practices have readily available professional interpreters, but many professionals are not adept at working with them efficiently and effectively. A reasonably good guide for doing so has been prepared by Mikkelson.[4] Further, health professionals, especially if working under time pressures, may resort to inappropriate choices for translation and utilize bilingual persons without medical knowledge or vocabulary; these may include patients' acquaintances, friends, relatives, or even patients' children.[5] These may result in inaccurate translation, health professional or patient discomfort in discussing questions about potentially embarrassing or sensitive subjects, and failure of patients to understand explanations and recommendations.

At times, because of a lack of immediate availability of translators, physicians may go on to other patients, leaving the patient with whom they do not share a language waiting for a translator to arrive. This is frustrating for patients; as a result, they may feel undervalued as persons by the clinic and professional.[6] These patients may perceive the lack of attention as racism, lack of interest, or lack of respect for them and their needs. This is especially true if there is no one readily available to explain that they are waiting for an interpreter. This frustration and perception of lack of respect may breed a lack of trust and confidence that their needs will be appropriately addressed.

Professionals are also frequently concerned about the accuracy of translation, even when provided by professional interpreters. The experience of asking a question or providing information, hearing a lengthy response in a language one does not understand, and having an interpreter provide a terse translation cannot help but leave one wondering what was omitted, what was lost in translation. The best response in such circumstance is to ask the interpreter to explain what was left out and why. But the experience necessarily affects one's confidence in translation.

There are times when face-to-face professional translation is simply not possible because of the small number of qualified interpreters in a community or because time is urgent and a professional interpreter is not immediately available. There are telephone interpretation services that provide access to many languages at all times; occasionally, though, a language used relatively rarely in Western societies is not immediately available. Telephonic interpretation services are excellent for some circumstances but less than optimal for others. Telephone interpretation is best avoided when providing mental health services, with hard-of-hearing patients, with children, when attempting to use visual aids for communication, and when several persons are in the conversation (e.g., when communicating with a patient and family).[7] Other means of bridging language gaps have been used, including the use of picture boards in emergency circumstances.[8]

Different languages are not the only barriers to communication between health professionals and patients and families. Communication can be impaired by failing to use terms that are understandable to those with whom one wishes to communicate. Different patients bring great variations in education, health literacy, idiom, vernacular, conceptualization and perception of wellness and illness, the existence of ethnic remedies, and notions of time and urgency to healthcare encounters. Even relatively simple terms may not convey understanding adequate to enable patients to deal reasonably and effectively with their problems and concerns.

Different cultures also have different styles of communication involving such things as "voice volume, tone, and intonations [and] nonverbal communications . . . ."[9] Health professionals should be sensitive to such differences, able to perceive whether or not their communication with any individual patient is effective and productive in serving the patient's interests.

These uncertainties of the quality of communication between providers and patients create concerns about the adequacy of understanding and its importance to ensuring truly informed consent, patients' participation in decision making, and patients' adherence to necessary care.[5]

It is essential that professionals know enough about each individual patient, or work with someone who does, to adapt their communication to cultural variables. The dominant model of health and disease in the United States is Western, science-based medicine, but it is not the only model. Some patients may consult with the medical care system in addition to, or to supplement, another tradition, or Western medicine may be a last resort for some whose traditional methods have not provided the relief they seek. If a professional does not appreciate how a person's culture and traditions affect their world view, perceptions, and expectations, then communication will not adequately inform the patient, patient satisfaction is likely to be decreased, the risks of poor or even adverse outcomes are enhanced, and the foundation of confidence and trust necessary for a therapeutic relationship is compromised.

Cultural Understanding

Conceptions of wellness and disease differ greatly among cultures. Many cultures have evolved and embrace diagnoses, etiologic and pathogenetic explanations, and practices and remedies that do not conform to the Western scientific medicine model.[10-12] The list is very long and differs among cultures. Many patients will have consulted folk healers and/or used folk remedies for symptoms before consulting health professionals trained in Western medicine. They may also continue to use folk methods simultaneous with consulting and following advice from health professionals. Many persons believe in the efficacy of prayer in healing and may ask their caregivers to join them.

The great many different cultural definitions of disease and therapeutic approaches to them render it practically impossible for health professionals to master them all. Health professionals will be most effective serving their patients if the health providers attempt to learn from the patients and their families about their perceptions of their problems and what causes them, and what they believe will be most effective in relieving those problems. It is also useful to consult with folk healers to gain understanding of concepts of disease and remedies, and even collaborate with them if it can benefit the patient. Most professionals will encounter enough persons of some cultures that they may develop reasonably comprehensive knowledge, but, unless they are steeped in the culture, it remains valuable to rely on others who are of the culture for interpretation, explanation, and guidance. Professionals should also ask for continuing education programs that inform and instruct them about different cultural conceptions of disease, folk healers, and remedies.

Most folk remedies or cultural practices are harmless or may be beneficial, even though unproven. Their value may derive from ingredients that are of use but have not been tested in Western medicine. They may also derive from what Western medicine calls the *placebo effect*. Unfortunately, some are harmful.[13–15] These can present a particular challenge to health professionals. Some instances, such as female genital mutilation (circumcision) or dermal burns from moxibustion ("cupping"), are or may be considered abuse in our society. In many states, professionals are required by law to report such instances to the police. This may result in children being removed from parents and put in foster homes—an outcome that may be more harmful to a child than the practice that led to it. In other instances, the harm may be the result of toxic substances in folk or home remedies (e.g., lead poisoning from treatments for *empacho*).

Health professionals should be aware of cultural and religious beliefs that may affect the way they relate to and care for some patients. Many physicians are unaware of the fact that many medications are derived from or contain animal products that are forbidden for some, such as medications containing or encapsulated in products derived from pork (Jews and Muslims) or beef (Hindus).[16] Other prohibitions include blood transfusions for Jehovah's Witnesses and unrelated men and women touching each other (some Muslims). Although most religious prohibitions may be suspended to avoid death or serious harm, it is important for health professionals to inform themselves about such beliefs of their patients and about the possibility of unknowingly violating these religious precepts. All patients with religious proscriptions should be informed about all potential treatment options and their wishes should be respected in prescribing medications or other therapies.

Different cultures deal with information management and decision making differently from the predominant American ethic.[17,18] Some cultures do not hold that individual autonomy is the appropriate model for decision making, relying on other loci of decision making—the head of family, elders, or some means of group consultation. Some cultures differ from the predominant model of truthfulness by withholding bad news about fatal diseases or dying. And there are different perceptions and practices regarding advance directives and different rituals that culturally competent professionals will take into consideration.

Two useful guides to relating effectively to persons of different cultures are the transcultural assessment model of Giger and Davidhizar[19] and the Purnell model for cultural competence.[20] But it is also important to recognize that respect for and consideration of the culture that a patient has been raised in and cultural practices to which they are accustomed does not excuse the health professional from considering the individuality of each patient and acting accordingly. Individuals adopt aspects of cultures different from that of their origins over time as they acculturate to or assimilate traits of other cultures with which they interact. This is clearly implied by the very fact that they resort to Western scientific medicine. Professionals must strive to know and accommodate others' cultural beliefs and practices while applying scientific medicine in patients' best interests. Professionals must know all patients as individuals, their beliefs, their expectations, and their desired outcomes of their encounters with the healthcare system.

Trust

Mutual trust between a health professional and patient is essential to the patient's well-being and a successful outcome of the relationship. Trust is necessary for the development of a *therapeutic alliance*, a relationship between patient and health professional based on mutual respect and confidence. It creates a collaboration between professional and patient so that they work in partnership to address a patient's concerns and problems. Professionals must rely on the veracity and completeness of information derived from patients to formulate effective diagnostic and treatment plans. Patients must trust professionals to be honest with them, providing information necessary for their understanding of problems and alternatives for dealing with them so that they may determine their best course of action. Such a relationship demands mutual trust.

Patients' trust of professionals is correlated with satisfaction and compliance with health care advice,[21–24] with good outcomes of care,[21,22] and more consistent use of preventive services.[25] It has also been shown that being trusting of others in general is correlated with better health and longevity.[26]

Health professionals must be acutely conscious of the need to develop a trusting relationship between themselves and each patient. And professionals should not tacitly assume that every patient they encounter brings trust to the relationship. Sad to say, about 20% of all patients do not have full trust in their physicians, a mistrust shared by most ethnic or racial groups but more pronounced in blacks and Hispanics than in whites.[27,28] Lack of trust is correlated with race or ethnicity, lower educational attainment, and low income.

Distrust can be based on group experiences, especially of minority populations that have been subjected to discrimination and other abuses; on individual experiences in which trust has been violated; or when one party in a relationship manifests distrust of the other. People tend to lack or lose trust in those whom they perceive to be untrusting.

Providers can take specific measures to engender trust by patients. A number of studies of characteristics or practices that correlate with patients' trust of health professionals have concluded that trust is earned by thorough, understandable communication, both verbal and nonverbal; provider knowledge of and interest in the patient; expressions of care by the provider; demonstrated listening skills; thoroughness of information seeking and examination; continuity of care by the provider(s); and referral to and coordination of specialty services.[21,24,25,27–32] It has also been demonstrated that continuity of care and coordination of care improve outcomes and decrease health disparities.[33]

There is also evidence that patients are more trusting of those with whom they share ethnicity, race, or gender, although the results are mixed. Race-concordant visits have been found to be longer and had higher patient ratings of satisfaction than race-discordant visits.[34] It has been reported that women, but not men, are more satisfied if their physician is of the same gender.[35] Another study found greater trust and patient satisfaction if patients share beliefs about information sharing and power with their provider. Patient concordance of belief with their physicians was correlated with being female, white, younger age and with education and income. College-educated, young, white middle-class women are more likely to have beliefs similar to those of their physicians.[36]

Health professionals must be aware that some patients enter into any encounter with a lack of trust. To engender trust, health professionals are advised to develop and demonstrate listening skills, to endeavor to understand clearly patient values and expectations, and to show respect and concern for patients by not "speaking down" to them or showing signs of impatience or being hurried. Make the effort to ensure that your patients understand and assimilate your explanations and can participate (and know that they can participate) in decision making regarding their care. Be prepared to refer as appropriate, perhaps even to ask if they prefer a professional of similar ethnicity, race, or gender. To the extent possible, encourage continuity of care and coordination of care provided by other professionals.

Actions by Others to Ensure Culturally and Linguistically Appropriate Care

Professionalism and the ethical duty to serve the best interests of patients is compelling enough reason for professionals and the institutions in which they practice to provide culturally appropriate care to all, to ensure effective communication, to understand their needs and desires as they understand them, and to develop a bond of trust with each patient. However, a history of failing to do so, the existence of great health disparities affecting primarily minority communities, and growing knowledge and concern about disparities have led to the development and adoption of laws, regulations, accreditation standards, and other measures intended to ensure culturally and linguistically appropriate care.

In 2000 the U.S. Department of Health and Human Services, in response to an executive order by President Bill Clinton, issued regulations requiring healthcare providers to establish practices and meet certain standards of culturally and linguistically appropriate services (CLAS) in health care.[3] Failure to adhere to these standards may result in loss of federal funds.

A number of states have enacted or are considering laws intended to ensure the cultural competence of professionals.[37] These laws generally affect licensing standards or impose obligations on educational institutions to implement courses in cultural competence. New Jersey led the way by enacting a law requiring evidence of a course in cultural competence for licensure or license renewal, thus affecting medical student and continuing medical education. California has also enacted legislation requiring evidence of continuing education in cultural and linguistic care to renew physicians' licenses. Illinois, New York, and Ohio have similar legislation pending. Washington has enacted SB 694, which requires that all health professions education programs (undergraduate and continuing education) integrate into their curricula instruction in "multicultural health" by July 1, 2008.

Accreditation bodies have also begun to require evidence of cultural competence. The Liaison Committee on Medical Education (LCME) has incorporated cultural competence requirements into its accreditation standards.[38] The Accreditation Council of Graduation Medical Education (ACGME) has also added cultural "sensitivity and responsiveness" to its general competencies for all graduate medical education programs.[39]

Other means of enforcing or providing incentives to provide culturally competent care include modifying payment mechanisms and standards, providing performance incentives, and assessing patient satisfaction.[40,41]

Experiences of Minority Professionals

A chapter on professionals' cultural competence and the challenges presented by cultural differences would be deficient if it did not mention the experiences of minority professionals, and their effects on those professionals, in a white-dominated healthcare system.[42] Minority professionals are acutely conscious of the fact that they are perceived as different and expected to be different. It affects their relationships with patients, patients' families, staff, and colleagues. Most often the experiences are negative: feeling "invisible," being mistaken for a nonprofessional (e.g., a maintenance or housekeeping employee), or being asked by a patient or family if they may see a different doctor or nurse. Less often is the experience positive, when minority patients express pride in being taken care of by a person of their race or ethnicity.

Minority professionals also often feel as though they are not integrated into the professional and social milieu of their institutions. They frequently feel a lack of mentoring or opportunity for career advancement and that they are put into or urged to accept stereotyped roles (e.g., as representatives of diversity or to relate to particular community). They often experience "racial fatigue," the "emotional and psychological sequelae of feeling isolated in [an] environment in which race regularly influences behavior but is consistently ignored."[42(p49)]

It behooves institutions and individual professionals in these environments to be aware and strive to adopt policies and behaviors that allow open discussion of race and its impact; to acknowledge that race matters; to be supportive of the aspirations of minority professionals, providing opportunities to realize them; and to avoid stereotyping.[43]

SUMMARY

The challenges of practicing a health profession in a diverse society can be daunting, especially when compounded by the pressures of a healthcare system that is market-based and values productivity and cost control more than quality and outcomes. Nonetheless, as professionals we have assumed fiduciary duties to serve our patients' best interests, not the interests of ourselves, our employers, those with whom we contract, or those who profit from our patient care.

It is essential that all health professionals recognize and understand cultural differences, value and respect persons whose cultures differ from theirs, learn to communicate effectively with persons of other cultures, and treat them with the respect and care that engender trust. Only by doing so are professionals able to ensure that their patients have the knowledge necessary to make good decisions and practice what will assist them to maintain the best health that they can. Understanding, communication, and trust produce the best outcomes and are the best way individual professionals have to reduce health disparities.

REFERENCES

1. Useem J, Useem R. (1963) Men in the middle of the third culture. *Human Org.* 1963;22(3):169–179.

2. Institute of Medicine. *Health Professions Education: A Bridge to Quality.* Washington, DC: National Academies Press; 2003.

3. U.S. Department of Health and Human Services, Office of Minority Health. National standards on culturally and linguistically appropriate services (CLAS) in health care. *Federal Register.* December 22, 2000;65(247):80865–80879.

4. Mikkelson H. The art of working with interpreters: A manual for health care professionals. *ACEBO.* April 2005. Available at: http://www.acebo.com/papers/artintrp.htm. Accessed September 11, 2007.

5. O'Brien RL, Kosoko-Lasaki O, Cook CT, Kissell J, Peak F, Williams EH. Self-assessment of cultural attitudes and competence of clinical investigators to enhance recruitment and participation of minority populations in research. *J Natl Med Assoc.* 2006;98(5):674–682.

6. Cook CT, Kosoko-Lasaki O, O'Brien RL. Satisfaction with and perceived cultural competency of health care providers: The minority experience. *J Natl Med Assoc.* 2005;97(8):1078–1087.

7. Kelly N. Telephone interpreting in health care settings: Some commonly asked questions. *Am Trans Assoc Chron.* June 2007;18–21. Available at: http://www.atanet.org/chronicle/feature_article_june2007.php. Accessed September 11, 2007.

8. Johnson LA. Picture Boards help bridge language gap in health emergencies. Associated Press Wire Service. September 2, 2007.

9. Purnell L. The Purnell Model for Cultural Competence. *J Transcultural Nurs.* 2002;12(3):193–196.

10. New Hampshire Governor's Office of Energy and Community Service. *Ethnic Community Profiles.* 2001. Available at: http://www.nh.gov/oep/programs/refugee/documents/ethnic_community_profiles.pdf. Accessed September 11, 2007.

11. Purnell LD, Paulanka BJ. *Guide to Culturally Competent Care.* Philadelphia: FA Davis; 2005.

12. Simons RC. Introduction to Culture Bound Syndromes. *Psychiatric Times.* November 2001;XVIII(11). Available at: http://www.psychiatrictimes.com/p011163.html. Accessed September 11, 2007.

13. Centers for Disease Control. Poisoning from Mexican folk remedies—California. *Morb Mortal Wkly Rep* 1983;32:554–555.

14. Baer R, Garcia de Alba J, Cueto L, et al. Lead based remedies for empacho: Patterns and consequences. *Soc Sci Med.* 1989;29:1373–1379.

15. Flores G. Culture and the patient–physician relationship: achieving cultural competency in health care. *J Peds.* 2000;136:14–23.

16. Sattar SP, Ahmed MS, Madison J, et al. Patient and physician attitudes to using medications with religiously forbidden ingredients. *Ann Pharmacotherap.* 2004;38(11):1830–1835.

17. Searight HR, Gafford J. Cultural diversity at the end of life: Issues and guidelines for family physicians. *Am Fam Physician.* 2005;71:515–522.

18. Giger JN, Davidhizar RE, Fordham P. Multi-cultural and multi-ethnic considerations and advanced directives: developing cultural competency. *J Cult Divers* .2006;13:3–9.

19. Giger JN, Davidhizar RE. The Giger and Davidhizar transcultural assessment model. *J Transcult Nurs.* 2002;13:185–188.

20. Purnell L. The Purnell model for cultural competence. *J Transcult Nurs*. 2002; 13:193–196.
21. Safran DG, Rogers WH, Kosinski M, Ware JE, Tarlov AR. Linking primary care performance to outcomes of care. *J Fam Pract*. 1998;47(3):213–220.
22. Thom DH, Kravitz RL, Bell RA, Krupat E, Azari R. Patient trust in the physician: relationship to patient requests. *Fam Pract*. 2002;19(5):476–483.
23. Hall MA, Zheng B, Dugan E, et al. Measuring patients' trust in their primary care providers. *Med Care Res Rev*. 2002;59(3):293–318.
24. Sheppard VB, Zambrana RE, O'Malley AS. Providing health care to low-income women: A matter of trust. *Fam Pract*. 2004;21(5):484–491.
25. O'Malley AS, Sheppard VB, Schwartz M, Mandelblatt J. The role of trust in use of preventive services among low-income African-American women. *Prev Med*. 2004;38(6):777–785.
26. Barefoot JC, Maynard KE, Beckham JC, Brummett BH, Hooker K, Siegler IC. Trust, health and longevity. *J Behavioral Med*. 1998;21(6):517–526.
27. Doescher MP, Saver BG, Franks P, Fiscella K. Racial and ethnic disparities in perceptions of physician style and trust. *Arch Fam Med*. 2000;9:1156–1163.
28. Keating NL, Gandhi TK, Orav EJ, Bates DW, Ayanian JZ. Patient characteristics and experiences associated with trust in specialist physicians. *Arch Int Med*. 2004;164:1015–1020.
29. Thom DH, Stanford Trust Study Physicians. Physician behaviors that predict patient trust. *J Fam Pract*. 2001;50(4):323–328.
30. O'Malley AS, Forrest CB. Beyond the examination room: primary care performance and the patient–physician relationship for low-income women. *J Gen Intern Med*. 2002;17:66–74.
31. Aruguete MS, Roberts CA. Participants' ratings of male physicians who vary in race and communication style. *Psychol Rep*. 2002;91(3 Pt 1):793–806.
32. Gordon HS, Street RL Jr, Sharf BF, Kelly PA, Souchek J. Racial differences in trust and lung cancer patients' perceptions of physician communication. *J Clin Oncol*. 2006;24(6):904–909.
33. Beal AC, Doty MM, Hernandez SE, Shea KK, Davis K. Closing the divide: How medical homes promote equity in health care. Results from the Commonwealth fund 2006 Health Care Quality Survey. The Commonwealth Fund, June 2007. Available at: http://www.commonwealthfund.org/usr_doc/1035_Beal_closing_divide_medical_homes.pdf?section=4039. Accessed September 11, 2007.
34. Cooper LA, Roter DL, Johnson RL, Ford DE, Steinwachs DM, Powe NR. Patient-centered communication, ratings of care and concordance of patient and physician race. *Ann Intern Med*. 2003;139(11):907–915.
35. Derose KP, Hays RD, McCaffrey DF, Baker DW. Does physician gender affect satisfaction of men and women visiting the emergency department. *J Gen Intern Med*. 2001;16:218–226.
36. Krupat E, Bell RA Kravitz RL, Thom D, Azari R. When physicians and patients think alike: Patient-centered beliefs and their impact on satisfaction and trust. *J Fam Pract*. 2001;50(12):1057–1062.
37. National Consortium for Multicultural Education for Health Professionals. Medical Cultural Competence Legislation and Regulation. Available at: http://culturalmeded.stanford.edu/news/laws.html. Accessed September 11, 2007.
38. Liaison Committee on Medical Education. Functions and structure of a medical school: Standards of accreditation of medical education programs leading to the

MD degree. June 2007. Available at: http://www.lcme.org/functions2007jun.pdf. Accessed September 11, 2007.

39. Accreditation Council on Graduate Medical Education. General Competencies. February 1999. Available at: http://www.acgme.org/outcome/comp/compFull.asp. Accessed September 11, 2007.

40. Angeles J, Somers SA. From policy to action: Addressing racial and ethnic disparities at the ground-level. Center for Health Care Strategies, Inc. August 2007. Available at: http://www.chcs.org/usr_doc/From_Policy_to_Action.pdf. Accessed September 11, 2007.

41. Casalino LP, Elster A, Eisenberg A, Lewis E, Montgomery J, Ramos D. Will pay-for-performance and quality reporting affect health care disparities? *Health Affairs* 2007;26(3):w405–w414. Available at: http://content.healthaffairs.org/cgi/reprint/26/3/w405. Accessed September 11, 2007.

42. Nunez-Smith M, Curry LA, Bigby JA, BergD, Krumholz HM, Bradley EH. Impact of race on the professional lives of physicians of African descent. *Ann Intern Med.* 2007;146(1):45–51.

43. Betancourt JR, Reid AE. Editorial: Black physicians' experience with race: should we be surprised? *Ann Int Med.* 2007;146(1):68–69.

Chapter 8

Cultural Competency Research: Description of a Methodology. Part I

Sade Kosoko-Lasaki, MD, MSPH, MBA
Cynthia T. Cook, PhD

Despite the overall improvement of health in the American population, studies have shown that there is a disparity in the health of certain racial groups. This pattern of disparity is evident in healthcare utilization and outcomes, and in the delivery of culturally and linguistically competent care.

Many of the determinants of well-being span the boundaries of health care and medicine; therefore, eliminating health disparities calls for new and nontraditional partnerships across diverse sectors of the community. The effort requires a new approach to research, especially if the subjects are of a diverse group and culture. The effort also calls for a fundamental change in how research is designed, conducted, and disseminated in collaboration with diverse racial and ethnic communities.

Minority populations harbor a distrust of the healthcare establishment and are reluctant to participate as subjects in clinical research projects. For clinical scientists to conduct research in this area, it is essential that they develop trusting relationships with members of minority communities. This requires that investigators understand the cultures they study and that minority populations understand and appreciate the value of participating in research.

To accomplish this, during the summer of 2003 a cultural proficiency study was convened. The purpose of this study was to assess the minority patient/client perception of the cultural competency of their healthcare providers within the Omaha, Nebraska, medical community and to have healthcare providers self-assess their ability to provide culturally competent care. Two instruments were developed, pilot tested, and administered during the summer and fall of 2003 for this purpose: the Community Assessment Instrument (CAI) and the Cultural Competency Instrument (CCI). The CAI assessed the cultural competence of healthcare providers by the minority community and the minority community's knowledge of medical research risks and benefits. The CCI assessed the cultural competence of healthcare providers and clinical investigators. This chapter focuses on the Community Assessment Instrument, while Chapter 9 focuses on Part 2, the Cultural Competency Instrument.

To date, to the best of our knowledge, no research has provided data that indicate cultural competency can reduce health disparities or improve health care.[1-7] In addition, there is limited data available on how to measure cultural competency.[8-14] Nevertheless, it is important to assess the cultural competency of healthcare providers and, more important, to determine if cultural competency has an impact on reducing health disparities.

We present a description of a methodology that we believe can effectively measure the cultural competency of healthcare providers. The results of the study have been previously detailed.[8-10] We encourage our reviewers and readers to replicate the study or improve and/or expand the research design in order to perfect the assessment instrument.

Background Information

In 1998, the Initiative to Eliminate Racial and Ethnic Disparities in Health (under the auspices of the U.S. Department of Health and Human Services) addressed the problem of health disparities. Six areas in which African Americans, Hispanics, and Native Americans have higher morbidity and/or mortality rates and/or access to preventive health measures were identified: cardiovascular disease, diabetes, infant mortality, HIV/AIDS, cancer screenings and management, and child and adult immunizations. The goal of eliminating these health disparities[15] has been embraced by policy makers, researchers, medical centers, managed care organizations, and advocacy organizations. Models and programs have been developed and partnerships have been formed by various advocacy groups, which include preventive care, community education, and case and disease management. In research, centralized data-collection models have been developed and sophisticated technologies have been employed for analyses and dissemination of results.

Significant barriers have been identified in establishing and implementing the new research agenda in conjunction with diverse communities. These barriers include:

Mistrust: Some members of racially and ethnically diverse groups shun participation in research studies because of historical mistrust due to past experiences with racism, bias, or exploitation in healthcare delivery systems.

Lack of identifiable benefits: Some diverse communities have not equitably benefited from their participation in research.

Conflict in values and benefits: Differing values and social, cultural, religious, and spiritual beliefs related to health may inhibit or prevent certain individuals and groups from participating in research protocols and studies.

Lack of relevance to research: Members of diverse racial and ethnic groups that are fairly new to this country may be neither accustomed nor willing to participate in research conducted according to traditional U.S. methodologies.

Methodologies do not reflect the "at-risk" population: Many faculty members within institutions of higher education neither use nor teach research approaches and methodologies that are based on culturally competent and participatory action.

Lack of guiding principles: Researchers have been slow to require principles of cultural competence, participatory action research designs, and advocacy-oriented approaches in the grants and contracts they support. Moreover, peer reviewers and contract officers often do not receive the necessary training to enhance their knowledge in this area.[16]

The racial/ethnic minority population that participated in the cultural competency study reiterated all of these concerns or barriers.[8,17] Until these barriers are overcome, low levels of minority participation in healthcare research will continue along with health disparities in morbidity and mortality rates. In this chapter we describe the research design used to collect the data in support of the eight hypotheses for the study that has been previously detailed.[8,10]

Research Design

Community Assessment Instrument (CAI): Methodology

The Community Assessment Instrument (CAI)[18-29] was an attempt to assess the Omaha minority community's perception of the cultural competency of

their healthcare providers and to assess their knowledge about the importance and their willingness to participate in healthcare research. Eight
hypotheses were formulated and 76 survey items developed to support or
refute the theory that healthcare providers in Omaha are not culturally competent and that minority members are not interested in participating in
healthcare research. The hypotheses are listed in **Table 8–1**. These are the
same hypotheses that were applied to the CAI pilot study.[10]

The CAI allowed select minority members to assess the cultural proficiency of healthcare providers and clinical investigators within the Omaha
medical community. The instrument attempted to identify those areas of
healthcare delivery that are proficient and those areas that need improvement. Through identification and rectification of problems associated with
cultural competency, healthcare providers and investigators hoped to establish trusting relationships with minority patients/clients that would lead to
their increased participation in healthcare research. The ultimate goal of
such participation is to reduce the health disparities that exist among the
racially and ethnically diverse population in the Omaha area, and within
the nation, by increasing their participation in healthcare and clinical
research.

The CAI was administered to eight ethnic/racial and/or gender groups
over a four-month period. **Table 8–2** lists the racial and/or ethnic and/or
gender group and the dates of their participation in the study.

Table 8–1 *Community Assessment Hypotheses*

1. Minority healthcare clients are not satisfied with health care in the Omaha community.
2. Minority clients are not able to communicate with healthcare providers in the Omaha community.
3. Minority clients prefer to be treated by healthcare providers who are of the same ethnic, racial, and/or cultural background.
4. Minority clients practice folk medicine.
5. Minority clients feel pressured to assimilate.
6. Minority clients have never participated in a healthcare study and do not want to.
7. Minority clients do not know the benefits of participating in a healthcare study and do not know anyone who has ever participated in one.
8. Minority clients do not know the leading cause of death for people in their ethnic/ racial group.
Adapted from the Community Assessment Instrument (CAI) Omaha.

Table 8–2 *Administration of Study by Race and/or Ethnicity and Time*

Ethnic/Racial Group	Date of Focus Group
Native American	August 20, 2003
Sudanese men	September 10, 2003
Hispanic men	September 17, 2003
African American	September 22, 2003
Sudanese women	September 29, 2003
Hispanic women	October 1, 2003
Vietnamese	November 9, 2003
White	November 24, 2003
Adapted from the Community Assessment Instrument (CAI) Omaha.	

Key organizations that had significant representation of a given ethnic or racial group in the Omaha community were contacted and asked to host a study session. However, not all organizations that were contacted participated. Hosting required the use of their neighborhood or local facility, providing refreshments that the study paid for, and recruiting 10 members as participants in the study. To get the minimum number at a study session, we solicited confirmation from at least 12 potential participants. All invited participants who arrived at the designated site were included in the study. If the study population's first language was not English, the host organization was responsible for providing interpreters. These trained interpreters stood next to the study presenter and focus group facilitator and interpreted every sentence to ensure consistency among all the study groups.

The Sudanese women's and men's groups, however, created the most challenge. Interpreters were needed for the Nuer, Dinka, and Arabic languages. In addition, many of the men and all of the women needed assistance in completing the questionnaire. Many of the female respondents had no formal education. As a result, we had similar answers to stated questions, possibly due to interpreter response bias. Similar problems on a smaller scale were found with the Hispanic groups and the Vietnamese population.

At the beginning of each study group, respondents were given an overview of the purpose of the cultural proficiency study. They were then asked to sign a consent form that was approved by Creighton University's Institution Review Board. When all the consent forms had been signed and collected, the CAI was distributed. Respondents were given approximately 30 minutes to complete the form. However, the time period varied with the study group's English language proficiency. It took approximately 90 minutes for the Sudanese women's group to complete the questionnaire. This was the only group that exceeded the allotted time period for completing the questionnaire and focus group discussion. Each woman needed the assistance of an interpreter to not only translate the question but to explain the possible answers and to record the correct answer on the questionnaire.

The Sudanese men's group had 15 people attend, but only 9 were part of the study. The 6 additional men were there to assist with completing the questionnaire as interpreters. When an announcement was made that only 9 men completed the consent form and we wanted 10, one of the interpreters agreed to be a participant. Only 3 of the Sudanese men who participated in this study did not need an interpreter.

All respondents were asked to answer the CAI questions to the best of their knowledge and ability and to hold their inquires and comments until the focus group was conducted. After the questionnaires were collected from all respondents, a trained and experienced facilitator (who was not affiliated with Creighton University) conducted the focus group. For the Vietnamese and Hispanic populations, the interpreter stood next to the facilitator and interpreted every sentence. For the Sudanese population, the interpreters stood or sat next to his or her language group. The Sudanese and Caucasian focus groups were held at Creighton University Medical Center in the same boardroom where the pilot studies were conducted in June 2003. In addition, the women's Sudanese group was moved to another location because they exceeded the time for use of the room, and three of the Arabic-speaking males were relocated to the cafeteria to complete the questionnaire while the focus group discussion began in the boardroom.

Furthermore, a Caucasian focus group was added as a reference group for the study to ascertain if whites had similar experiences with the Omaha medical community as the minorities interviewed. The facilitator was a white female (who was affiliated with Creighton University Medical Center). Respondents were paid $50 for travel expenses. The host organization was compensated $250 for its assistance.

The CAI assessed the strengths and the weaknesses of the Omaha medical community in providing culturally competent and/or proficient health care to an ethnically and racially diverse client/patient population. It identified the areas that can be used as models for developing, improving, and maintaining cultural competency and/or proficiency within the medical community. It also identified areas that the Omaha minority community perceives as needing improvement through self-awareness and/or cultural sensitivity training. In addition, the instrument assessed how well the ethnically and racially diverse Omaha community members were informed about their particular group's healthcare needs and their knowledge of and willingness to participate in healthcare or clinical studies.

Immediately after the focus group meeting, a post-CAI questionnaire was administered. The purpose of the post-CAI questionnaire was to assess the changes in the knowledge of participants concerning the health care of the given ethnic and/or racially diverse group and their willingness to participate in healthcare or clinical studies.

Descriptive and inferential statistics were used to analyze the data. The results of the pre- and post-CAI survey have been detailed in the *Journal of the National Medical Association.*[8] **Appendices 8–A and 8–B** are the Pre- and Post-Community Assessment Instrument.

REFERENCES

1. Anderson LM, Scrimshaw SC, Fullilove MT, Fielding JE, Normand J. Culturally competent healthcare systems. A systematic review. *Am J Prev Med.* 2003;24(suppl 3): 2,3,8,9.

2. Brach C, Fraser I. Can cultural competency reduce racial and ethnic health disparities? A review and conceptual model. *Med Care Res Rev.* 2000;57(suppl 1):181–217.

3. Betancourt JR. Cultural competency: Providing quality care to diverse populations. *Consult Pharm.* 2006;21(12):988–995.

4. Betancourt JR, Green AR, Carrillo JE, Ananeh-Firempong, O. Defining cultural competence: A practical framework for addressing racial/ethnic disparities in health and health care. *Public Health Rep.* 2003;118:293–302.

5. Rosa UW. Impact of cultural competence on medical care: Where are we today. *Clin Chest Med.* 2006;27(3):395–399.

6. Gonzalez-Espada, WJ, Ibarra, MJ, Ochoa, ER, Vargas, PA. Multicultural medical encounters: The experience at a pediatric clinic. *J. Ark Med Soc.* 2006;102(8): 227–229.

7. Gregg J, Saha S. Losing culture on the way to competence: The use and misuse of culture in medical education. *Acad Med.* 2006;81(6):542–547.

8. Cook CT, Kosoko-Lasaki O, O'Brien RL. Satisfaction with and perceived cultural competency of health care providers: The minority experience. *J Natl Med Assoc.* 2005;97(8):1–10.

9. O'Brien R, Kosoko-Lasaki O, Cook CT., Kissell J, Peak F, Williams EH. Self assessment of cultural attitudes and competence of clinical investigators to enhance recruitment and participation of minority population in research. *J Natl Med Assoc.* 2006; 98(5):674–682.

10. Kosoko-Lasaki O, Cook CT, O'Brien RL, Kissell J, Purtilo R, Peak F. Promoting cultural proficiency in researchers to enhance the recruitment and participation of minority populations in research: Part 1, Development and refinement of survey instruments. *Eval Progr Planning.* 2006;29(3):227–235.

11. Arthur TE, Reeves I, Morgan O, et al. Developing a cultural competence assessment tool for people in recovery from racial, ethnic, and cultural backgrounds: the journey, challenges and lessons learned. *Psychiatr Rehabil J.* 2005: 28(3):243–50.

12. Robins LS, White CB, Alexander GL, Gruppen LD, Grum CM. Assessing medical students' awareness of and sensitivity to diverse health beliefs using a standardized patient station. *Acad Med.* 2001;76(1):76–80.

13. Frusti DK, Niesen, KM, Campion JD. Creating a culturally competent organizaton: Use the diversity competency model. *Nurs. Admin.* 2003;33(1):31–38.

14. Hobgood C, Sawning S, Bowen J, Savage K. Teaching culturally appropriate care: A review of educational models and methods. *Acad Emerg Med.* 2006;13(12): 1288–1295.

15. Healthy People 2010. U.S. Department of Health and Human Services. 2000. www.healthypeople.gov.

16. Policy Brief 3, Cultural competence in primary health care: Partnerships for a research agenda. National Center for Cultural Competence. Creighton University Center for Child & Human Development.

17. Cook CT, Kosoko-Lasaki O, O'Brien RL. Minority attitudes and perception of health care: A comparison of comments from a cultural competency questionnaire and focus group discussion. In: Kosoko-Lasaki O, Cook CT, O'Brien RL, eds. *The Role of Cultural Proficiency in Eliminating Health Disparities.* Sudbury, MA: Jones and Bartlett; 2009.

18. The Community Assessment Instrument (CAI) terms and definitions are adapted from: Blue, AV. *The Provision of Culturally Competent Health Care.* Department of Family Medicine, Medical University of South Carolina College of Medicine, 2000. www.musc.edu/deansclerkship/rccultur.html. Accessed February 26, 2003.

19. Oncology Nursing Society. Oncology Nursing Society Multicultural Outcomes: Guidelines for Cultural Competence, by the Society, 1999, Pittsburgh, PA: Author.

20. Cross TL, Bazron BJ, Dennis KW, et al. *Towards a Culturally Competent System of Care.* CASSP Technical Assistance Center: Georgetown University Child Development Center. 1989;1.

21. Edgar E, Patton JM, Day-Vines N. Democratic dispositions and cultural competency. *Remedial Spec Educ.* 2002;23(4):231–242.

22. Glenn-Vega A. Achieving a more minority-friendly practice. *Fam Prac Manag.* June 2002. www.aafp.org/fpm.

23. Hanley JH. Beyond the tip of the iceberg: Five stages toward cultural competence: Reaching today's youth. *Community Circle Caring J.* 1999;(3)2:9–12.

24. Jackson VH. Cultural Competency. *Behav Health Manag.* March/April 2002:20–26.

25. Mason JL. *Cultural Competence Self-Assessment Questionnaire: A Manual for Users.* Research and Training Center on Family Support and Children's Mental Health. Portland State University. 1995.

26. National Center for Cultural Competence. *Promoting Cultural Diversity and Cultural Competency: Self-Assessment Checklist for Personnel Providing Services and Supports to Children with Special Health Needs and Their Families 2002.* www.georgetown.edu/research/gucdc/nccc7.html. Accessed February 26, 2003.

27. Outcomes and Accountability Alert. Performance measures reflect how well systems serve diverse populations. 1999;4(1):1. Available at: scilib.univ.kiev.ua/doc .php?6384634. Accessed on April 7, 2002.

28. Rose VL. Cultural competency in health care. *Am Fam Phys.* 1998; 57(11): 2882.

29. Sue, DW. A model for cultural diversity training. *J Counsel Devel.* 1991;70: 99–105.

Appendix 8–A. Community Assessment Instrument (Pre-Test)

Case Number _____

Identifying Data

1. Gender/sex
   a. male
   b. female
2. Marital status
   a. single
   b. married
   c. divorced
   d. widowed
   e. separated
3. What is your age? _____
4. How many children do you have?
   a. 0_____
   b. 1_____
   c. 2_____
   d. 3_____
   e. 4_____
   f. 5 or more (specify) _____
5. How many children are under age 19?
   a. 0
   b. 1
   c. 2
   d. 3
   e. 4 or more
6. What are their ages?
7. What is the highest grade or degree that you have completed?
   a. some high school
   b. high school/GED graduate
   c. some college
   d. associate's degree
   e. bachelor's degree
   f. some graduate work
   g. master's degree
   h. PhD, JD, MD
   i. other (specify) _____

8. What is your occupation?
9. What is your race and/or ethnic group?
   a. African American/Black
   b. Caucasian/White
   c. Hispanic/Latin
   d. Native American
   e. Sudanese
   f. Vietnamese
   g. Other (specify) _____
10. What is your religion (optional)?
    a. Protestant
    b. Catholic
    c. Native American
    d. Buddhist
    e. Muslim
    f. Judaism
    h. Other (please specify) _____
11. Is English your first (mother) language?
    a. yes
    b. no
12. If no, what is your first language? _____

Health Care

13. Have you ever been treated at a Creighton University hospital or clinic?
    a. yes
    b. no
    c. don't know
14. I would like for you to think about the **last time** you or a family member was sick or ill. Did you or the family member:
    a. go to an emergency room
    b. go to a clinic or HMO
    c. go to a doctor's office/private physician
    d. treat yourself or family member at home
    e. other (specify) _____
15. If you answered a, b, or c in question 14, was the health facility or healthcare provider affiliated with Creighton University Medical Center?
    a. yes
    b. no
    c. don't know

16. The **last time** you went to the emergency room (ER), clinic, or doctor's office, were there forms or papers that you had to complete?
    a. yes
    b. no
    c. don't know

17. If you said yes in question 16, were you able to complete the forms?
    a. yes
    b. no

18. If no, can you explain why you were not able to complete the forms?

    _____

19. How would you rate the care you received from the nurses at your last visit to the emergency room, clinic, or doctor's office?
    a. excellent
    b. good
    c. adequate/satisfactory
    d. below adequate
    e. unsatisfactory

20. If you answered a, b, or c in question 19, can you explain why you were **satisfied** with the nursing care?

    _____

21. If you answered d or e in question 19, can you explain why you were **dis-satisfied** with the nursing care?

    _____

22. How would you rate the care you received from the doctor at your last visit?
    a. excellent
    b. good
    c. adequate/satisfactory
    d. below adequate
    e. unsatisfactory

23. If you answered a, b, or c in question 22, can you explain why you were **satisfied** with the medical care or the visit?

    _____

24. If you answered d or e in question 22, can you explain why you were **dis-satisfied** with the medical care or the visit?

    _____

25. Did you go to another healthcare provider within two months before your last doctor's visit for the same condition or illness?
    a. yes (if yes, go to question 26)
    b. no (if no, skip to question 30)
    c. don't know

26. This person was a:
    a. medical doctor
    b. nurse practitioner
    c. physician assistant
    d. religious person
    e. spiritualist (a person who prayed for you)
    f. folk healer (a person who treated you with herbs/plants)
    g. other (specify) _____

27. How would you rate the care or treatment you received from the person who treated you in question 26?
    a. excellent
    b. good
    c. adequate/satisfactory
    d. below adequate
    e. unsatisfactory

28. If you answered a, b, or c in question 27, can you explain why you were **satisfied** with the medical care or visit?

    _____

29. If you aswered d or e in question 27, can you explain why you were **dissatisfied** with the medical care or visit?

    _____

30. Did you have contact with any other healthcare personnel during your last visit?
    a. yes (if yes, please specify job title _____)
    b. no (if no, skip to question 34)
    c. don't know

31. If you answered yes to question 30, how would you rate the care or treatment that you received from this healthcare personnel?
    a. excellent
    b. good
    c. adequate/satisfactory
    d. below adequate
    e. unsatisfactory

32. If you answered a, b, or c in question 31, can you explain why you were **satisfied** with the care or treatment?

    _____

33. If you answered d or e in question 31, can you explain why you were **dissatisfied** with the care or treatment?

    _____

34. Did the doctor ask you what you thought caused your illness?

    a. yes

    b. no

    c. don't know

35. Did the doctor ask you what treatment you thought you should receive?

    a. yes

    b. no

    c. don't know

36. Did the doctor ask you if there was someone else who could help with your illness?

    a. yes

    b. no

    c. don't know

37. If yes, who did you say could help with your illness?

    _____

38. Did the doctor ask you what your family or friends thought about your illness?

    a. yes

    b. no

    c. don't know

39. If yes, how did your friends or relatives perceive your illness?

    _____

40. Can you tell me why you went to the doctor? What was wrong with you?

    _____

41. Did you receive medication or an injection for the illness or condition?

    a. yes

    b. no

    c. don't know

42. Did you need an interpreter when you visited the emergency room, clinic, or doctor's office?

    a. yes

    b. no (skip to question 47)

    c. I brought a relative or friend to interpret for me.

43. If you answered yes to question 42, did you have to wait long for an interpreter?

    a. yes

    b. no

    c. don't know

44. If you answered yes to question 43, how long did you have to wait?

    _____

45. Do you think the interpreter did an adequate job of explaining your illness/condition to the primary care provider?
    a. yes
    b. no
46. If you answered no to question 45, please explain.

    _____

47. Did the healthcare provider make an attempt to communicate with you in language or through gestures?
    a. yes
    b. no
    c. don't know
    d. not applicable
48. Did the healthcare provider use visual aids to communicate? For example, did the healthcare provider show you a picture of your heart, lungs, digestive system, etc., when explaining your condition or illness?
    a. yes
    b. no
    c. don't know
    d. not applicable
49. The healthcare provider (physician)
    a. spoke to me at my level
    b. used too many big words that I didn't understand
    c. spoke down to me
    d. b and c
    e. don't know
50. Were you able to talk to the **nurse** about your illness?
    a. yes
    b. no
    c. yes, but he/she _____
    d. don't know
    e. not applicable
51. Were you able to talk to the **doctor** about your illness?
    a. yes
    b. no
    c. yes, but he/she _____
    d. don't know
    e. not applicable

52. Were you able to talk to the other healthcare personnel who care for or treated you?
    a. yes
    b. no
    c. yes, but he/she _____
    d. don't know
    e. not applicable
53. Were you comfortable with the healthcare provider's medical knowledge of your illness?
    a. yes
    b. no
    c. don't know
54. If you answered no to question 53, please explain.

    _____

55. Do you think the healthcare provider was familiar with your cultural background well enough to treat someone of your ethnic, racial, or cultural group?
    a. yes
    b. no
    c. don't know
56. If you answered no to question 55, please explain.

    _____

57. Are there certain illnesses or conditions that you think can be better treated by someone of the same ethnic, racial, or cultural group as you?
    a. yes
    b. no
    c. don't know
58. If you answered yes to question 57, please explain or state what conditions you think can be better treated by someone of the same ethnic, racial, or cultural group as you.

    _____

59. When you are ill, are there cultural practices (such as prayer, herbal medicine, food, drink, and/or tonic) that you perform or take before going to a healthcare provider?
    a. yes
    b. no
60. If you answered yes to question 59, please explain or give examples.

    _____

61. When you visit a healthcare provider, do you feel uncomfortable because you talk, dress, or look different from other people sitting in the doctor's office?
    a. yes
    b. no
62. If you answered yes to question 61, please explain.

    _____

63. When you visited the emergency room, clinic, or doctor's office, were you pressured to accept treatment or therapy that you did not want?
    a. yes
    b. no
64. If you answered yes to question 63, can you explain what the treatment or therapy was and why you did not want it?

    _____

65. When you visited the emergency room, clinic, or doctor's office, did you feel pressured to behave or act in a way that is different from your culture?
    a. yes
    b. no
    c. don't know
66. If you answered yes to question 65, please explain.

    _____

67. If you had to return to the emergency room, clinic, or doctor's office, would you want to see the same healthcare provider or a different one?
    a. same provider
    b. different provider
68. If you answered different provider for question 67, please explain why.

    _____

69. Have you ever been asked to participate in a healthcare research study?
    a. yes (specify or name the study) _____
    b. no (skip to question 71)
70. If you answered yes to question 69, why did you participate in the healthcare study?

    _____

71. If you were asked, would you participate in a healthcare study?
    a. yes
    b. no
    c. don't know
72. Please give a reason for your yes or no answer in question 71.

    _____

73. Do you see any benefits to you, your family, or your ethnic/racial community to participating in a healthcare study?

    a. yes

    b. no

    c. don't know

74. Please explain your yes or no answer in question 73.

    _____

75. Do you know anyone who has participated in a healthcare research study?

    a. yes (if yes, who? _____)

    What relationship are they to you? _____

    b. no

76. Do you know the leading cause of death or illness for someone of your ethnic/racial background?

    a. yes (specify) _____

    b. no

Appendix 8–B. Community Assessment Instrument (Post-Test)

Case Number _____

1. Gender/sex
   a. male
   b. female
2. Marital status
   a. single
   b. married
   c. divorced
   d. widowed
   e. separated
3. What is the highest grade level or degree that you have completed?
   a. some high school
   b. high school/GED graduate
   c. some college
   d. associate's degree
   e. bachelor's degree
   f. some graduate work
   g. master's degree
   h. PhD, JD, MD
   i. other (specify)
4. What is your occupation? _____
5. What is your race and/or ethnic group?
   a. African American/Black
   b. Caucasian/White
   c. Hispanic/Latin
   d. Native American
   e. Sudanese
   f. Vietnamese
   g. Other (specify) _____
6a. Is English your first (mother) language?
   a. yes
   b. no
6b. If no, what is your first language? _____
7. What are the leading causes of death for someone in your ethnic and/or racial group?
   Please list

8. What are the advantages to participating in a healthcare study? Please list:

9. What are the disadvantages to participating in a healthcare study? Please list:

10a. Have you participated in a healthcare study?
   a. yes
   b. no

10b. If no, would you consent to participating in a healthcare study?
   a. yes
   b. no

   Please, explain your yes or no answer:

We have described the CAI instrument that was designed and used in a cultural proficiency study in Omaha, Nebraska. The results from this study have been published in peer-reviewed journals. However, we welcome additional comments and suggestions regarding refining this instrument, and we hope that you will utilize this instrument to better assess the cultural competency of healthcare providers and patient/client willingness to participate in healthcare research in your community.

Chapter 9

Cultural Competency Instrument: A Description of a Methodology. Part II

Sade Kosoko-Lasaki, MD, MSPH, MBA
Cynthia T. Cook, PhD

*C*ultural competence has been defined as "a set of congruent behaviors, attitudes, and policies that come together in a system, agency, or among professionals and enable that system, agency, or those professionals to work effectively in cross-cultural situations"[1]; "the ability to work effectively across cultures in a way that acknowledges and respects the culture of the person or organization being served"[2]; and/or "as an ongoing and interactive process, based on respect of others' customs, beliefs and values."[3] Cultural competency may be related to patient outcome, that is, to persons who receive services from culturally competent providers achieve better outcomes.[4] Culturally competent providers may reduce the health disparities that exist among racially and ethnically diverse populations within the community. Culturally competent providers may also be instrumental in encouraging racially and ethnically diverse healthcare consumers to participate in healthcare research. To improve the delivery of healthcare services to an ethnically and racially diverse population, Creighton University needs to know the level of cultural competency and/or proficiency of their healthcare providers and clinical investigators. The Cultural Competency Instrument (CCI) that is presented in this chapter is designed to identify the six levels of cultural competency and/or proficiency of primary care providers in the Creighton University medical research community.

Background

The CCI identifies six levels of cultural competency. The first or lowest level, *cultural destructiveness*, occurs when individuals and groups do not recognize cultural differences in their population and when differences exhibited by a racial/ethnic group are perceived as deviant and/or inferior. For instance, culturally destructive providers may use children as interpreters for adult patients or may refer ethnic or minority patients with no recognizable medical symptoms to a mental health provider. The second level, *cultural incapacity*, disregards the differences that exist among racially and ethnically diverse populations but does not label these differences as deviant. In this case, illness is not considered deviant but is dismissed; the provider assures patients with no medical symptoms that they are healthy and sends them on their way. Another example of cultural incapacity occurs when facilities offer only English-speaking healthcare providers.

The third level of competency is *cultural blindness*. The organization claims it is an "equal opportunity provider" but ignores cultural differences and considers cultural/color blindness a desired state. A culturally blind facility assumes that all patients have assimilated the dominant culture and promotes itself as capable of treating all patients regardless of age, gender, race, or ethnicity. Organizations that practice at the levels of cultural destructiveness, cultural incapacity, or cultural blindness do not recognize the value of diversity in their multicultural community; as a result, these providers have been associated with poor patient outcomes and decreased minority worker retention.

Cultural precompetence, the fourth level, is accomplished when healthcare providers acknowledge cultural differences in their client population and seek to sensitize their staff through training, retention, and recruitment of minority personnel. An example of this level is staffing healthcare personnel who are knowledgeable about the language and culture of the ethnic or racial population served. *Cultural competence*, the fifth level, is achieved when providers have learned to value cultural differences, have obtained knowledge of the local minority population, and have retained and continued to recruit minority personnel based on continual facility or community needs assessment. The sixth level is *cultural proficiency*; providers are supportive of and promote minority culture through minority-friendly legislation, minority organizations, and minority healthcare research. This is the highest level in the cultural competency continuum. The providers and/or institutions that meet these criteria are deemed cultural competent or proficient in the delivery of healthcare services to a racially and ethnically diverse patient population.

The last three levels of the continuum acknowledge the importance of communication between the healthcare provider and the patient/client. These levels indicate that the healthcare provider is attempting to understand the beliefs, attitudes, and practices of its ethnically and racially diverse client/patient population for better communication and patient outcome. Some researchers suggest that valuing diversity, conducting self-assessments, being aware of the dynamics of differences, acquiring knowledge of culture, and adapting to a different culture facilitates cultural competency.[5] Moreover, having interpreter services (for speakers of languages other than English), recruitment and retention policies, cultural sensitivity training, conferences with traditional healers, community/minority health workers as liaisons, culturally competent health promotions, family and/or community members participate in healthcare decisions and treatment, staff immersed into another culture to combat ethnocentrism, and administrative and organizational accommodations (i.e., making sure healthcare facilities are near enrollees, that transportation is available, and that linguistic competency exist throughout the patient's encounters) will also facilitate cultural competence.[6]

Research Design

Community Competency Instrument (CCI): Methodology

The second part of the cultural proficiency study dealt with healthcare providers' and clinical investigators' self-assessment of their departments or clinics, sensitivity to cultural differences of the patient/client population. Their cultural competency was measured by the Cultural Competency Instrument (CCI). For the purposes of the study, *cultural competency* is defined as healthcare providers being aware of the cultural uniqueness of their patient/client population and acknowledging this cultural uniqueness when interacting with this patient population, while always being cognizant that it is the health and welfare of the patient that is of the utmost important. The CCI that was administered to 37 healthcare providers and researchers at Creighton University Medical Center (CUMC) was designed to identify areas of patient/provider interaction that may need clarification or discussion in order to maintain or improve quality of care to minority and/or ethnically and/or racially diverse populations and to encourage this population to participate in healthcare research. Only one hypothesis is addressed in this section of the study: Creighton healthcare providers and researchers are not culturally competent. Twenty-six survey items were developed to support or refute this hypothesis.

All department heads at CUMC were contacted via letter, e-mail, and/or telephone during the summer of 2003 and asked to participate or nominate members of their staff to participate in one of three focus groups that were held on October 22, 30, and November 3, 2003. The only criterion for participation was that the nominee be someone responsible for providing service to racially and/or ethnically diverse patients through healthcare or clinical research. Focus groups were originally limited to 10 participants. However, all who applied were accepted for whatever time they indicated. Persons who participated in the previous pilot study on June 16, 2003, were ineligible.

At each CCI study session, respondents were given an overview regarding the purpose of the cultural proficiency study. They were then asked to sign a consent form that had been pre-approved by the Creighton University Institution Review Board (IRB). When all consent forms had been signed and collected, the CCI instrument was distributed to the study participants. Respondents were given approximately 30 minutes to complete the form. As with the Community Assessment Instrument (CAI) group participants, there were many inquiries and comments about the instrument. Respondents were asked to answer the questions to the best of their knowledge and ability and to hold their questions and comments until the focus group was conducted.

The focus group was conducted after the questionnaire had been collected by the same trained and experienced facilitator who conducted the focus group for the CAI pilot, main CAI, and CCI pilot. Respondents were paid $50 for travel expenses, even though most of the participants were at their place of work and had been given time off to attend. Unfortunately, transcripts are only available for the October 22 and November 3 focus groups. The transcriptionist was not available for the October 30 focus group.

SUMMARY

The CCI instrument sought to measure how well the items described (**Appendix 9–A**) were integrated into the delivery of health care for an ethnically and racially diverse population. The results allow administrators and/or healthcare providers to identify areas or levels of cultural competency that may need improvement and/or to develop policy with respect to how a given ethnic and/or racial group should be treated when they exhibit cultural patterns that may differ from the accepted or dominant group. Knowing the level of competence allows facilities and providers to begin discussions on how to improve services to a racially and ethnically diverse population or to recognize their limitations[7]; that is, the facility is competent to provide services to a monocultural or bicultural population only. To facilitate this understanding, we have identified survey items that measure cultural competence (CC), not culturally competent (not CC), or no assessment (NA). This classification is based on a variety of literature that can be found in the References.[8–15] **Figure 9–1** further clarifies the six levels.

Cultural Destructiveness

1. Ethnic patient has no recognizable medical symptoms, but patient and relatives acknowledge an "illness."

2. Health providers are only able to provide care to English- or Spanish-speaking patients. Have target minority population that they feel competent to serve, but discourage others from using the facility.

3. Encourage women to make decisions without consulting spouses or family members.

4. Use children and relatives as interpreters for non-English-speaking patients.

5. Voice or indicate disapproval of certain indigenous or cultural practices like female circumcision (FGM), early/adolescent marriages, large families.

6. Think immigrant children should learn the U.S. culture as soon as possible because of harmful indigenous or foreign cultural practices.

7. Health providers have a paternalistic attitude with ethnic patients because of the patients' low educational levels.

Cultural Incapacity

1. No qualified interpreter on staff. Not familiar with the local/target minority groups culture.

2. Ethnocentrism, dominant culture is the best culture.

3. Dismiss folk illness as unimportant. No knowledge of folk illness or community folk healers.

4. Encourage minority patients to seek care elsewhere.

5. No minorities on staff due to lack of funds or knowledge of their importance.

Cultural Blindness

1. Is equal opportunity provider: treat everyone the same. No attempt to differentiate clientele/patients based on color, gender, age, ethnic group, education, or religion.

2. Assumes all people/patients have assimilated.

3. Assumes patient lack of education causes health problems.

4. Facility expects and adheres to middle-class norms.

5. Posters, booklets, and pamphlets show white women as opposed to women of color. May discourage women of color from seeking care at facility. No pictures of them.

6. Assumes two-parent household. Don't recognize other adults may be part of the family.

continues

Figure 9–1   *Guide to Interpreting the Cultural Competency Instrument**
*The guidelines for interpreting the CCI and the instrument itself were developed based on the literature presented in the reference section.

Cultural Precompetence

1. Recognize that it is only competent to treat a specific minority/ethnic group.

2. Attempts to recruit more minority and ethnic healthcare providers.

3. Provides cultural sensitivity training for staff.

4. Performs needs assessment regularly.

Cultural Competence

1. Respects cultural differences.

2. Accumulates continually knowledge of local minority communities.

3. Recruits and retains minority staff.

4. Performs needs assessment continually.

5. Trains all staff for cultural sensitivity.

6. Recognizes multicultural world.

Cultural Proficiency

1. Supports minority culture by participating in community activity.

2. Supports minority-friendly legislature.

3. Makes charitable contributions to minority group organizations.

4. Provides role models for other healthcare providers.

5. Conducts research on minority culture for the benefit of improving the health status of the minority population. Shares the result with the community and asks for its input before and after the research.

6. Uses or explores the use of new or existing therapeutic approaches based on the culture.

7. Publishes results of research.

8. Hires specialist on minority culture.

Figure 9–1 *Guide to Interpreting the Cultural Competency Instrument (continued)*

REFERENCES

1. Cross TL, Bazron BJ, Dennis KW, Isaacs MR. *Towards a Culturally Competent System of Care*. CASSP Technical Assistance Center: Georgetown University Child Development Center. 1989;1.
2. Hanley JH. Beyond the tip of the iceberg: Five stages toward cultural competence: Reaching today's youth. *Community Circle Caring J*. 1999;3(2):9–12.
3. Rose VL. Cultural competency in health care. *Am Fam Phys*. 1998;57(11):2882.
4. Outcomes and Accountability Alert. Performance measures reflect how well systems serve diverse populations. 1999;4(1):1. Available at: scilib.univ.kiev.ua/doc.php? 638634. Accessed on April 7, 2002.
5. Edgar E, Patton JM, Day-Vines, N. Democratic dispositions and cultural competency. *Remedial Spec Educ*. 2002;23(4):231–242.
6. Brach C, Fraser I. Can cultural competency reduce racial and ethnic health disparities? A review and conceptual model. *Med Care Res Rev*. 2000;57(1):181–217.
7. O'Brien RL, Kosoko-Lasaki O, Cook CT, Kissell J, Peak F, Williams EH. Self assessment of cultural attitudes and competence of clinical investigators to enhance recruitment and participation of minority population in research. *J Natl Med Assoc*. 2006;98(5):674–682.
8. Glenn-Vega A. Achieving a more minority-friendly practice. *Fam Pract Manage*. June 2002. www.aafp.org/fpm.
9. Anderson LM, Scrimshaw SC, Fullilove MT, Fielding JE, Normand J. Culturally competent healthcare systems. A systematic review. *Am J Prev Med*. 2003;24(3): 2–3, 8–9.
10. Jackson VH. *Cultural Competency*. March/April 2002:20–26.
11. Mason JL. *Cultural Competence Self-Assessment Questionnaire: A Manual for Users*. Research and Training Center on Family Support and Children's Mental Health. Portland State University. 1995.
12. National Center for Cultural Competence. *Promoting Cultural Diversity and Cultural Competency: Self-Assessment Checklist for Personnel Providing Services and Supports to Children with Special Health Needs and Their Families*. 2002. www.georgetown.edu/research/gucdc/nccc7.html. Accessed February 26, 2003.
13. Oncology Nursing Society. Oncology Nursing Society Multicultural Outcomes: Guidelines for Cultural Competence, by the Society, 1999, Pittsburgh, PA: Author.
14. Blue AV. *The Provision of Culturally Competent Health Care*. Department of Family Medicine, Medical University of South Carolina College of Medicine 2000. www.musc.edu/deansclerkship/rccultur.html. Accessed February 26, 2003.
15. Sue DW. A model for cultural diversity training. *J Counsel Devel*. 991;70:99–105.

Appendix 9–A. Cultural Competency Instrument (CCI)*

Identifying Data (To be completed by facility administrator and/or health care provider or clinical investigator)

Name of Facility _____

Name of Administrator _____

Exact Title _____

Age _____

Education/Degrees _____

Race/Ethnicity _____

How long have you had this position? _____

Multiple-Choice Questions

1. Ethnic or minority patients with no recognizable medical symptoms are
   a. referred to mental health providers (cultural destructiveness).
   b. assured that they are healthy and sent on their way (cultural incapacity).
   c. reassessed using cultural-specific diagnostic instruments (cultural competency/proficiency).
   d. given a battery of tests to ensure that nothing is missed in the diagnosis or prognosis (cultural precompetence/competence).
   e. referred to facility or institution that is better equipped to deal with this segment of the population (cultural incapacity).

2. Primary healthcare providers at this facility are competent to treat
   a. all patients regardless of language and cultural background (cultural blindness or cultural proficiency).
   b. only English-speaking patients (cultural incapacity).
   c. only English- and Spanish-speaking patients (cultural incapacity).

3. If we need an interpreter for a patient
   a. a relative will be used regardless of age, e.g., children (cultural destructiveness).
   b. we will ask another patient to translate for us (cultural incapacity).
   c. we will use healthcare personnel who know the language (cultural precompetence/competence).
   d. we will use a professional interpreter (cultural competence/proficiency).

*The guidelines for interpreting the culturally competent instrument and the instrument itself were developed based on the literature presented in the reference section.

4. Ethnic or minority women
   a. are encouraged to make medical decisions after consultation with their doctors (cultural destructiveness).
   b. are encouraged to make medical decisions after consulting with their doctors and spouses and/or relatives (cultural competence).
   c. are encouraged to accept the doctor's decision regarding treatment (cultural destructiveness).
   d. would probably prefer a female physician or to have another female present during their visit (cultural competence).
5. This facility does needs assessment
   a. annually (cultural precompetence/competence/proficiency).
   b. biannually (cultural precompetence/competence/proficiency).
   c. only when needed for additional beds and equipment (cultural destructiveness/incapacity).
   d. never (cultural destructiveness/incapacity).

True/False

6. This facility does not condone aberrant cultural practices and reports suspected cases to the proper authorities. (true = cultural destructiveness; false = cultural precompetence/competence).
7. Based on my experience and knowledge, assimilation is good because it prevents children from learning harmful indigenous or cultural practices. (true = cultural destructiveness; false = cultural precompetence/competence/proficiency)
8. It is for the good of the ethnic/minority patient that healthcare providers take a paternalistic attitude with him/her. (true = cultural destructiveness; false = cultural precompetence/competence/proficiency)
9. This facility, consistent with the needs of the community, has several qualified interpreters on staff (i.e., Spanish, Sudanese, French, etc.). (true = cultural competence/proficiency; false = cultural destructiveness/incapacity/blindness)
10. This facility, consistent with the needs of the community, has several specialists on staff who are familiar with minority/ethnic folk illnesses and practitioners. (true = cultural competence/proficiency; false = cultural destructiveness/incapacity/blindness)
11. This facility is not equipped to treat minority/ethnic folk illnesses and refers patients to a facility that is equipped. (true = cultural incapacity; false = cultural competence/proficiency)
12. This facility has no minority on staff because it is difficult to find qualified minority healthcare providers. (true = cultural incapacity; false = cultural competence/proficiency)

13. This facility has no minority on staff because we do not have the funds for additional personnel. (true = cultural incapacity; false = cultural precompetence/competence/proficiency)

14. This facility is an equal opportunity healthcare provider; we treat everyone. We do not differentiate clients/patients based on age, gender, color, race, ethnicity, education, or income. (true = cultural blindness; false = precompetence/competence/proficiency)

15. This facility assumes that all patients have assimilated or are in the process of assimilating. We support and encourage assimilation. (true = cultural blindness; false = cultural precompetence/competence/proficiency)

16. Based on my experience and knowledge, patients' health problems are usually related to lack of education. (true = cultural blindness; false = cultural precompetence/competence/proficiency)

17. This facility's posters, booklets, and pamphlets include pictures of people of color as well as whites to indicate the diversity of our clientele and providers. (true = cultural precompetence/competence/proficiency; false = cultural blindness)

18. This facility recognizes that other adults in the household, besides spouses and parents, may have to be consulted before any medical decisions can be made regarding a patient. (true = cultural precompetence/competence/proficiency; false = cultural destructiveness)

19. This facility recognizes it is competent to treat only one or two ethnic/minority groups based on its staffing (i.e., minority health provider, social worker, and/or interpreter on staff). (true = cultural precompetence)

20. This facility is making an aggressive attempt to increase the number of ethnic/minority healthcare providers. (true = precompetence)

21. This facility provides cultural sensitivity training to its nonethnic/nonminority staff. (true = cultural incapacity/blindness; false = cultural precompetence/competence)

22. This facility supports and participates in the organizing of ethnic/minority cultural events. (true = cultural proficiency)

23. This facility supports legislature that provides for additional funding for ethnic/minority based health care. (true = cultural proficiency)

24. This facility has and continues to support research on ethnic/minority groups for the purpose of improving the delivery of healthcare services to that group. (true = cultural proficiency)

25. This facility has utilized ethnic/minority therapeutic approaches in its treatment of ethnic/minority patients. (true = cultural competence/proficiency)

26. This facility makes a charitable contribution to ethnic/minority organizations. (true = cultural proficiency)

Chapter 10

Statistical Models in Health Disparities Research

Gleb Haynatzki, DSc, PhD
Vera Haynatzka, PhD

S tatistics is a science that studies different approaches to making inference about one or more populations of like individuals based on samples drawn from these populations. Because the Health Resources and Services Administration (HRSA) of the U.S. Department of Health and Human Services defines *health disparities* as "population-specific differences in the presence of disease, health outcomes, or access to health care," it follows that statistics is an appropriate approach to analyzing health disparities. Sometimes it may be possible to study *health disparities measures* involving whole populations, but very often it is more practical to sample populations followed up by calculating sample statistics, which are then used to draw inference on the true population parameters (**Figure 10–1**).

Ideally, in order to generate reliable and accurate inferences about the populations, such samples should be random and sufficiently large to decrease the likelihood of chance affecting the observed results. There are different ways to draw random samples, depending on the *study design*. The study design also determines the relevant **statistical models** for analyzing the generated data on health disparities. On the other hand, such models should be kept in mind while finalizing the study design. Thus, health disparities measures, study design, and statistical models are mutually dependent and should be dealt with in parallel when putting together a research study. In particular, statistical modeling can and should be used to evaluate effectively all aspects of health disparities: (1) disease-specific disparities, (2) disparities in access to health care, (3) disparities in healthcare delivery,

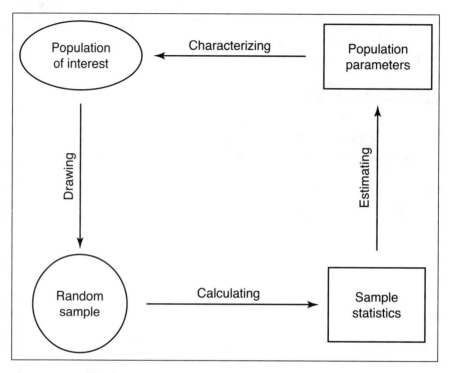

Figure 10–1   *Flow diagram of drawing a random sample from a population that is followed up by calculating sample statistics, which are then used to draw inference on the true population parameters*

and (4) disparity-reduction programs. **Figure 10–2** shows a flow diagram of a typical health disparities research study. The topics and activities in bold font are discussed in this chapter, including a brief overview of study design while expanding more on health disparities measures and statistical models for health disparities research. Reporting the results of the data analysis and their interpretation are shown mainly as part of concrete examples.

Study Design

Researchers often would have the data already generated and even cleaned for them, without having to conduct a study or choose health disparities measures, but then be left to deal only with the choice and performance of appropriate statistical methods of data analysis. However, adequate knowledge of study design is required in such cases because the design determines

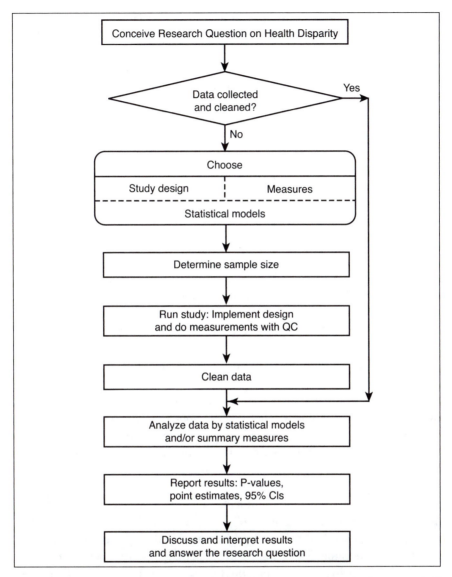

Figure 10–2   *Flow diagram of a typical health disparities research study. Activities in bold font are discussed in this chapter (QC = quality control).*

the relevant statistical approaches to data analysis. Therefore, we will provide a brief summary of design considerations and refer the reader to texts that expand more on study design.

After a research question has emerged and the health disparities measures of interest determined, the choice and implementation of an appropriate study design is the next and most important step in conducting good research. Inappropriate design can ruin even the most well-intended health disparities research. If a study is not designed to minimize bias and increase precision, subsequent statistical analysis may not be able to fix it. Designs are usually classified as experimental (i.e., involving some intervention controlled by the researcher) versus observational (i.e., without any intervention), longitudinal (i.e. with follow-up in time) versus cross-sectional (i.e., at a single point in time); if longitudinal, then they may be prospective (i.e., forward in time) or retrospective (i.e., backward in time). The most popular and basic study designs of interest to health disparities research are the *case series*, *case-control*, *cross-sectional*, *cohort*, and *randomized controlled trials*. More complex designs are usually combinations of the basic ones and comprise more than one phase. Each design has its specific strengths and weaknesses, and should be carefully chosen according to the situation at hand. As simple and obvious as it may seem that a comparison is needed for a definitive health disparities statement or any other causal relationship between a risk factor and a disease or a treatment and a cure, the need for comparison is sometimes overlooked, which leads to study invalidation and rejection (e.g., by peer review). Except for the case series design, all other designs focus on one or more comparisons.

The most rigorous of the preceding five designs is the randomized controlled trial (experimental design), followed by the cohort study design, the case-control and cross-sectional designs, and the case series. Whereas every study may be *biased* (i.e., its results may not reflect the truth) in assessing health disparities factors or therapeutic interventions, a randomized controlled trial is less susceptible to bias than the observational studies. It is therefore recommended that randomized controlled trials be used whenever possible (which is the case when rigorous medical research is conducted for treatment comparisons). We focus the exposition next on health disparities measures and statistical methods for data analysis, and refer the reader to statistics and epidemiology texts for more on designs.[1-5]

Health Disparities Measures

The choice of quantitative health disparities measures follows from our definition of health disparities, which is linked to ethical perspectives and derives from our values. Therefore, both simple and more sophisticated measures as those discussed in Harper and colleagues[6] may be modified or replaced by others in the future. Currently, the definition of health disparities in *Healthy People 2010* focuses on gender, race or ethnicity, education or income, disability, geographic location, and sexual orientation.[7]

The recommendations in Harper and colleagues[6] for measuring health disparities gradually move from inspecting tables and graphs of raw data, and conducting simple pairwise comparisons, to more sophisticated summary measures. Although aimed at the area of cancer research, these recommendations are equally relevant to most other areas. In particular, if a social group has a natural ordering (e.g., defined by level of education and income), Harper and colleagues recommend using either the Slope Index of Inequality (SII)[8] or the Absolute Concentration Index (ACI)[9–11] as a measure of absolute health disparity, and either the Relative Index of Inequality (RII)[12,13] or the Relative Concentration Index (RCI)[14] as a measure of relative disparity. However, when comparisons across multiple groups that have no natural ordering (e.g., race/ethnicity) are needed, the recommendation is to use the Between-Group Variance (BGV)[15] as a summary of absolute disparity and the general entropy class of measures—more specifically, the Theil index[16] and the Mean Log Deviation (MLD)[16]—as measures of relative disparity. We refer the reader to Table 5 in Harper et al.,[6] which lists the advantages and disadvantages of many different summary health disparities measures, and where the authors emphasize the primacy of absolute over relative health disparity.

In general, the summary measures of health disparities are ends in and of themselves, but such measures often could be included in statistical models for further comparisons and analysis. Moreover, the more sophisticated health disparities measures are themselves based on statistical and probabilistic models, and are essentially probability metrics.[17,18] For example, the SII and RII are derived through linear regression, whereas the BGV is derived through an analysis of variance (ANOVA)–like model. Although summary measures of health disparities are more sophisticated, they are sometimes difficult to interpret when there are more than two groups because they detect an overall disparity without showing exactly which groups differ. In such cases, it is necessary to follow up with pairwise comparisons.

Next we discuss descriptive statistics and some simple measures of disparity, as well as pairwise comparisons, first for continuous response variables, then for categorical ones.

Continuous Response: Descriptive Statistics

Mean values and standard deviations are common measures for location and variability in the case of continuous measurements. However, these statistics are not always appropriate. When the dataset is asymmetric or has outliers (measurements that are far apart from the bulk of the data), the median is more meaningful than the mean because it is less affected by outliers. The median has the property that half of the sample has measurements below it, and the other half has measurements above it. The median is reported as a measure of variability in combination with the inter-quartile range (IQR), that is, the difference between the third and first quartiles that contain the middle 50% of the sample. Histograms and stem-and-leaf plots by group on the same measurement scale provide good detailed description of the distribution patterns in different groups. The box plots (or box-and-whiskers plots) present graphical summaries, and are particularly useful when the number of observations is large.[1,2] Example 10–1 demonstrates the application of these concepts.

Continuous Response: Tests for Statistically Significant Differences between Two Groups

When characterizing disparities, in addition to comparing group means, standard deviations, and/or medians and IQRs, it is important to determine how much of the observed differences between groups could be explained by chance alone. There are two types of statistical tests that compare group disparities: parametric (or ANOVA-type) tests that are appropriate for symmetric data and the so-called nonparametric tests (e.g., the Kruskal-Wallis test, median test, and Kolmogorov-Smirnov test) that compare the ranks of the observations in the ordered dataset. Parametric tests are relevant under stricter assumptions about the data distribution than nonparametric tests. Such assumptions should be verified before selecting a parametric test for group comparison. The advantage of the parametric tests is that they provide easy estimates of the actual disparity——the mean difference between groups, together with a confidence interval (CI) for that difference, usually a 95% CI (see Example 10–1).

Continuous Response: Estimating Disparity between Two Groups with 95% CIs

Estimating disparities by a point estimate of a population parameter based on a selected sample from the population produces results that differ from sample to sample due to random fluctuations. The smaller the sample size, the bigger the difference between the obtained point estimates. Either the sample size should be increased considerably, which is costly, or the confidence interval approach should be employed. A $(1 - \alpha)\%$ CI is built for a true population parameter (e.g., the population mean) based on any random sample. In most cases, $\alpha = 5\%$ and the respective 95% CI is computed, with the true population mean falling in the computed 95% CI for about 95% of all possible samples. Reporting the point estimates of a disparity in combination with a CI provides information not only about the magnitude of the disparity but also about the *precision of the estimate*. The wider the confidence interval, the less reliable the estimate. Suppose that samples of large sizes n_1 and n_2 are selected from two population groups for which a disparity measure is compared in just one pairwise comparison. Denote the sample averages by $\bar{x}$ and $\bar{y}$, and the sample standard deviations by s_x and s_y, respectively. Then the 95% CI for the difference $(\bar{x} - \bar{y})$ is given by the formula $(\bar{x} - \bar{y}) \pm 1.96 \sqrt{s_x^2/n_1 + s_y^2/n_2}$. The number 1.96 is derived from the normal distribution and corresponds to a selected confidence level of 95%, whereas the expression involving the radical is actually the standard error for the difference. The two group means are equal only when their difference is zero. If the 95% CI for the group mean difference contains zero, the means are considered equal with 95% confidence. In the terminology of hypothesis testing, the disparity is not considered statistically significant at the 5% level of significance.

Continuous Response: Multiple Comparison Tests

When the number of population groups is greater than two, it is usually of interest to compute all pairwise differences among the group means. Computing 95% CIs for these pairwise differences is carried out in a way similar to the one for two population groups, but uses the pooled standard deviation from all groups (obtained from the ANOVA computations) to account for the variability of the point estimate. Some statistical schools advise controlling for multiple comparisons (using, e.g., the Tukey or Bonferonni adjustments) in order to maintain the preselected level of significance (usually 5%). Others advise against this approach, concerned about the loss of power in detecting real differences. Because the number of population groups in disparity studies is usually small, it is often possible to compute the pairwise differences without multiple comparison adjustments. Another option is to compare all groups under study to the prevalent group (usually the group hypothesized to have above average outcome), either without adjustment or by using Dunnett's test.[1,2]

Example 10–1

Consider a dataset adapted from the results of the California Men's Health Study.[19] Four samples, each consisting of 300 adult males (ages 45–69 years) from each of the four main race/ethnic groups in a community (African Americans, Asian/Pacific Islanders [PI], white Hispanics, and non-Hispanic Whites), have been selected. The histogram plots for percent calories from fat in the four samples are presented in **Figure 10–3**, whereas the corresponding box plots are in **Figure 10–4**. The data distribution is quite symmetric by race/ethnicity, with somewhat larger spread for the African American and Hispanic groups.

The box plot suggests lower fat consumption in the Asian/Pacific Islanders sample. Both the parametric F-test and the nonparametric Kruskal-Wallis test detect significant difference in percent fat intake

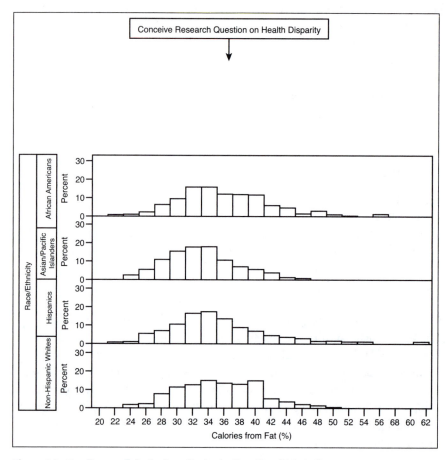

Figure 10–3   *Percent Calories from Fat in the Four Race/Ethnic Groups*
Adapted from Enger SM, Van Den Eeden SK, Sternfeld B, et al. California Men's Health Study (CMHS): A multiethnic cohort in a managed care setting. *BMC Public Health*. 2006;6:172; http://www.biomedcentral.com/1471-2458/6/172.

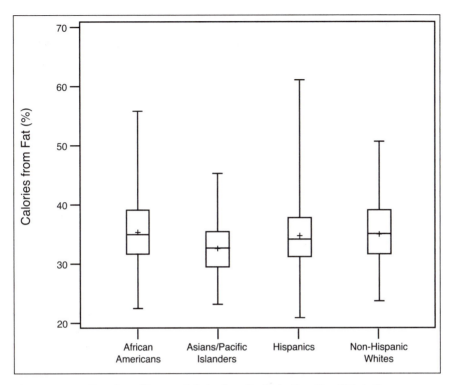

Figure 10–4   *Box-plots of Percent Calories from Fat in the Four Race/Ethnic Groups*
Adapted from Enger SM, Van Den Eeden SK, Sternfeld B, et al. California Men's Health Study
(CMHS): A multiethnic cohort in a managed care setting. *BMC Public Health*. 2006;6:172;
http://www.biomedcentral.com/1471-2458/6/172.

between groups. **Table 10–1** shows summary of the results helps to identify where the disparities are.

The 95% CIs for difference between the average fat intake in the corresponding race/ethnicity group and the reference group, non-Hispanic Whites (NHW), were produced using a standard deviation estimate equal to 4.5% that was obtained after pooling the whole dataset. The upper confidence limit for the fat intake in Asian/PI is less than the lower confidence limit for all other three groups. Compared with NHW, only this group shows significant difference (the CIs for the other two differences contain zero). Additional testing of pairwise comparisons confirms that fat intake in the Asian/PI sample is significantly lower than in all other groups and that the differences among the other three groups are not significant (results not shown).

Table 10–1 *Average Fat Intake by Race/Ethnicity*

Race/Ethnicity	Mean (SD)	Difference from NHW
African Americans	35.6% (5.2%)	0.28% (–0.53, 1.10%)
Asians/Pacific Islanders	32.9% (4.4%)	–2.43% (-3.24, –1.61%)
Hispanics	34.8% (5.7%)	–0.44% (–1.26, 0.37%)
Non-Hispanic Whites	35.3% (4.9%)	***

Adapted from Enger SM, Van Den Eeden SK, Sternfeld B, et al. California Men's Health Study (CMHS): A multiethnic cohort in a managed care setting. *BMC Public Health*. 2006;6:172; http://www.biomedcentral.com/1471-2458/6/172.

Categorical Response: Descriptive Statistics, Difference between Two Groups, CIs

Generally, categorical data are reported as counts and percentages (out of total) by category. The report could be in a form of cross-tabulation by population group and category. Because many of the statistical tests for this type of situation are valid only when there are enough counts in each group by category cell, the first descriptive step in the analysis is very important. When the number of cells is small, it is a good idea to collapse several categories into one in a *meaningful* way; otherwise, *Simpson's paradox* may occur,[20,21] or the paradoxical observation that low-birth-weight children born to smoking mothers have a lower infant mortality rate than the low-birth-weight children of nonsmokers.[22] In addition to the cross-tabulation, pie and column charts are appropriate for visualizing categorical data. There is a variety of tests to identify differences among categorical measures. The Pearson chi-square is the most popular among significance tests for such data. This test works best when there are enough expected counts in each test cell (usually at least five). For smaller sizes, the Fisher exact test for two-by-two tables is more reliable, although it is also more computationally intense and thus difficult to use for large sample sizes.

Dichotomous (or binary) measures are categorical measures with only two levels (e.g., having or not having a certain health condition or being of a particular race and not of any other). For dichotomous measures, one of its two conditions is fixed and is referred to as the "event" (e.g., death or disease). The goal of the data analysis is to compare the occurrence of this event among population groups. When the samples from the population groups have been selected at random (as in cohort or cross-sectional studies), the results are summarized by computing the proportion of persons for whom the event has occurred divided by the total sample size for each group. This proportion estimates the probability of the event by group.

Table 10–2 shows the dichotomous variable X with two levels: $X = 1$ and $X = 0$. There are two population groups with sizes $(a + b)$ and $(c + d)$, respectively. Fixing $X = 1$ as the event of interest, the probability for the event $(X = 1)$ in Group I is estimated by $r_1 = a/(a + b)$, and in Group II by $r_2 = c/(c + d)$. The disparity between the two groups could be measured in two ways: by the absolute risk difference $r_2 - r_1$, or more often by the relative risk (RR) r_2/r_1. As in the continuous case, we should consider obtaining the 95% CIs for the observed disparities. Provided that a, b, c, and d are sufficiently large, the 95% CI for the risk difference is computed as $(r_2 - r_1)$ $\pm 1.96\sqrt{r_1(1 - r_1)/(a + b) + r_2(1 - r_2)/(c + d)}$.

Because of the skewness of the relative risk r_2/r_1, it is easier to build 95% CI based on the normal approximation for the logarithmic transformation of r_2/r_1. Then, to derive back the confidence interval for r_2/r_1, we have to exponentiate the obtained confidence interval to get $(r_2/r_1)exp[\pm 1.96\sqrt{1/a - 1/(a + b) + 1/c - 1/(c + d)}]$. Again, these are large sample estimates and should only be used for sufficiently large values of a, b, c, and d. When measured by risk difference, a disparity is not considered significant at the 5% level of significance if the confidence interval contains zero. When measured by relative risk, the disparities would not be significant if the confidence interval contains the number 1.

In case-control studies, there may be no random sampling from the population groups, particularly when matching is employed. Instead, the sums $(a + c)$ and $(b + d)$ are fixed. In such cases, it is not possible to estimate the probability of the event in each group. Still, it is possible to estimate the odds for those with the event (i.e., $X = 1$) to be from Group I rather than Group II as $a{:}c$, and the odds for those without the event (i.e.. $X = 0$) to be from Group I as $b{:}d$. Then the odds ratio $(a{:}c)/(b{:}d) = ad/bc$ is greater than 1 if the odds for a person from Group I to be among the events are higher than to be among the nonevents. Thus, the odds ratio is another measure of association between population groups and the outcome measure. This measure is more difficult to interpret than the relative risk, which com-

Table 10–2 *A 2-by-2 Contingency Table*

Group	X = 1	X = 0	
I	a	b	a + b
II	c	d	c + d

pares probabilities of events instead of odds. So, although odds ratios could measure disparities in all kinds of study designs, they are used mainly in the case-control setting, when the relative risk is not available. Importantly, when the probability of the event in the population is small (<10%), the odds ratio is a good approximation of the relative risk. The formula $(ad/bc)exp[\pm 1.96\sqrt{1/a + 1/b + 1/c + 1/d}]$ provides 95% confidence interval for the odds ratio (ad/bc). Notably, when logistic regression is used, odds ratio is the measure analyzed, not relative risk.

Categorical Response: Multiple Comparison Tests

The previously described analytic methods are easily extended for the case of more than two population groups. See Example 10–2.

Example 10–2

Returning to the data for percent fat intake in the four samples by race/ethnicity, let us categorize the outcome variable. We define a dichotomous variable with values 0 if the percent calories from fat are less than 30% (current dietary guidelines established by the U.S. Department of Agriculture) and 1 otherwise. **Figure 10–5** shows that although the percentage of persons consuming more than 30% of their calories from fat is large in all four groups, it is the lowest for the Asian/PI group, and highest for African Americans. The difference between groups is significant (with chi-square test P-value of 0.024).

Rate differences and ratios together with their confidence intervals are listed in **Table 10–3**. As with Example 10–1, only the Asian/PI population differs from the other three, with 13% more men consuming recommended percentage calories from fat compared with the non-Hispanic White population.

The situation in which a person designates himself or herself as belonging to several racial/ethnic groups when answering questionnaires cannot be handled by traditional methods, and special approaches are needed. One approach for handling only the association between categorical multiresponse variables (without adjustment for continuous covariates) has been recently developed by Bilder and Loughin.[23]

Statistical Models

A statistical model is the mathematical representation of the relationship between the outcome (response) variable and one or more explanatory (predictor or factor) variables. There are different types of models depending on

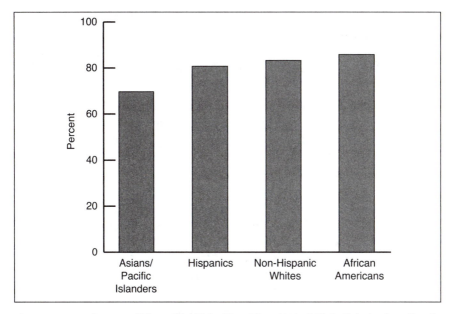

Figure 10–5   *Percent of Those Who Take More Than 30% of Their Calories from Fat, by Race/Ethnic Group*
Adapted from Enger SM, Van Den Eeden SK, Sternfeld B, et al. California Men's Health Study (CMHS): A multiethnic cohort in a managed care setting. *BMC Public Health*. 2006;6:172; http://www.biomedcentral.com/1471-2458/6/172.

Table 10–3 *Absolute or Relative Risks and Odds Ratios by Race/Ethnicity*

Race/Ethnicity	*Count (%)*	*Risk Difference*	*Relative Risk*	*Odds Ratio*
African Americans	262 (87.3%)	2.3% (−3.2%, 7.9%)	1.03 (0.96, 1.10)	1.22 (0.76, 1.94)
Asians/Pacific Islanders	216 (72.0%)	−13.0% (−19.5%, −6.5%)	0.85 (0.78, 0.92)	0.45 (0.30, 0.68)
Hispanics	246 (82.0%)	−3.0% (−8.9%, 2.9%)	0.96 (0.90, 1.04)	0.80 (0.52, 1.24)
Non-Hispanic Whites	255 (85%)	***	***	***

Adapted from Enger SM, Van Den Eeden SK, Sternfeld B, et al. California Men's Health Study (CMHS): A multiethnic cohort in a managed care setting. *BMC Public Health*. 2006;6:172; http://www.biomedcentral.com/1471-2458/6/172.

whether the outcome variable is continuous (e.g., temperature, height, blood sugar level) or categorical (e.g., smoking status, race, ethnicity) and whether the explanatory variables are (1) all categorical, (2) all continuous, or (3) a mixture of both. Similar combinations of explanatory variables are possible when the outcome variable is categorical. An important phenomenon, *interaction*, arises sometimes in models with two or more predictors, when one of them modifies the effect of another on the outcome variable. For example, the effect of (the same amount of) smoking on risk of lung cancer is different in men and women, being more pronounced for women (i.e., gender modifies the relationship between smoking status and lung cancer).

The correct use of (linear) statistical models allows us to detect statistically significant differences between groups (with usual choice at level of significance 5%), as well as whether slopes of linear relationships are different from zero (i.e., upward or downward), and to find estimates for such entities in terms of their mean values and 95% CIs. However, it is important to remember that a statistical model is of no use if it cannot be interpreted in terms of health disparities and that clinical (or other health-disparities-relevant) significance is more important than statistical significance alone. For example, if a particularly large study finds that drinking at least 20 cups of green tea a day significantly (and statistically) decreases a person's relative risk for stomach cancer (SC) by 50% (lowering the absolute risk from 0.04% to 0.02%), that person should first consult his or her physician before beginning to drink green tea regularly in such quantities only because of the fear of contracting stomach cancer. This example touches on both statistical versus clinical significance and the absolute versus the relative risk.

Confounders, Causality, Collinearity, and Sample Size

All existing knowledge on the research question should be used to decide how to design the study (if not designed yet) and what statistical methods to apply for data analysis. Such knowledge includes, in particular, plausible *confounders* (i.e., variables that are associated with both the predictor and outcome and that may account for the apparent causal relationship between the predictor and the outcome variables) and how to handle them in the new study. The confounding phenomenon is inherently connected to the *causality-versus-association* question.

Consider the following simple example. A researcher decides to investigate whether excessive alcohol drinking causes lung cancer in one or more of the race/ethnic groups. A study has been conducted, the data collected and analyzed, and the results clearly indicate that there is an association between excessive alcohol drinking and cancer of the lungs. It is then concluded that alcohol drinking is the cause for lung cancer. The problem with the found causality is that those who smoke also tend to overindulge in alcohol drinking, but the researcher had not taken into account the smoking habits of the study subjects. The true cause for lung cancer—smoking—has been overlooked. In this case, smoking is a confounder, and if it were measured and incorporated in the statistical model (i.e., *adjusted for* or *controlled for* in the model), alcohol drinking would have not been found to be significant. In most situations, we have more than one confounder, and the (design and) analyses have to account for them carefully. A trivial fact is that if we do not suspect a confounder or do not measure it, then it is impossible to account for it. It is therefore important to found the study on as much previous knowledge about the research question as possible.

In the health disparities setting, race/ethnicity may be heavily confounded by socioeconomic status (SES). In particular, it may be SES and not race that is a risk factor for a particular disease or healthcare issue. The best way to distinguish the effect of race from that of SES is to start with a good design and employ statistical analyses that incorporate both factors. However, when SES is not accounted for in the design (e.g., by stratifying for it) but only in the statistical model, it may give rise to a collinearity problem that has to be resolved when interpreting the results. *Collinearity* refers to a situation in which two or more predictor variables in the same statistical model are strongly correlated (i.e., are in a linear relationship) with one another. For example, race and SES are very strongly correlated, and so are height and weight. For prediction, collinearity does not create problems (rather, the more predictors the better), but for causal relationships it creates serious problems with the interpretation of results. There are different approaches to resolve collinearity issues. For example, in the case of height (Ht) and weight (Wt), they can be replaced in the model with a widely used "combo" variable, body mass index (BMI), which is defined by the formula $BMI = Wt / (Ht)^2$. A ready-made solution like BMI does not exist in most cases, and common sense and other statistical approaches, like principal components or factor analysis, should be followed.[24,25]

Another important issue is the sample size. Whereas the sampling procedure is determined by the study design, the sample size depends on the chosen statistical model and should guarantee certain level of statistical power (i.e., the conditional probability of finding difference if such exists) and is often set at 80% or higher. Intuitively, the larger the sample, the more statistical power there is. The use of statistical methods assumes some sort of random sample that, if large enough, also meets the natural expectation that the sample is representative of the population under study.

Two frequently used types of random sample are the (*simple*) *random sample*, when everybody in a population has an equal chance of being selected, and the *probability sample*, when everybody in a population has a known (not necessary equal) probability of being selected. For example, when health disparities research is conducted, minority groups may be *oversampled* (which is a version of probability sampling with larger probability for members of such groups than for nonminority groups) in order to achieve adequate enrollment of them. Insufficient data of good quality on minorities is a persistent problem and a serious restriction on documenting the nature of disparities in health care and developing strategies that eliminate disparities.

Statistical Models for Continuous Outcome Data

When the response variable is continuous and all explanatory variables are categorical, we deal with an analysis of variance (ANOVA) model (1); when all explanatory variables are continuous, we deal with a (multivariate-) *linear regression* model (2); and when some explanatory variables are continuous while others are categorical, we deal with an analysis of covariance (ANCOVA) model (3). Obviously, (3) is a generalization of (1) and (2) and is more complex than each of them, although none is straightforward. One or more of these linear statistical models could be used for analyzing any of the previously discussed designs (case-control, cross-sectional, cohort, and randomized controlled trial) depending on whether the response variable is continuous. It is reasonable to expect that at least one of the explanatory variables in at least one of the analyses for a particular health disparities study will be categorical (e.g., race, ethnicity). Moreover, even continuous variables like annual income are often categorized (e.g., below $30,000, $30,000–49,999, $50,000–74,999, $75,000–99,999, above $100,000) and are used as categorical variables in the analyses. On the other hand, we should not exclude the possibility of modeling a continuous response on one or more continuous explanatory variables (e.g., annual income as a function of years of education). An example of a continuous response modeled on one or more categorical and one or more continuous explanatory variables is when annual income is modeled as a function of race and years of education. Example 10–3 discusses the use of ANOVA and ANCOVA to study the effect of race/ethnicity on cardiovascular disease risk and adjustment for covariates.

Example 10–3

Wendel and colleagues[26] have studied racial and ethnic disparities in the control of cardiovascular disease risk factors in insulin-treated Southwest American veterans with type 2 diabetes in the Diabetes Outcomes in Veterans Study. They conducted a *cross-sectional* study on 338 randomly selected veterans: Hispanics (H), African Americans (AA), and non-Hispanic whites (NHW). They tested two models for each continuous response variable: glycemic control (hemoglobin A1C), insulin dose, lipid levels, and blood pressure control. These models are (1) ANOVA when testing only race (which is categorical) in the model and (2) ANCOVA when testing the effect of race but with *adjustment for* covariates (age, BMI, oral hypoglycemic medications, socioeconomic barriers, attitudes about diabetes care, diabetes knowledge, depression, cognitive dysfunction, and social support).

An ANOVA yielded that the mean (standard deviation [SD]) hemoglobin A1C differed significantly by race/ethnicity: NHW 7.86 (1.4)%, H 8.16 (1.6)%, AA 8.84 (2.9)%. The corresponding multivariate-adjusted ANCOVA has yielded that A1C was significantly higher for AA (+0.93%) relative to NHW. Further, another ANOVA has shown that insulin doses (unit/day) also differed significantly: NHW 70.6 (48.8), H 58.4 (32.6), and AA 53.1 (36.2). The corresponding ANCOVA yielded that multivariate-adjusted insulin doses were significantly lower for AA (-17.8 units/day) and H (-10.5 units/day) compared with NHW. Decrements in insulin doses were even greater among minority patients with poorly controlled diabetes (A1C $\geq 8\%$). The disparities in glycemic control and insulin dose could not be explained by differences in any of the covariates *adjusted for* in the ANCOVA models. No significant racial/ethnic differences in lipid or blood pressure control were found. The authors found that in their sample of insulin-treated minority veterans, African Americans in particular had poorer glycemic control and received lower doses of insulin than non-Hispanic whites. However, they found no differences for control of other cardiovascular disease risk factors and concluded that the diabetes treatment disparity could be due to provider behaviors and/or patient behaviors or preferences.

Statistical Models for Categorical Outcome Data

When the response variable is categorical and, in particular, binary and all explanatory variables are either categorical or continuous, we deal with a (multivariate-) *logistic* regression model. Logistic regression could be used for analyzing any of the previously discussed designs (case-control, cross-sectional, cohort, and randomized controlled trial) depending on whether the response variable is categorical and, more generally, on the situation at hand. An example of a categorical response modeled on one or more categorical and one or more continuous explanatory variables is when dichotomized annual income (High versus Low) is modeled as a function of race and years of education. The *odds ratio* is the measure analyzed by logistic regression, and it could be a good approximation of a more useful measure, *relative risk* (RR), when the event of interest is a rare one (<10% prevalence). (Relative risk and odds ratio were discussed already in the categorical response sections.) The Cochran-Mantel-Haenszel method estimates the relative risk and its 95% CI when all predictors are categorical only.[27] For investigating the association between categorical multiresponse variables (e.g., one person self-designating as multiple race/ethnicity categories) without adjustment for continuous covariates, see Bilder and Loughin.[23] Example 10–4 discusses the use of logistic regression and adjustment for covariates for the effect of race/ethnicity on the risk of developing congenital syphilis.

Example 10–4

Black and Hispanic infants are 19.9 and 10.3 times more likely, respectively, than white infants to develop congenital syphilis, a disease that is preventable with timely prenatal screening and treatment. Fowler and colleagues[28] have examined racial/ethnic group differences in prenatal syphilis screening among pregnant women with equal financial access to prenatal care through Medicaid. They have used Florida claims data to examine (1) any, (2) early, and (3) repeat screening among non-Hispanic white, non-Hispanic black, and Hispanic women with Medicaid-covered deliveries in fiscal year (FY) 1995 ($n = 56,088$) and FY2000 ($n = 54,073$). They estimated screening rates for each group and used *logistic regression* to assess whether screening disparities remained after controlling for other factors (including Medicaid enrollment characteristics and prenatal care source) and associations between access-related factors and screening odds for each group. They found that between FY1995 and FY2000, rates of any and early syphilis screening increased, while repeat screening rates decreased. In FY1995, any, early, and repeat rates were highest for blacks and lowest for Hispanics. In FY2000, any and early screening rates were highest for whites and lowest for blacks, while repeat screening rates were similar across groups. Racial/ethnic differences in any and early screening remained for non-Hispanic blacks after adjustment. In general, Medicaid enrollment early in pregnancy, primary care case management participation, and use of a safety net clinic were associated with higher screening odds, although results varied by test type and across groups. The authors concluded that unexplained racial/ethnic disparities in prenatal syphilis screening remain for blacks, but not Hispanics, and that individual, provider, and program factors contribute to differences across and within groups.

Example 10–5 discusses the use of logistic regression and adjustment for both categorical and continuous covariates for the effect of race/ethnicity and socioeconomic status on osteoporosis screening after hip fracture.

Example 10-5

Racial and socioeconomic disparities have been suspected in osteoporosis screening. Neuner and colleagues[29] conducted a study to determine whether racial and socioeconomic disparities in osteoporosis screening diminish after hip fracture. They studied a retrospective cohort study of female Medicare patients in the entire states of Illinois, New York, and Florida. The study participants were female Medicare recipients aged 65 to 89 years old with hip fractures between January 2001 and June 2003. Measured were differences in bone density testing rates by race/ethnicity and ZIP-code-level socioeconomic characteristics during the 2-year period preceding and the 6-month period following a hip fracture. It was found that among all 35,681 women with hip fractures, 20.7% underwent bone mineral density testing in the 2 years prior to fracture and another 6.2% underwent testing in the 6 months after fracture. In a *logistic regression* model *adjusted for* age, state, and comorbidity, women of black race were about half as likely (RR = 0.52, 95% CI = 0.43–0.62) and Hispanic women about two-thirds as likely (RR = 0.66, 95% CI = 0.54–0.80) as white women to undergo testing before their fracture. They remained less likely (RR = 0.66, 95% CI = 0.50–0.88, and RR = 0.58, 95% CI = 0.39–0.87, respectively) to undergo testing after fracture. In contrast, women residing in ZIP codes in the lowest tertile of income and education were less likely than those in higher-income and educational tertiles to undergo testing before fracture, but were no less likely to undergo testing in the 6 months after fracture. The authors concluded that racial, but not socioeconomic, differences in osteoporosis evaluation continued to occur even after Medicare patients had demonstrated their propensity to fracture, and that future interventions may need to target racial/ethnic and socioeconomic disparities differently.

Statistical Models for Time-to-Event Outcome Data

A time-to-event (i.e., survival or lifetime) study is conducted when a set of subjects is observed from a well-defined point in time, followed for a substantial period of time, and then the times at which events are occurring are recorded. The "event" of interest could be death, bone fracture, cancer diagnosis, or any other event. While recording time-to-event, not everyone may experience the event, or different mutually exclusive subtypes of the event may be of interest (e.g., death from cancer or from heart attack), or sometimes multiple occurrences of the event to the same subject are recorded during study (e.g., several fractures or cancer recurrences); the latter requires specialized methods for analysis. The study subjects may be followed-up in time prospectively by the researcher or retrospectively when they (or their proxies) are asked to recall the timing of past events. The retrospective design is much less reliable because of recall bias and ascertainment bias. Specific models of survival analysis are preferred over conventional methods (ANCOVA, linear or logistic regression) because the latter cannot handle data with censoring (those not experiencing the event are "censored" at the end of their follow-up) and time-dependent covariates (some covariates remain constant during study—e.g., gender, race, age at baseline—but others may change—e.g., treatment group). The models of survival analysis include life tables (i.e., actuarial method), the Kaplan-Meier (estimator) for one curve, the log-rank test comparing two (or more) survival curves, the Cox proportional-hazards model incorporating covariates, and its extensions. Example 10–6 discusses the use of Kaplan-Meier survival curve analysis and Cox proportional hazards models with covariates on survival from head and neck squamous cell carcinoma.

Example 10–6

Black patients are reported to have a higher incidence of advanced disease and increased mortality from head and neck squamous cell carcinoma (HNSCC) but constitute the minority of patients in large-scale studies investigating the effect of race on outcome. Gourin and Podolsky[30] sought to determine if racial disparities exist between black and white patients with HNSCC treated at a single large institution in the South with a high proportion of black patients. The authors conducted a nonrandomized retrospective cohort analysis. The tumor registry was used to identify patients diagnosed with HNSCC from 1985 to 2002. The medical records of non-Hispanic white and black adult patients were retrospectively reviewed. Median household income, percentage of population below poverty level, and education level based on census tract and block information were obtained from U.S. Census 2000 data. Kaplan-Meier survival curve analysis and Cox proportional hazards models were used to analyze the effects of covariates on survival.

A total of 1,128 patients met study criteria (478 black, 650 white). Compared with white patients, black patients were significantly younger (mean age, 53.9 versus 56.4 years, $P < 0.0001$), were male (81.2% versus 72.3%, $P = 0.0005$), more commonly abused alcohol (88.0% versus 74.3%, $P < 0.0001$), and were significantly less likely to have insurance (8.6% versus 21.7%, $P < 0.0001$). There was no difference in the incidence of tobacco use (91.7%), advanced comorbidity (35.9%), or primary tumor site. Black patients had a significantly greater incidence of stage IV disease (65.7% versus 46.6%, $P < 0.0001$) and nonoperative treatment (48.7% versus 30.8%, $P < 0.0001$), which was performed for inoperable disease in 57.1% of black compared with 31.0% of white patients ($P < 0.0001$). Black patients resided in census block groups with significantly lower mean education level, median income, and a higher percentage of population below poverty compared with white patients. The 5-year disease-specific survival differed significantly between black (29.3%) and white (54.7%) patients (P < 0.0001).

Cox proportional hazards models revealed that alcohol abuse, advanced TNM (i.e., tumor, node, metastasis) stage, high tumor grade, nodal disease, extracapsular spread, advanced comorbidity, and regional or distant metastatic disease were associated with poorer survival for all patients. An interaction with race was found for insurance status, nonoperative treatment, and extracapsular spread. Stepwise variable selection adjusting for patient, tumor, and treatment characteristics showed a significant effect only for race by payor status on disease-specific survival (P = 0.0228). Insurance status, treatment, and extracapsular spread differentially affected the survival of black patients compared with white patients. Only insurance status had a significant effect on survival in black patients after controlling for other variables. These data suggest that racial differences in HNSCC outcomes are primarily related to differences in access to health care.

Statistical Multilevel Models

Multilevel (or hierarchical) statistical models account for data heterogeneity due to the clustering by incorporating variables that are not defined at the subject level but at cluster level.[31] In health disparities research, such models are often needed when the sampling has been carried out in a hierarchical manner. For example, it may not be practical or meaningful to select a random sample from the total population of a large city; rather, a hierarchical sample of various exposure sources and activity areas can be used to sample areas with a high prevalence of elevated blood lead in children.[32] The size of area and the average level of lead pollution from source are variables that are not defined at the subject level but are incorporated in a multilevel model. Another example of the appropriate application of multilevel modeling is combining individual studies (meta-analysis). Example 10–7 discusses the use of hierarchical linear models in order to regress self-rated health on county-, neighborhood-, and individual-level racial and socioeconomic variables.

Example 10–7

Robert and Ruel[33] examined whether racial segregation is associated with poorer self-rated health among older adults and whether racial segregation helps explain race disparities in self-rated health between black and white older adults. Multilevel data was used at the individual, neighborhood (tract), and county levels, from two national surveys: the Americans' Changing Lives (ACL) survey and the National Survey of Families and Households (NSFH). Hierarchical linear models were used in order to regress self-rated health on county-, neighborhood-, and individual-level racial and socioeconomic variables.

In the NSFH, there was an association between county racial segregation and poorer self-rated health among white but not black older adults (net of county percent black and percent poverty). In the ACL, there was no statistically significant association between racial segregation and self-rated health. In the NSFH, there was some indication that black older adults had better self-rated health when living in neighborhoods with a higher percentage of black residents than the county percentage. Although aggregate-level studies demonstrate associations between racial segregation and mortality rates, the multilevel analyses with two national datasets suggest only weak associations between racial segregation and self-rated health. However, socioeconomic status at multiple levels contributes to race disparities in health.

Example 10–8 discusses the use of a three-level hierarchical logistic regression models in order to decompose individual, spatial, and temporal variance in self-rated health.

Example 10–8

Browning and colleagues[34] used the Metropolitan Community Information Center—Metro Survey (a serial cross section of adults residing in the City of Chicago, conducted from 1991 through 1999) in combination with 1990 Census data to simultaneously examine the extent to which self-rated health varies across Chicago neighborhoods and across time. Three-level hierarchical logistic regression models are employed to decompose individual, spatial, and temporal variance in self-rated health. Results indicate that variations in self-rated health across neighborhoods are explained, in part, by variations in the level of neighborhood affluence. Neighborhood-level poverty, however, is not a significant predictor of self-rated health. Community-level affluence, moreover, accounts for a substantial proportion of the residual health deficit experienced by African Americans when compared with whites (after controlling for individual-level SES). The effects of affluence hold when controlling for spatial autocorrelation and when considered in primarily African American neighborhoods. Findings also indicate that individuals living in the City of Chicago became significantly healthier over the decade of the 1990s, and that this improvement in health is explained largely by the increasing education and income levels of Chicago residents.

SUMMARY

The exposition in this chapter touched on different aspects of health disparities research while keeping the main focus on the proper use of statistical models. However, it is important to keep in mind that health disparities measures, study design, and statistical models are mutually dependent and should be dealt with in parallel when putting together a research study. It is also obvious from the examples, taken from recent publications, that there is a long way to go before health disparities are eliminated.

REFERENCES

1. Bland M. *An Introduction to Medical Statistics*, 3rd ed. New York: Oxford University Press; 2000.
2. Altman DG. *Practical Statistics for Medical Research*. Boca Raton, FL: Chapman & Hall/CRC Press; 1991.
3. Rothman KJ, Greenland S. *Modern Epidemiology*, 2nd ed. Philadelphia: Lippincott Williams & Wilkins; 1998.
4. Gordis L. *Epidemiology*, 3rd ed., Philadelphia: Elsevier Saunders; 2004.
5. Woodward M. *Epidemiology: Study Design and Data Analysis*, 2nd ed. Boca Raton, FL: Chapman & Hall/CRC Press; 2004.
6. Harper S, Lynch J. *Methods for Measuring Cancer Disparities: A Review Using Data Relevant to Healthy People 2010 Cancer-Related Objectives*. Report to Division of Cancer Control and Population Sciences of the National Cancer Institute, NIH [T-074] Pub. No. 05-5777, 2005, http://seer.cancer.gov/publications/disparities/.
7. U.S. Department of Health and Human Services. *Healthy People 2010: Understanding and Improving Health*. Washington DC: U.S. Department of Health and Human Services; 2000.
8. Preston SH, Haines MR, Pamuk E. Effects of industrialization and urbanization on mortality in developed countries. In: *International Union for the Scientific Study of Population*. International Population Conference, Manila, 1981: Solicited Papers. Vol. 2. Leige: Ordina Editions, 1981;233–254.
9. Dorschner J. The minority health crisis. *Miami Herald*. September 13, 2004:22G.
10. Wagstaff A. The bounds of the concentration index when the variable of interest is binary, with an application to immunization inequality. *Health Econ*. 2005;14:429–432.
11. Wagstaff A. Inequality aversion, health inequalities and health achievement. *J Health Econ*. 2002;21(4):627–641.
12. Pamuk ER. Social-class inequality in infant mortality in England and Wales from 1921 to 1980. *Eur J Popul*. 1988;4:1 21.
13. Kunst AE, Mackenbach J. International variation in the size of mortality differences associated with occupational status. *Int J Epidemiol*. 1994;23(4):742–750.
14. Kakwani N, Wagstaff A, Vandoorslaer E. Socioeconomic inequalities in health: Measurement, computation, and statistical inference. *J Econom*. 1997;77(1):87–103.
15. Chakravarty SR. The variance as a subgroup decomposable measure of inequality. *Soc Indic Res*. 2001;53(1):79–95.

16. Theil H. *Economics and Information Theory*. Amsterdam: North-Holland; 1967.
17. Rachev ST, Haynatzka VR, Haynatzki GR. Probability metrics and limit theorems in AIDS epidemiology. In Rao MM, ed. *Real & Stochastic Analysis: Recent Advances*. Boca Raton, FL: CRC Press, 1997:159–223.
18. Rachev ST. *Probability Metrics and the Stability of Stochastic Models*. New York: John Wiley & Sons; 1991.
19. Enger SM, Van Den Eeden SK, Sternfeld B, et al. California Men's Health Study (CMHS): A multiethnic cohort in a managed care setting. *BMC Public Health*. 2006;6:172; http://www.biomedcentral.com/1471-2458/6/172.
20. Simpson EH. The interpretation of interaction in contingency tables. *J Royal Statistical Soc, Ser. B*. 1951;13:238–241.
21. Freedman D, Pisani P, Curves R. *Statistics*, 3rd ed. New York: W. W. Norton; 1998.
22. Wilcox A. The perils of birth weight—A lesson from directed acyclic graphs. *Am J Epidemiol*. 2006;164(11):1121–1123.
23. Bilder CR, Loughin TM. Modeling association between two or more categorical variables that allow for multiple category choices. *Commun Stats: Theory Meth*. 2007;36(2):433–451.
24. Everitt BS, Dunn G. *Applied Multivariate Data Analysis*. 2nd ed. New York: Oxford University Press, A Hodder Arnold Publication; 2001.
25. Johnson RA, Wichern DW. *Applied Multivariate Statistical Analysis*, 6th ed., Upper Saddle River, NJ: Prentice Hall; 2007.
26. Wendel CS, Shah JH, Duckworth WC, Hoffman RM, Mohler MJ, Murata GH. Racial and ethnic disparities in the control of cardiovascular disease risk factors in Southwest American veterans with type 2 diabetes: The Diabetes Outcomes in Veterans Study. *BMC Health Serv Res*. 2006 May 23;6:58.
27. Jewel NP. *Statistics for Epidemiology*. Boca Raton, FL: Chapman & Hall/CRC Press; 2004.
28. Fowler CI, Gavin NI, Adams EK, Tao G, Chireau M. Racial and ethnic disparities in prenatal syphilis screening among women with Medicaid-covered deliveries in Florida. *Matern Child Health J*. July 18, 2007—Epub, ahead of print.
29. Neuner JM, Zhang X, Sparapani R, Laud PW, Nattinger AB. Racial and socioeconomic disparities in bone density testing before and after hip fracture. *J Gen Intern Med*. 2007 Sep;22(9):1239-1245. Epub June 27, 2007.
30. Gourin CG, Podolsky RH. Racial disparities in patients with head and neck squamous cell carcinoma. *Laryngoscope*. 2006 Jul;116(7):1093–1106.
31. Goldstein H. *Multilevel Statistical Modeling*, 2nd ed., London: Edward Arnold; 1995.
32. Ericson JE, Gonzalez EJ. Hierarchical sampling of multiple strata: An innovative technique in exposure characterization. *Environ Res*. 2003 Jul;92(3):221–231.
33. Robert SA, Ruel E. Racial segregation and health disparities between Black and White older adults. *J Gerontol B Psychol Sci Soc Sci*. 2006 Jul;61(4):S203–S211.
34. Browning CR, Cagney KA, Wen M. Explaining variation in health status across space and time: implications for racial and ethnic disparities in self-rated health. *Soc Sci Med*. 2003 Oct;57(7):1221–1235.

Chapter 11

Addressing Health Disparities: The Hispanic Perspective

Ann V. Millard, PhD
Margaret A. Graham, PhD
Nelda Mier, PhD
Isidore Flores, PhD
Genny Carrillo-Zuniga, MD, ScD
Esmeralda R. Sánchez, MPH

Inadequate preventive and curative healthcare services exacerbate Hispanic health disparities in many ways. The development of adequate services requires training healthcare providers as one of several approaches to improving access to care. Reduction of health disparities further requires attention to social and economic structural factors that sustain high rates of poverty in many Hispanic subpopulations. We will focus on documenting Hispanic health disparities and give brief attention to the training needs for healthcare providers.

In this chapter, we use *Hispanic* and *Latino* synonymously to mean people with ancestors from Latin America, Puerto Rico and the rest of the Spanish-speaking Caribbean, and the Iberian Peninsula. *Hispanic* is a term so defined by the U.S. Census Bureau to designate an ethnic group defined as multiracial. Many scientific problems exist with these categories[1-3]; however, they are used in many government documents and databases, and their social salience links to the various forms of discrimination and racism that play a key role in determining the distribution of resources in our society. Some prefer to be called *Latino*, perhaps partly in resistance to government-imposed categories. (Latina[s] is the feminine form; Latino[s] includes men or both men and women.)

As a major ethnic group, Latinos comprise the fastest growing population in the United States. The Mexican-descent population is the largest and fastest growing subpopulation, including two-thirds of all Hispanics, with relatively high rates of fertility and immigration **(Table 11–1)**.[4-8] Puerto

Table 11–1 *Sociodemographic Characteristics of Hispanics*

	Hispanics	Non-Hispanic Whites
Hispanic or Latino (2006)[4]	47.5 million	
In the 50 states	43.7 million	
Commonwealth of Puerto Rico	3.8 million	
Population not Hispanic or Latino	255.4 million	
Total U.S. population (50 states) (2006)	299.1 million	
Hispanic subpopulations (2006)[5]		
Mexican Americans	66.0%	
Puerto Ricans	9.4%	
Central Americans	7.8%	
South Americans	5.2%	
Cuban Americans	4.0%	
Other Hispanics	7.6%	
Age		
Median age, Hispanics (2007)[6]	27.4 years	40.5 years
≥ 65 years (2005)[7]	6%	15%
Education, completed high school or more (2004)[5]	58.4%	90%
Income: families with annual earnings < $35,000[8]	50.9%	26%

Sources: U.S. Bureau of the Census. *2005 Puerto Rico Survey* (B03001-3-EST); 2006b; U.S. Bureau of the Census. The Hispanic Population in the United States: March 2004. *Current Population Reports*, Data Tables including Educational Attainment in the United States, Detailed Tables (PPL-169) (does not include Commonwealth of Puerto Rico). Internet release, last revised March 2004; U.S. Bureau of the Census. *Annual Estimates of the Population by Sex, Race, and Hispanic or Latino Origin for the United States: July 1, 2006* (NC-EST 2005-03); May 17, 2007b; U.S. Bureau of the Census. 65+ in the United States: 2005. *Current Population Reports*; 2005c; and U.S. Bureau of the Census. *Current Population Survey, Annual Social and Economic Supplement*. Ethnicity and Ancestry Statistics Branch, Population Division (does not include the Commonwealth of Puerto Rico); 2004b.

Ricans are the next most numerous subpopulations (9.4%) followed by those of Cuban descent (4.0%).[9] The countries of Central and South America, when aggregated, contribute more descendants than Puerto Rico, and they are immigrating in increasing numbers.

Variations of health disparities exist among Hispanic subpopulations and also vary according to age, gender, and socioeconomic status.[10,11] Important determinants of variations between Hispanic subpopulations are national origin, culture, and relationship to immigration status (e.g., nonimmigrant, first-generation immigrant, second-generation, [a child of immigrants], etc.).

In some instances, Hispanic subpopulations are healthier than the non-Hispanic white population. These include birth outcomes, cardiovascular disease, cancer, and mental health; they are known as the Hispanic epidemiological paradox.[12–14] Hispanic immigrants also tend to have better health than U.S.-born Hispanics, suggesting that some aspects of life in the United States harm the health of Hispanics and, by extension, that of others as well. If the causes of the dimensions of variability were understood, it would be possible to deal more effectively with health problems of Hispanics and the entire U.S. population.

As an ethnic minority population in the United States who suffer from discrimination, Hispanics include higher percentages of poor families, uninsured adults, and employees exposed to dangerous working conditions than do non-Hispanic whites.[1] Hispanics thus suffer higher death rates from diabetes, asthma, HIV/AIDS, and work-related injuries **(Table 11–2)**.[15] These higher death rates could be substantially reduced by regular medical care, safer working conditions, and alleviation of poverty, which shapes health behavior, health literacy, and educational accomplishment.[11] There are also disparities in immunization of Hispanic children and elders;[16] this could be improved by enhanced access to preventive medical care. Hispanics have a higher incidence of cancer of the cervix and the stomach compared with non-Hispanic whites,[15] problems that could be reduced by prevention, screening, and early treatment.

Hispanics also exceed non-Hispanic whites in prevalence of obesity.[17] The rise in obesity increases risks of developing cardiovascular disease, type 2 diabetes, and some types of cancer. The tendency of those descended from Hispanic immigrants to develop less healthy behavior as they become more acculturated to the United States also increases disease risk. For example, among eighth graders, more Hispanics smoke (28.0%) than non-Hispanic whites (23.7%) or non-Hispanic blacks (25.3%).[18] The increased risk factors foretell even greater disparities in the future. These health disparities are heavily dependent on cultural and behavioral factors; thus an informed and empowered Hispanic populace can reduce these risk factors and diminish the toll taken by chronic disease.

Table 11–2 *Examples of Health Disparities among Hispanic Americans*

Health Issue (Year Data Collected)	
Subpopulation	**Rate**
Diabetes mortality rate per 100,000 (2000)	
Puerto Ricans	172
Mexican Americans	122
Cubans	47
Asthma mortality rate per million in the northeast U.S. (1993–1995)	
Hispanics/Latinos	34
Whites	15.1
HIV/AIDS mortality rate per 100,000 (1999)	
Puerto Ricans living on the U.S. mainland	32.7
Non-Hispanic whites	2.4
National average	5.4
Work-related fatal injuries among foreign-born workers (1995–2000)	
Mexican-born workers	69%
Cuban-born workers	6%
El Salvadoran-born workers	5%
Guatemalan-born workers	4%
Dominican Republic-born workers	4%
Adult immunization, 65+ years (2002)	
Influenza vaccination	
Hispanics/Latinos	46.7%
Whites	70.2%
Pneumococcal vaccination	
Hispanics/Latinos	23.8%
Whites	60.6%
Cancer of the cervix (2000)	
Hispanic incidence higher than that of non-Hispanic whites by	152%

Table 11–2 *Examples of Health Disparities among Hispanic Americans*
(Continued)

Health Issue (Year Data Collected)	
Subpopulation	**Rate**
Cancer of the stomach (2000)	
Males: Hispanic incidence higher by	63%
Females: Hispanic incidence higher by	150%
Overweight among Hispanics 20 to 74 years of age	
Males: Hispanic incidence higher than in non-Hispanic whites by	11%
Females: Hispanic incidence higher by	26%
Obesity, 20 to 74 years of age	
Males: Hispanic incidence higher by	7%
Females: Hispanic incidence higher by	32%

Source: Centers for Disease Control and Prevention. *Fact Sheet: Hispanic Health Disparities, 2004.*
http://www.cdc.gov/od/oc/Media. Accessed October 3, 2007.

As a result of these and other health inequities, Hispanics have disparities in years of potential life lost. Calculated as years lost before age 75, the loss of life because of diabetes, stroke, chronic liver disease and cirrhosis, HIV, and homicide among Hispanics is substantially higher than in non-Hispanic whites **(Table 11–3)**. Hispanics also have less coverage by health insurance, less access to regular medical care, and fewer vaccina-

Table 11–3 *Dispartities in Years of Potential Life Lost before Age 75*

Diabetes	41%
Stroke	18%
Chronic liver disease and cirrhosis	62%
HIV	168%
Homicide	128%

Percentage of higher loss of life among Hispanics/Latinos compared with non-Hispanic whites (per 100,000)
Source: Centers for Disease Control and Prevention. *Fact Sheet: Hispanic Health Disparities, 2004.* http://www.cdc.gov/od/oc/Media. Accessed October 3, 2007.

tions of children and elders than non-Hispanic whites[15] **(Table 11–4)**. Only 66% of Hispanics have health insurance, compared with 87% of non-Hispanic whites.[20-22] This disparity exists despite similar employment rates.[19] Hispanic death and disability could be substantially reduced by improving access to preventive medical care and alleviating poverty.

Access to Care

Access to health care can be described in three tiers listing specific barriers along the pathway.[23] This approach allows researchers to delineate "where along the continuum toward obtaining quality health care specific barriers may exist."[23-24]

The first tier, *primary access*, is defined as simply having health insurance. Numerous studies indicate that Latinos have a higher rate of being uninsured, a barrier to even starting on the path to health care.[25] In most instances, health insurance is tied to employment opportunities and socioeconomic status. Among the employed, those least able to afford health insur-

Table 11–4 *Disparities in Health Care Access*

	Hispanics	Non-Hispanic Whites
Health insurance and regular health care		
Those under the age of 65 years with health insurance	66%	87%
Children with health insurance (2005)[6]	78%	87%
Those with a regular source of ongoing health care	77%	90%
Employment rates, working-age adults (2004)[19]	69%	65%
Vaccinations[15]		
Children aged 19–35 months who are fully vaccinated (2002)	73%	78%
Adults 65+ years who had influenza and penumococcal vaccination in the preceding 12 months	49%	69%

Sources: U.S. Bureau of the Census. Annual Estimates of the Population by Sex, Race, and Hispanic or Latino Origin for the United States: July 1, 2006 (NC-EST 2005-03); May 17, 2007b; Centers for Disease Control and Prevention. Fact Sheet: Hispanic Health Disparities, 2004. http://www.cdc.gov/od/oc/Media. Accessed October 3, 2007; and U.S. Bureau of Labor Statistics. Civilian Labor force participation rates by sex, age, race, and Hispanic origin, 2004. http://www.bls.gov. Accessed on December 7, 2005.

ance are also the least likely to be covered as employees; this is particularly true of Latino day laborers, gardeners, and household service workers.

Those with health insurance often face barriers at another tier, *secondary access*. Those who may be insured may deal with "institutional, organizational, or structural" barriers."[23] These may include long wait times for referrals, lack of access to after-hours advice and services, access to specialists, and problems making appointments.[26-28]

The final tier, *tertiary access*, refers to cultural barriers that include language and communication.[23,27,29-33] Even when Latinos are insured and able to secure appointments, cultural barriers affect their care and their understanding of the medical visit.[27,29,34,35]

Immigration and Acculturation

Hispanic immigration to the United States is a complex process differing by nationality, historical period, and social class. A few examples illustrate the complexity. In the mid-19th century, the Treaty of Guadalupe-Hidalgo at the end of the Mexican-American War ceded about one-third of Mexican territory to the United States; with the land came Mexican citizens, who could choose U.S. citizenship according to the treaty. Their descendants point out that "We did not cross the border; the border crossed over us." A similar process occurred in other regions that were formerly Spanish colonies, later absorbed into the United States. These segments of the Hispanic population are not the descendants of immigrants to the United States. Puerto Rico was seized by the United States and is now a commonwealth where birth confers U.S. citizenship and freedom to travel to the 50 states. Most statistics on U.S. Hispanic health omit those who live in Puerto Rico and include only Puerto Ricans living on the mainland. When Puerto Rico is included with the United States, those who live in Puerto Rico constitute more than 12% of the total number of Hispanics, 47.5 million people (2006 data). (See Table 11–4.)

Mexico today is one of the largest Latin American countries and the biggest trade partner of the United States. Mexico has a 1,950-mile-long border with the United States, surplus labor, and a minimum wage that is approximately one-sixth that in the United States.[36] These factors make migration to the United States attractive to low-income Mexicans. Many other Mexicans travel to the United States to study or conduct business, and some decide to stay. In general, overstaying a visa is a more common way for immigrants to gain a foothold in the United States than entering the country illegally, despite the popular image of the Mexican immigrant who sneaks across the border without official documents. Generally, the attraction of large numbers of low-income Mexican immigrants to the United States is the promise of better wages.[37]

At various points during the 20th century, people from Mexico moved to the United States to escape violence (e.g., the Revolution of 1910 in Mexico) or political oppression.[38] The latter is also a common reason for past migration from several Central American and Caribbean countries to the United States. From all Latin American countries, there is also a brain drain—highly educated people immigrate to the United States, whether in pursuit of higher income or professional opportunity.

Most Hispanics are in the United States legally, and that includes most people of Mexican descent. There are also millions of Hispanics, especially Mexican Americans, who are "undocumented"; that is, they lack authorization to live and work in the United States. Periodically during the 20th century, the United States had official channels for importing Mexican laborers until an economic downturn occurred, whereupon the United States sometimes would deport Mexicans, especially when Mexicans were made into scapegoats and blamed for poor economic conditions in the United States; this was true during a recession in the early 1920s and the Great Depression of the 1930s.[38]

Acculturation is one of several factors affecting the health status of Latinos. The definition of acculturation is complex and has various dimensions.[39–42] This summary draws heavily from the insightful synthesis of Lara and colleagues.[14] In simple terms, acculturation can be viewed as the level of immersion in the new culture or how far people have deviated from their cultural origins[41,43,44] in adopting features of the new or dominant culture. "Cultural maintenance is the degree to which an individual continues to value and adhere to the norms of the culture of origin."[14(p.370)] The level of acculturation varies and depends on such aspects as knowledge of cultural traditions, cultural history, dietary patterns, television and radio choices, language use and preference, and social affiliations.[14,33,39,40,42,45] One of the most simplified measures of acculturation is language, including the ability to read, write, and speak, although there are strong critics of using language as a reliable measure.[46] Other factors important to acculturation are the age of a person at the time of immigration, the generation of someone descended from an immigrant, and education. Furthermore, it is important to consider the society and social class from which the immigrant originated. Societal factors, educational opportunities, and employment status in the country of origin are important factors.[14]

The effect of "assimilation to mainstream U.S. culture" on the health behavior and outcomes of Latinos is a complex matter that is not clearly understood.[14] Assimilation results in both positive and negative health trends, but overall, according to Lara and colleagues, acculturation has a negative effect on Latino health.[14] Some evidence shows that more acculturated Latinos will use preventive services such as cancer screening,[47,48] but acculturated women have a greater tendency toward substance abuse than less acculturated Latinas.[49–51]

Negative health effects of acculturation have also been observed in use of alcohol, smoking, nutrition, and birth outcomes.[14,51–53] Breastfeeding has been associated with lower levels of acculturation, although research shows mixed results, with higher rates of breastfeeding among educated women. Greater levels of acculturation are associated with higher rates of insurance coverage, increased use of preventive services by women, and increased access to services.[14,47,48,54]

Health across the Life Course

For the U.S. Latino population in general, rates of poverty and population growth are high, with related health effects at all ages. The rate of poverty among Latino children is the fastest growing among all children in the country.[55] Lack of health insurance is a problem for many Latino children, as are obesity, type 2 diabetes, asthma, substance abuse, violence, depression, and suicide.[56,57] The household context is also important to children's health; for example, exposure to pesticides in agricultural communities can depend on household practices, housing locations, and parental employment.[58–60] Reproductive health disparities vary; Latinas have relatively high rates of birth and better than expected birth outcomes.[61,62]

On the other hand, both women and men are more likely to be diagnosed with specific types of advanced cancer because they tend to lack access to regular health care, including regular screening, because of their lack of health insurance.[62] Elderly Latinos also face barriers in accessing health care, and in many cases because of their earlier lack of health insurance, have advanced disease by the time they qualify for Medicare. Those lacking documents for U.S. residency cannot qualify for Medicare at all and tend to become reliant on hospital emergency rooms on the rare occasions when they do access medical attention. Hospital emergency departments provide care that is expensive, inefficient, and episodic, making it particularly inappropriate for elders suffering from chronic disease.

Reproductive Health

Latina women have the highest birth rates among the major racial/ethnic groups in the United States. In 1998, their rate was 24.3 live births per thousand compared to 12.1 for non-Latino whites.[63,64] The high birth rates are related to the younger population profile of the Latino population as well as their relatively large families. Mexican American women have a particularly high fertility rate; those from 20 to 24 years of age in 1998 had 197.6 births per thousand, compared with 90.7 for white women. Among Latinas, there is considerable diversity in birth rates, and Cuban women have the lowest fertility rate (50.1) of all racial and ethnic groups in the United States.[63]

Teen births and births out of wedlock are increasing in different Latino groups, especially among women born in the United States.[63,64] Latinas receive relatively little sex or health education and little information about birth control and sexually transmitted diseases.[65,66] They tend to have low use of contraceptives and low rates of voluntary abortion.[66] Among women aged 15 to 19 in the late 1990s, Latinas had an abortion ratio of 27.5% (the rate of abortion per 100 pregnancies); whites had a ratio of 32%; and African Americans, 40.8%.[66]

The low Latino rate of ongoing coverage by health insurance means that during pregnancy, Latinas tend to delay prenatal care and have relatively low access to sophisticated medical technology, such as ultrasound.[65,67,68] Additionally, Latinos report experiencing unfair treatment in the medical system, another disincentive to visiting the doctor.[22]

Latinas are unlikely to experience complications during delivery,[64] even though a significant number develop gestational diabetes. Latinas have twice the risk of developing this condition as do whites. Puerto Ricans have the highest rate of gestational diabetes, 34.7 per 1000; Mexican Americans, 25.4; African Americans, 24.9; and whites 25.6.[69] Latinas have a slightly lower rate of cesarean delivery than whites (20.6% compared with 21.2%).[70] On the other hand, Cuban American mothers born in the United States have the highest rate of cesarean delivery, 33.7%.[64]

Latino birth outcomes as measured by birth weight are comparable to those of whites;[64] this equivalence is termed an *epidemiological paradox* because, on average, Latinas have more risk factors for low-birth-weight babies. Latinas tend to be much less well educated and have more limited incomes, lower rates of coverage by health insurance, and less involvement in prenatal care. On the other hand, Mexican American women tend to drink little alcohol, particularly those who are immigrants, and they tend to have other good health habits.[71] In 2006, low-birth-weight births occurred in only 6.8% of Hispanic babies compared with 7.1% of non-Hispanic white babies and 13.4% of non-Hispanic black babies.[61] Among Hispanics, low birth weight affected 6.4% of Mexican American babies, 6.5% of Central and South American babies, 7.7% of Cuban babies, and 9.8% of Puerto Rican babies.[61] Racial/ethnic differences in infant mortality rates have a pattern similar to that of birth weight. Per 1000 live births in 2003, the infant mortality rate was 5.6 among Hispanic babies, 5.7 among non-Hispanic white babies, and 13.5 among non-Hispanic black babies.[61]

Immigrant Latinas had slightly better birth outcomes than those born in the United States. According to one study, higher acculturation was correlated with higher prenatal stress, which linked to tendencies toward preterm delivery, substance abuse, and low social support.[53] A possibly related differential is the greater rates of low birth weight among Puerto Rican babies,[63] because Puerto Rico has considerable influence from the U.S. mainland.

Immigrant Latina women breastfeed at higher rates than U.S. women, but by the third generation, Latinas breastfeed at the same rate as others in the same socioeconomic group.[65] In 2005, 79.0% of Hispanic babies were breastfed compared with 75.7% of non-Hispanic white babies and 59.6% of non-Hispanic black babies.[16]

The Health of Latino Elderly

Rapid growth of the Latino elderly population is expected in the next 30 years. While the population of people age 65 and over is expected to jump by 93%, the Latino elderly population is expected to grow much faster, by 555%.[72] By 2050, it is estimated that the elderly (age 65 and over) will be composed of 15% Latinos, 7% Asians, 10% African Americans, and 67% whites.[72] Elderly Latinos are poorer than whites, with 22.5% living in poverty and another 36.3% living in near poverty.[72] Unmarried elderly women are the most vulnerable, with about 50% living in poverty in 1990.[72]

Elderly Latinos are more likely to report poor health, and approximately 85% reported having at least one chronic condition.[73] Major health problems reported by elderly Latinos include arthritis, cognitive impairment, diabetes, cardiovascular disease, depression, hypertension and cerebrovascular problems.[72,74] Many of these chronic conditions result in long-term disability and difficulties performing activities of daily living that may result in higher levels of dependency and need for assistance with daily activities.[72,75,76] Overall, the health status of elderly Latinos is poor in the areas of functioning and certain chronic diseases.[72] Elderly Latinos are more likely to be cared for by family members who may themselves be economically disadvantaged.[72,77] Much of the information on the health of elderly Latinos is based on studies with Mexican Americans[77]; thus basic data on other subpopulations are needed to broaden our knowledge of Latino health experiences in old age.

Rates of adult immunization for influenza and pneumonia are lower for elderly Latinos compared with non-Hispanic whites. In 2002, 70.2% of white adults 65 years and older received influenza vaccine while only

46.7% of elderly Latinos did. Pneumococcal vaccination shows a wider gap—60.6% for whites and 23.8% for Latinos.[15,16]

Chronic and Communicable Disease

The risk factors for chronic and communicable disease are the same for the Hispanic population as other population groups. Extension of public health measures and access to medical care could assist Hispanics and the rest of the population to enjoy better health. Rates of several communicable diseases are reported to be higher in Latinos than in whites, although the higher percentages of Latinos receiving health care at public clinics may be responsible for this difference, as public clinics take more responsibility in reporting diseases.[78] For example, according to the National Health and Nutrition Examination Survey (NHANES), which carries out physical exams on participants, rates of genital herpes infection were the same in 20- to 29-year-old Mexican Americans and whites. In contrast, Latinos are widely reported to have higher rates of sexually transmitted disease, as noted in the later section on social and behavioral health. Reported rates include the following comparisons of Latinos with other groups: higher rates of new AIDS cases than whites; higher rates of gonorrhea and syphilis than among whites; higher rates of chlamydia and pelvic inflammatory disease than among whites.[78] The extent to which bias from reporting differences is responsible for this variation is unclear.

Other disparities in communicable diseases include food-borne hepatitis A (24.2 per 100,000 in Latinos compared with 7.3 in whites).[78] Latino rates of tuberculosis are also higher than among whites (13.6 per 100,000 in Latinos, twice as high as among whites).[78] This difference may be due in part to immigration from countries with higher TB rates; HIV co-infection in the United States; and poor access to screening, treatment, and case management among Latinos.[79]

Obesity

Obesity has attained epidemic proportions in the United States and is correlated with a number of health problems including type 2 diabetes, cardiovascular disease, hypertension, arthritis, depression, and cancer.[80-84] The NHANES 2003–2004 data show that 66.3% of adults (20 years of age and older) are overweight or obese,[17] a two-fold increase compared to the obesity rate in 1988–1991 (33.4%).[85] Also, 17.1% of children and adolescents aged 2 to 19 were overweight in 2003–2004.[17]

There are continuing ethnic disparities in the prevalence of obesity[86–89] with more pronounced disparities in women.[17,86,87,89] In 2003–2004, Latino adults and children (2 to 19 years of age) had a higher prevalence of overweight or obesity (75.8% and 41.4%, respectively) than white adults and children (64.2% and 35.4%, respectively).[17] Complex interactions of genetic, social, cultural, behavioral, and environmental factors may explain the higher prevalence of obesity in the Latino population.[89,90]

Cardiovascular Disease

Latino cardiovascular death rates have tended to be lower than those for whites and African Americans.[91] This differential is reflected for Cuban Americans, Mexican Americans, and Puerto Ricans in deaths from heart disease and stroke. In one study, for example, heart disease mortality rates among people born in Cuba, Mexico, and Puerto Rico and residing in the United States between 1979 and 1981 were lower than the rates among whites. Rates among Latino men were 15% to 30% lower than among white men; women showed a similar pattern with a slightly smaller difference.[92] Known risk factors across all populations include smoking, high lipid and cholesterol levels, and hypertension; these factors account for 60% of cardiovascular mortality. In a cohort study in San Antonio, risk scores were higher among 3,301 Mexican Americans 25 to 65 years of age compared with 1,877 whites.[93] Subsequent studies have supported the existence of this differential, which constitutes another epidemiological paradox. Based on risk factors, greater incidence and prevalence of cardiovascular disease and symptoms in Latinos than non-Latino whites can be predicted, but Latinos have lower rates of actual disease.[76,94–96]

Fewer detailed studies of cardiovascular disease and clinical treatment have been done of Latinos than of African Americans, and further research on all these areas is needed. In 2006, rates of high serum cholesterol among Mexican American men (16.9%) were slightly higher than among non-Hispanic white men (16.0%), but among women, Mexican Americans had lower rates (14.0%) compared with non-Hispanic whites (17.4%).[61] In the 5 years before 2006, only 47.6% of Mexican American adults were screened for high blood cholesterol, compared to 62.5% of non-Hispanic whites and 57.7% of non-Hispanic blacks.[61] Mexican Americans with limited incomes and low educational levels tended to have low cholesterol levels, and their diets commonly emphasized rice, beans, and corn or flour tortillas. Those whose diet more closely resembled that of the prevailing culture had higher cholesterol levels.[61]

Diabetes

Diabetes is the sixth leading cause of death in the United States, and its increasing prevalence has reached epidemic proportions.[97,98] In 2005, 20.6 million people or 9.6% of all people aged 20 years and older had diabetes. Most of these cases are type 2 diabetes, as less than 5% of cases are type 1.[99] Between 1991 and 2001 there has been a positive trend in the prevalence of diabetes from 6.3% to 8.8%, and it is expected to increase to 14.5% in 2031.[98]

Ethnic disparities in diabetes are pronounced, but the etiology of the differences is not clearly understood. The interaction of genetic, lifestyle, and socioenvironmental factors influences the increased risk and prevalence of diabetes in Latinos.[100–103] Diabetes affects disproportionately more Latinos than whites. In 2005, an estimated 2.5 million (9.5%) Latinos aged 20 years and older had diabetes.[104] Mexican Americans, the largest Latino subgroup, have almost twice the prevalence of whites.[105] Moreover, it is projected that ethnic disparities in diabetes will continue to persist, and by 2031 more than 20% of the Latino adult population will suffer from this chronic disease.[98] At the United States–Mexico border, ethnic disparities in diabetes are even more prominent. The diabetes death rate for Latinos living in U.S. counties along the border (46.7 age-adjusted per 100,000 population) is three times the rate for whites (16.3 age-adjusted per 100,000 population).[106] One study found that in border counties, age-adjusted diabetes hospital discharge rates are significantly higher (130%) in Latinos (28.4 per 10,000; 95% CI, 27.6–29.1) than in non-Latinos (12.4 per 10,000; 95% CI, 12.0–12.8).[107] In nonborder counties, Latinos had intermediate rates (23.5 per 10,000; 95% CI, 23.1–23.8).

Diabetes is a leading cause of cardiovascular disease, stroke, blindness, end-stage renal disease, and lower extremity disease.[108] With respect to diabetes complications and ethnic disparities, the literature is inconsistent. Macro-vascular complications include coronary artery disease, myocardial infarction, stroke, and congestive heart failure. Two studies report similar prevalence in macro-vascular consequences in Latinos and whites.[109,110] Other studies, however, show lower prevalence rates of myocardial infarction among Latinos than whites.[111,112] Still other research found higher risk for micro-vascular complications (retinopathy and renal disease) in Latinos compared with whites,[110,111,113,114] while another study reported a smaller risk for Latinos.[115] The prevalence of lower extremity disease was found to be higher in Mexican Americans than whites in one study,[116] but similar in other research.[110]

Cancer

Cancer data are limited for Latino populations as well as for other ethnic minority populations.[117] The primary sources for U.S. cancer research data are the

Centers for Disease Control and Prevention state cancer registries and the National Cancer Institute's Surveillance, Epidemiology, and End Results (SEER) program.[117,118] Cancer incidence rates have been available since 1992.[118]

According to the National Center for Health Statistics, cancer was the second leading cause of death after heart disease for Latinos (both sexes, all ages) in 2003.[119] Malignant neoplasm represents 19.7% of total deaths, while heart disease accounts for 23.2% of total deaths.[119]

Registry data show that Latinos experience lower cancer incidence and death rates than non-Latino whites.[118] The incidence rates of the major cancers (prostate, breast, lung, colon, and rectum) are lower than those for non-Latino whites. Latinos have higher rates for cancers of the stomach, liver, cervix, and gallbladder and for acute lymphocytic leukemia.[118]

Comparison of Cancer Rates between Latinos and Non-Hispanic Whites

Lower Rates among Hispanics

Although breast cancer is the most commonly diagnosed cancer and the leading cause of cancer death for Hispanic women, the incidence of breast cancer is about 40% lower than the rate for white women.[117,118] Hispanic women, however, are less likely to be diagnosed at the earliest stage[118] and are more likely to be diagnosed with larger tumors than white women.[120] Compared with non-Hispanic white women, Latinas are about 20% more likely to die of breast cancer diagnosed at similar age and stage.[121] The incidence of breast cancer has changed very little in Latina women between 1994 and 2003.[122] Death rates declined by 2.2% per year during the same period,[122] a decrease seen in non-Hispanic white women as well.

A similar situation exists for Latino males and prostate cancer. It is the leading cancer diagnosis for Latino males—30% of all new cases expected for 2006—but its incidence rate is about 20% lower than that for white men.[117,118] It is the third leading cause of cancer death for Hispanic men, but the death rate has dropped by 3.2% per year in Hispanic men and by 4.1% in non-Hispanic white men.[122]

Colorectal cancer is the second most commonly diagnosed cancer for both Latino males and females. The rate of colorectal cancer is 20% to 30% lower among Latino males and females than among whites.[118] Rates of colorectal cancer are higher among U.S. Hispanics than in Spanish-speaking countries in Central and South America and in countries where physical activity levels are low and diets are high in fat, refined carbohydrates, and animal protein.[118]

Lung cancer is the third most commonly diagnosed cancer for Hispanic males and females, and the leading cause of cancer death for males and the second among Latinas.[118] Compared with whites, both male and female Latinos have lower rates of lung cancer. For males, the incidence rates are 40% to 50% lower. For females, the rates of lung cancer incidence are 50% to 70% lower.[117] This lower risk is attributed primarily to lower rates of cigarette smoking among Latinos.[117,118]

Higher Rates among Hispanics

Hispanics have higher incidence and death rates of stomach, uterine, cervical, and liver and biliary tract cancers than do non-Hispanic whites. The rates are highest for first-generation immigrants.[123.124]

Although incidence rates of stomach cancer have declined among all ethnic groups, Latinos have rates at least 70% higher than non-Hispanic whites.[118] Dietary factors such as smoked, salted meats or fish, infection *(H. pylori)*, and low socioeconomic status are associated with high risk of stomach cancer.[117,118]

Incidence rates of cervical cancer are high for Latinas, about double those of non-Hispanic white women in 2000–2003.[122] Mortality rates for cervical cancer are about 50% higher than for non-Hispanic whites.[122] Higher mortality rates for cervical cancer are thought to be related in part to lower use of screening Pap tests among both insured and uninsured Latinas.[118,125,126]

Latinos have incidence and death rates of liver cancer double those for non-Hispanic whites.[117,118] Between 1994 and 2003, death rates increased by 1.5% per year in Latino men and 2% per year in women.[118] Chronic infections (hepatitis B and C), alcohol use, aflatoxin-contaminated grains and organic solvents in agriculture are associated with liver cancer. Finally, gallbladder cancer incidence and mortality are pronounced in Hispanics, especially females. Incidence rates for Latino men and women are more than double those for non-Hispanic whites.[118,122]

Cancer Screening

Rates of cancer screening for breast and cervical cancers are increasing among Hispanic women. In 2003, 66.1% of Hispanic women 40 and older had a mammogram within the past two years compared with 70.8% of non-Hispanic whites.[118] Rates of participation in cervical cancer screening are also improving. Mexican American women are the least likely among Hispanic populations to have had a recent mammogram or Pap test. Despite these improvements, access to cancer screening and care continues to be the number-one priority for Latino cancer control efforts in the United States.[127]

Mental Health

Mental health statistics on Latinos are incomplete, and studies of rates and trends are contradictory; however, there is some evidence of a Latino epidemiological paradox in mental health. According to sources that are the most inclusive and consistent, the need for mental health treatment is lower among Mexican Americans and Cubans than among non-Latino ethnic groups.[128,129] Other nondiagnostic studies showed the opposite,[130] which may be due to the transient nature of symptoms.

Measuring major depressive episodes (MDEs) among adults at the population level is of great interest because it is associated with social dysfunction in many areas of life; indeed, it is responsible for the highest burden of disease among illnesses in developing countries.[131] A number of studies using the Diagnostic Interview Schedule (DIS),[132] and the Composite International Diagnostic Interview (CIDI)[133] produced evidence that Latinos born outside the United States have lower rates of major depression than U.S.-born Latinos or European Americans.[128,129,134–137] Mexican immigrants, for instance, suffer mental health problems at a rate of 3.3% in comparison with 6.3% of U.S.-born Mexican Americans. These ratios also hold true for alcohol and substance abuse. Although substance abuse appeared negligible among Latina women, they had higher rates of MDEs than men in all of the studies.

Poverty and low educational achievement are associated with higher illness rates, but not for Latinos.[138] Immigrants from many Spanish-speaking countries have fewer mental health problems[13] than non-Hispanic white immigrants,[139] in comparison with U.S.-born Latinos and non-Latino whites. Latino immigrants leave behind family and community ties that provide social and institutional support. After their arrival, the carry-over effects of those cultural protective factors begin to wane with time.[140] Most Latino groups begin to lose their lead in good health in successive generations,[128,141] but generally they retain some lead over non-Hispanic white immigrants.[139]

Other interesting issues that have a bearing on mental health for Latinos include several crucial points. Latino Medicaid recipients receive only about 35% per patient of funds spent on members of the majority culture,[142] which reflects the level of services consumed. Latinos continue in mental health treatment at greater rates if their therapists are of the same ethnicity.[143,144] Managed care has neither helped nor hindered the utilization rates of mental health services among Latinos.[145]

It appears that culture is a protective factor against mental and substance abuse problems among Latinos,[50,52] while acculturation is a risk factor for both Latino and non-Latino immigrants.[139,146] Addressing mental health disparity requires attention to healthcare discrimination,[147] vigorous education efforts encouraging access to treatment,[148] and other environmental issues.[136,141]

Occupational and Environmental Health

Farm Workers

Latinos make major contributions to the farm labor force in much of the United States, as well as to related enterprises such as food packing, processing, and butchering. Other rural enterprises such as forestry and mining also involve significant numbers of Latino workers. These jobs are physically difficult and tend to be low-wage, lack health benefits, and involve considerable turnover in the work force. By gaining access to the Food Stamp Program, many Latino farm workers are able to sustain their households through times of unpredictable and fluctuating wages earned in the fields. Contrary to popular impression, Food Stamps, not Temporary Aid to Needy Families, are the main poverty program used by migrant farm workers.

Primary occupational hazards of Latino farm workers are pesticide exposure, sun exposure, injuries, and poor field sanitation.[59,149,150] The ergonomic aspects of farm work have received relatively little attention from researchers, and they involve considerable stress from working in awkward positions, repetitive motion, and carrying heavy loads. Secondary occupational hazards involve structural and institutional problems, including lack of access to health care, adequate housing, and clean water as well as lack of health insurance and weak enforcement of safety and health standards.[149] In some rural areas, workers have access to migrant and community health clinics supported by federal funds and services to patients who are eligible for Medicaid and Medicare.[151,152] Migrant clinics have the advantage of providing medical care regardless of patients' ability to pay and their legal status in the United States. In addition, many organizations serving Latino farm workers employ community health workers *(promotores)* who are from the Latino population, are able to speak Spanish, have basic health literacy, and can assist farm workers in accessing medical care.[153]

Urban Workers

The health status of U.S. workers continues to improve with time. The 2004 edition of the National Institute for Occupational Safety and Health (NIOSH) *Worker Health Chartbook* reports that the rates of fatal occupational injuries and nonfatal occupational injuries and illnesses have declined significantly, and Americans are living longer, healthier lives.[154-156] Despite these positive trends, occupational safety and health surveillance faces significant challenges. The data NIOSH reported attest to the depth of current surveillance programs, but a comprehensive and integrated surveillance program remains a long-term goal.[157] Current survey and surveillance programs do not adequately track occupational illnesses because of problems in recognition, recording, and reporting. These limitations hinder a complete and accurate assessment of the nation's occupational injury and illness burden.

The most common occupational injuries involve the musculoskeletal system, with more than 1 million workers sustaining back injuries each year.[158] Many studies of injury reporting systems in industry indicate that occupational injuries are grossly underreported. Nonetheless, injury rates have declined as a result of fundamental changes in U.S. industry and employment patterns. The service sector is growing (e.g., restaurants, sale of groceries and clothing, banking, insurance) and is generally safer than labor or trade work with heavy equipment and mechanized processes. The major causes of occupational death are work-related motor vehicle accidents, falls, trauma, and electric shocks. Higher rates of fatal injury occur in construction, agriculture, mining and quarrying.

The Hispanic/Latino work force grows daily as a result of immigration. The U.S. Immigration and Naturalization Service reports that as of January 2006, there were an estimated 11.6 million unauthorized immigrants living in the United States.[159] Nearly 4.2 million had entered in 2000 or later, and an estimated 6.6 million of the 11.6 million unauthorized residents were from Mexico.

In March 2006, the Current Population Survey (CPS), a national sample survey of about 60,000 households conducted monthly for the Bureau of Labor Statistics by the U.S. Census Bureau, reported that 23% of Hispanic or Latino families were maintained by women.[160] On average, Hispanic immigrants have less formal education, and many of them do not speak English. They reported that the most common occupation that Hispanic male immigrants find upon arrival is construction. Wages are the lowest for the Hispanic population with high-risk jobs. Lower educational attainment, fewer job skills, and, in some cases, lack of proficiency in the English language may contribute to this trend. Workers born in Mexico were reported as two of every five fatally injured, foreign-born workers (41%).[161]

Construction Workers

Construction is one of the largest industries in United States and the most dangerous, accounting for 20.3% or 1,121 of all occupational deaths in 2002. Since 1992, Hispanic construction workers have had markedly higher fatal occupational injury rates than their non-Hispanic counterparts. In 2001 (the most recent year measured), the rate of work-related deaths from construction injuries for Hispanics was 19.5 per 100,000 full-time workers—62.5% higher than the rate of 12.0 for non-Hispanic construction workers. During 1990–2001, Hispanic employment in construction increased greatly, from 649,800 in 1990 to 1.5 million (or 15.6% of the construction work force) in 2001.[157]

Hispanic workers accounted for 10.2% of employed U.S. workers in 2000 but 17.1% of all nonfatal injury and illness cases in 2001. White, non-Hispanic workers accounted for 74.1% of employed U.S. workers in 2000 but 68.2% of nonfatal injury and illness cases with days away from work in 2001.[162] Many work-related injuries are due to the lack of knowledge of English. For example, a worker slipped off a wet roof, broke his back and was paralyzed. His supervisor might have been able to prevent the accident but did not speak Spanish. Another serious injury was due to the inability to read a label prohibiting the use of carbon monoxide in a closed space.[163]

The Pew Hispanic Center reported that the Hispanic labor force added 867,000 workers in the second quarter of 2006 compared with the second quarter of 2005, accounting for about 40% of all workers added to the U.S. labor force.[161] In 2001, white workers accounted for 83.8% of the civilian labor force, black workers for 11.3%, and Hispanic workers for 10.9%.[164] As the percentage of white workers decreases, there is corresponding job growth for minority groups; black workers are projected to account for 12.7% of the labor force and Asian and other workers, excluding Hispanics, for 6.1% by 2010. The percentage of Hispanic workers is projected to more than double during this period, increasing from 5.7% in 1980 to 13.3% in 2010.

A number of Hispanics are temporary workers due to their undocumented status; therefore, their status poses a challenge when trying to reduce and control exposures due to occupational hazards. They enter the construction trade by working first as laborers; with experience, they can become carpenters and painters. Due to a lack of documented status, many construction workers cannot develop a long-lasting relationship with their employers. Hispanic workers come to the United States with a different cultural and work background; they bring with them their own beliefs, traditions, and cultural inheritance, and some are illiterate. They work in poor physical environments; are exposed to dangerous tools, machines, and equipment; have non-Spanish-speaking supervisors; and lack adequate personal protective equipment. There is a critical need to develop educational and training resources dealing with safety on the job. Educating those workers will decrease the rate of injuries and deadly accidents; adequate linguistically and culturally appropriate training targeting Hispanic workers will be beneficial because they will learn how to avoid hazardous exposures in their environment.[165]

Maquiladoras

Maquiladoras are manufacturing plants with special legal status along the U.S.–Mexico border. They are designed to have some operations on the U.S. side and some on the Mexican side of the border with an international agreement that no import duties or taxes are charged to make the goods competitive. The original concept was to provide employment along the northern border of Mexico to slow immigration into the United States and to assist Mexican economic development. The North American Free Trade Agreement (NAFTA) was implemented by the Mexican, U.S., and Canadian governments in 1993. NAFTA proponents promised that the agreement would help alleviate many of the current border problems caused by the existing free-trade zone. NAFTA would also help improve working conditions, better enforce environmental laws, and decrease the high maquiladora concentration along the border.[166] Many provisions were made to ensure safe working conditions, safe disposal of toxic substances produced in the plants, and reasonable wages; however, enforcement has been lax. The 948,658 Mexicans who work in the maquiladoras must endure terrible working environments that include inadequate training, exposure to many potentially hazardous materials, and inadequate information and protective equipment.[167]

Household Health

More than 1 million children 14 years of age and younger die from unintentional injuries annually. Among children less than 5 years old, 90% of all unintentional morbidity and 50% of all deaths caused by unintentional injury take place in their homes.[168] The home setting accounts for about 33% of all injuries; however, insufficient evidence exists for the effectiveness of safety items and lack of cultural competency training among a mobile minority group.[169] Perhaps less well known is the economic toll of unintentional injury costs on society. In 2000, unintentional injuries and deaths of children less than 15 years of age cost society $58 billion in medical bills, lost wages of the children's caregivers, and the future productivity of the children who died prematurely.[170] Among children in this age group, during the summer of 2004, more than 2.4 million emergency room visits were due to unintentional injury,[104] and 2,143 children died.[171]

Scalds are one of the most common mechanisms of burn injury for young children consistently reported for the last 30 years. Children older than 6 months of age and younger than 5 years have the highest incidence and percentage of scald admissions to hospitals. Mortality rates are the highest among young children.[168] It is known that those accidents occur in the home and are related to daily activities such as bathing, cooking, and eating. Normally, injuries occur when there is a brief lack of parental supervision. Many home water heaters are set at dangerously high levels, as often happens in low-income homes where water heaters tend to have a relatively small capacity per capita, and household members tend to turn up the heat as the heater ages, begins to fill with sediment, and becomes less efficient. Experts advise that the water heater should be set at less than 120°F (49°C) measured by a meat thermometer under a running hot water tap. Public education needs to be improved.

House fires are another major cause of burns to children; cigarettes are the number-one cause of these fires. Many parents and other family members are unaware of the fire-related dangers of smoking. The elderly are statistically more likely to smoke as well as to have a smoking accident. Another important prevention tool is a home smoke detector. The presence of a functioning detector has been shown to decrease the risk of death by fire by 60%. Studies show that community-based, smoke detector "give-away" programs also reduce the incidence of fire-related injuries. Families should be educated to develop an escape plan that parents and children practice regularly. Parents should also learn about and teach "stop, drop, and roll" techniques to their children so that the children know what to do if they should ever find their clothing ablaze. While there is no replacement for vigilant supervision, proactive childproofing can go a long way toward preventing accidents.

Social and Behavioral Health

As noted in the preceding sections, the Latino population varies in health status and risk factors according to gender, age, social class, immigration status, and acculturation. Latino subpopulations also vary in these dimensions. The epidemiological paradoxes of Latinos noted earlier are hypothesized to relate largely to cultural differences from non-Latino whites. Examples of social and behavioral domains where some of these changes come into play are physical activity, eating patterns, and sexually transmitted diseases.

Physical Activity and Eating Behaviors

Adequate physical activity and healthy eating are critical to healthy living and reduce the risk for cardiovascular disease, cancer, diabetes, high blood pressure, and stroke. Healthy lifestyle behaviors contribute to weight control; healthy bones, muscles, and joints; depression and anxiety reduction; and fewer hospitalizations and medications.[172-175] Physical inactivity among the increasing Latino population is a notable public health concern. National surveys indicate that more whites (50.9%) than Latinos (41.1%) meet the recommended guidelines of 30 minutes per day of moderate-intensity physical activity at least most days of the week.[176] NHANES 1988–1994 data reveal that the prevalence of leisure time inactivity in Latino adults (40%) is more than twice the rate in white adults (18%).[177] Physical inactivity is also more prevalent among Latino adolescents (14 to 18 years of age) than their white counterparts (58.5% versus 65.2%).[178]

The National Cancer Institute's 5 A Day for Better Health Program recommends eating five or more servings of vegetables and fruit daily for better health.[179] Research examining fruit and vegetable intake in Latinos, however, has yielded inconsistent findings. Data from the 2000 National Health Interview Survey indicate that Latinos have higher intakes of fruit, vegetables, and fiber, and a lower percentage of energy consumption from fat, than whites.[180] The 2005 Behavioral Risk Factor Surveillance System, on the contrary, shows similar intake levels of fruit and vegetables for both Latinos and whites.[181] Another large study analyzing data collected in seven study centers found that Latinos consume fewer daily servings than whites.[182] Additional studies exploring ethnic differences in caloric, carbohydrate, total fat, and fiber intake also show conflicting results.[180,183-185] Research assessing micronutrient intake differences found that whites reported higher mean intakes in calories, calcium, magnesium, potassium, phosphorous, riboflavin, niacin, zinc, vitamin A, and vitamin C than did Latinos.[186] Another study on folic acid consumption found that a lower proportion of Latinas than white females were meeting recommendations.[187] Data discrepancy among studies may be attributable to variations in databases, dietary methodologies and measurements, population characteristics, and participants' income level.[183,184] Further research is needed to better understand nutrition-related ethnic disparities.

Although the causal web of influences on ethnic disparities in physical activity and eating patterns are not clearly established, studies indicate that gender, socioeconomic level, acculturation, immigration status, and environmental factors influence lifestyle behaviors in Latinos.[177,183,188-197]

Sexually Transmitted Diseases

Ethnic disparities in sexually transmitted diseases (STDs) are also prominent among Latinos. In 2004, HIV/AIDS was the fourth leading cause of death among Latinos aged 35 to 44 and the sixth for whites.[198] Moreover, Latinos have the second highest rate of AIDS diagnoses for adults and adolescents (24.0 cases per 100,000) after blacks (68.7). The Latino rate is more than three times the rate among whites (6.9/100,000).[198] Latinos are more likely than whites to be diagnosed during the late stages of HIV infection or when they already developed AIDS, an indication that more Latinos are probably being tested at a later stage of the disease.[198–200] Ethnic disparities are also reflected in HIV education efforts. Nationwide, white students in grades 9 to 12 are significantly more likely than Latino students (91.1% and 80.5%, respectively) to have been taught about AIDS and HIV infection in schools.

Additional STDs for which marked ethnic differences also exist include chlamydia, gonorrhea, and syphilis. It is estimated that 19 million new infections of sexually transmitted diseases occur each year affecting mostly young individuals ages 15 to 24 (50% of cases) and minority groups.[201,202] Chlamydia is the most commonly reported infectious disease in the United States and has greater health consequences for women than men. Chlamydia prevalence rates are three times higher among Latinas (733.2/100,000) than among white females (237.2). One study found a higher prevalence of chlamydia among Latinas in the 15- to 19-year-old group (11%) than comparable white females (5%).[203] The Latino population also has higher rates of reported gonorrhea and syphilis when compared with whites.[201,202] The Latino prevalence of gonorrhea (74.8/100,000) is more than two-fold that of whites (35.2).[201]

Ethnic differences in STDs may be explained by high-risk behaviors, limited access to quality health care, and poverty in Latinos.[201,204] Another factor is the validity of the data as noted earlier: a higher percentage of Latinos receive health care at public clinics that have higher rates of reporting sexually transmitted diseases than nonpublic providers.[78]

How to Address Health Disparities among Hispanics

Addressing health disparities among Hispanics requires a multidimensional approach recognizing the importance of barriers to accessing medical care as well as the importance of social, cultural, and economic conditions in shaping health. Hispanic health disparities vary with social class and acculturation; better educated, higher-income Hispanics face fewer barriers to health care than the less educated with lower incomes. Better educated Hispanic health professionals can provide a bridge to health care for those who are less educated; their training about health disparities and how to diminish them should differ from that of non-Hispanics who lack familiarity with the culture and language of the patients.

The training of healthcare providers to communicate well with patients, taking account of cultural background and other social characteristics, is fundamental to addressing health disparities in underserved populations.[176,205] Public health interventions also require the incorporation of cultural sensitivity to be effective in reaching different populations and subpopulations.

Cultural Proficiency: Approaches to Training Healthcare Providers

An important advance in training healthcare providers, the LEARN model, was developed in California in a residency program dealing largely with low-income Hispanic patients.[206] Berlin and Fowkes, a nurse-medical anthropologist and a physician, approached training through daily, hands-on efforts to improve health care of the underserved Hispanic population. Their approach provides practical steps for clinical encounters. The LEARN mnemonic summarizes the steps:

L   Listen with sympathy and understanding to the patient's perceptions of the illness.

E   Explain your perception of the problem.

A   Acknowledge and discuss the differences and similarities.

R   Recommend treatment to the patient.

N   Negotiate treatment with the patient.

These steps proved effective with the Mexican American patient base of the clinic where they were developed. They were valuable in enhancing rapport and adherence to medical recommendations for various patients. The approach encourages dialogue between doctor and patient, opening the door for the patient to explain any reasons for not following doctor's instructions, and discussion by doctor and patient about how the patient's problem will be treated.

Respect is important in Mexican American culture, and these steps reflect that cultural value by showing that patients' ideas and experiences are taken into account by healthcare providers in discussing diagnoses and treatment recommendations. Negotiating treatment is crucial; it gives the patient an opportunity to explain any reasons for rejecting recommendations. For example, a Mexican American patient refused an appointment for surgery recommended by his doctor. The LEARN approach, however, elicited his belief that he needed to build up his strength for 2 weeks beforehand by getting sufficient rest and eating well. Having learned his rationale, his doctor was able to negotiate a schedule for the surgery following a 2-week rest period, and the patient was content to follow the recommended course of treatment.

Further recommendations for training healthcare providers include a list of questions from which residents could choose to ensure that they carried out the LEARN steps. Suggested key questions for patient–practitioner dialogue are as follows:

1. How would you describe the problem that has brought you to me?
2. What do you think is wrong? What do you think is causing your problem?
3. Why do you think this problem happened to you?
4. Why do you think it started when it did?
5. What do you think your sickness does to you? How does it work?
6. How bad (severe) do you think your illness is? Do you think it will last a long time, or will it get better soon, in your opinion?
7. Why did you decide to come to me for treatment?
8. Apart from me, who else do you think can help you get better?
9. What do you think will help clear up your problem?
10. What are the most important results you hope to get from treatment?
11. Are there things that make you feel better or give you relief that doctors don't know about?
12. Has anyone else helped you with this problem?
    a. What did that person say was wrong with you?
    b. What did that person say you should do for this problem?
    c. Do you agree?
    d. Did you try it?
13. What are the chief problems your illness has caused you?
14. Does it cause problems for your family?
15. What worries you most about your sickness?
16. Is there anyone else you would like me to talk to about your problem?
17. Is there anything else you would like to discuss?

Finally, healthcare providers are advised to compile information about cultural aspects of their patients. Berlin and Fowkes advise medical residents to record observations in loose-leaf notebooks to use as references in the future. If a Mexican American mother brought her child in with a case of what she called *empacho*, a Mexican American folk illness, for example, the residents were instructed to record the way she explained it and what treatment seemed appropriate to her. This process of compiling information can allow physicians and nurses to build a foundation of cultural information that improves communication with other patients who raise the same issue.

The approach recommended by Berlin and Fowkes is particularly strong in providing a framework for physicians to take an individualistic approach with each patient and yet to take that person's cultural background and personal situation into account. The approach avoids cultural stereotyping and provides the opportunity for patients to express their own concepts that may aid or hinder the acceptance of treatment.

Components of Culturally Sensitive Interventions in Physical Activity and Nutrition

The persistence of health disparities in lifestyle behaviors affecting Latinos demands a culturally sensitive approach in the design and implementation of behavioral interventions. Health interventions adapted to the social and cultural context of ethnic minority populations are more likely to increase an intervention's external validity[207] and to accelerate advances in minority health.[208] According to a comprehensive literature review by Mier and colleagues,[209] components of culturally sensitive interventions targeting Latinos to improve diet and physical activity include:

- Utilization of delivery agents or facilitators who are Latinos and bilingual. The intervention materials should also be prepared in English and Spanish using an acceptable translation technique that will ensure language transparency and cultural equivalency. Intervention materials should also meet the literacy level of participants.

- Application of the *promotoras* model approach. *Promotoras* (community health workers) are effective in recruiting and retaining intervention participants and also in delivering and facilitating programs.

- Inclusion of participants' families and social networks in intervention activities.

- Intervention design and implementation based on formative research and Latino cultural values. Formative research may include health assessments, focus groups, literature searches, and interviews. These formative research techniques are useful to tailor an intervention culturally to Latinos' attitudes, beliefs, language use, and health behaviors. For example, *familism*, one of the most critical Latino cultural values, means that an individual has a strong identification with and attachment to their nuclear and extended families. Familism also includes feelings of loyalty, reciprocity, and solidarity with the family.[210]

- Acknowledgment of the diversity and immigration status of the Latino population in the intervention design.

Many of these points should be taken into account in the clinical care of Latinos as well.

Additional Ways of Addressing Hispanic Health Disparities: Language and Health System Literacy

In the case of Hispanic patients with poor English skills, language difficulties can be a major impediment, and clinics should ensure the availability of bilingual staff in regions with many Hispanic patients. The availability of interpreters can also provide significant support to Hispanic patients. In addition, over the long term, courses in English as a Second Language can allow Hispanic immigrants to increase their skills in communicating and help to empower them in accessing health care. Ideally, healthcare providers and patients will improve their communication skills, including studying another language, to enhance mutual understanding.

Informing Hispanics of their rights can further empower them so they can access health care effectively and efficiently. Information about how to access local healthcare resources will increase their healthcare system literacy and their understanding of how to navigate the patchwork medical system in the United States.

SUMMARY

Major health disparities of Hispanics in access to preventive health care, early detection, early treatment of disease, and problems from chronic disease result in a greater disease burden. Compared with non-Hispanic whites, a greater percentage of Hispanics are uninsured, are poor, and work under dangerous conditions. The result is that Hispanics have higher rates of death from work-related injuries, diabetes, asthma, and HIV/AIDS than non-Hispanic whites. Additionally, Hispanics have higher rates of stroke, chronic liver disease, cirrhosis, and homicide. A lower percentage of the Hispanic population receives vaccinations compared with non-Hispanic whites. A higher percentage of Hispanic teenagers lack sex education, and teen pregnancy is an increasing problem. Obesity, cancer of the cervix, and cancer of the stomach are all problems of higher percentages of Hispanics than of non-Hispanic whites. Food-borne hepatitis A and tuberculosis affect higher percentages of Hispanics as well. Because many of these conditions can be addressed through adequate medical care, increasing access to care that is culturally sensitive is important in eliminating these disparities.

The epidemiological paradox, in which Hispanics suffer less disease than would have been predicted on the basis of risk factors, is a fascinating puzzle. The paradox includes birth outcomes, cardiovascular disease, cancer, and mental health, all conditions for which Hispanics on average have greater risk factors but fewer health problems than non-Hispanic whites. The Latino epidemiological paradox implies that U.S. culture is harmful for Latino health and, by extension, the health of others as well.

By pursuing research that includes social, cultural, and economic factors and compares different Latino subgroups, it should be possible to elucidate the causes of the paradox. Culture change is an ongoing phenomenon that can respond to health education and health-promoting behavior change. Research into the causes of the epidemiological paradox has the potential to benefit Hispanics and the rest of the U.S population as well.

Approaches for addressing Hispanic health disparities can be formulated in relation to the three types of barriers to accessing health care that deprive the population of preventive care and thus intensify disparities. Primary access to care deals with health insurance, which many low-income Hispanic workers lack. They therefore tend to receive diagnoses of cardiovascular disease, type 2 diabetes, and cancer at advanced stages, leading to higher morbidity and mortality rates than among those who receive regular screening. In some cases, increasing understanding of the healthcare system can reduce barriers by showing low-income Hispanics how health insurance works, what preventive care does, and where to access low-cost medical care. In addition, courses in English as a Second Language can empower low-income immigrant Hispanics and reduce the barriers they face. Barriers to primary access can also be addressed through policy making to extend care to more people. These changes can greatly improve access to preventive health care, early screening, and treatment.

Barriers to secondary access, that is, impediments due to institutional, organizational, or structural issues, can be diminished by providing trained staff to assist with after-hours advice and making appointments. Bilingual staff members are crucial in improving secondary access for Hispanic patients. Tertiary access to health care deals with cultural barriers faced by Hispanics when dealing with healthcare providers during a clinical appointment. More bilingual healthcare providers are called for, even in communities on the U.S.–Mexico border that train bilingual nurses, because the local bilingual nurses are recruited by healthcare providers elsewhere. In addition, Latino mental health providers are needed because Latino patients tend to stay in treatment longer if their therapist matches their ethnicity and language ability. Training healthcare providers in cultural sensitivity is crucial to improving tertiary access to care.

Well-trained, culturally sensitive providers can assist in reducing Latino health disparities through their own interactions with patients and by shaping the policies of healthcare organizations. Staff with the same ethnicity and language abilities as Hispanic patients can be a tremendous resource in this effort; however, they, too, need training in working with Hispanic patients. Once having received medical education, members of any ethnic group are likely to have discarded many traditional understandings as unscientific, and many need to learn to respect their cultural traditions to work successfully with their patients. Mutual respect of providers and Hispanic patients is a fundamental requisite for building rapport and trust in the clinical setting. The approach recommended through the LEARN model of clinical interaction emphasizes respect for patients, their culture, and their decision-making abilities. A multifaceted approach can extend culturally sensitive and fully accessible medical care, including prevention and health education, to all Latinos and thus reduce health disparities significantly. Insights into the causes of health disparities and the epidemiological paradox have the potential to improve Hispanic health status and to contribute to the health of the entire U.S. population as well.

REFERENCES

1. Millard AV, Chapa J, McConnell ED. "Not racist like our parents": Anti-Latino prejudice and institutional discrimination. In: Millard AV, Chapa J, with Burillo C et al., eds. *Apple Pie and Enchiladas: Latino Newcomers in the Rural Midwest*. Austin: University of Texas Press; 2004:102–124.
2. Hahn RA, ed. *Anthropology in Public Health: Bridging Differences in Culture and Society*. New York: Oxford University Press; 1999.
3. Bibeau G, Pedersen D. A return to scientific racism in medical social sciences: The case of sexuality and the AIDS epidemic in Africa. In: Nichter M, Lock M, eds. *New Horizons in Medical Anthropology: Essays in Honor of Charles Leslie*. New York: Routledge; 2002:141–171.
4. U.S. Bureau of the Census. *2005 Puerto Rico Survey* (B03001-3-EST); 2006b.
5. U.S. Bureau of the Census. The Hispanic Population in the United States: March 2004. *Current Population Reports*, Data Tables including Educational Attainment in the United States, Detailed Tables (PPL-169) (does not include Commonwealth of Puerto Rico). Internet release, last revised March 2004.
6. U.S. Bureau of the Census. *Annual Estimates of the Population by Sex, Race, and Hispanic or Latino Origin for the United States: July 1, 2006* (NC-EST 2005-03); May 17, 2007b.
7. U.S. Bureau of the Census. 65+ in the United States: 2005. *Current Population Reports*; 2005c.

8. U.S. Bureau of the Census. *Current Population Survey, Annual Social and Economic Supplement.* Ethnicity and Ancestry Statistics Branch, Population Division (does not include the Commonwealth of Puerto Rico); 2004b.

9. Falcón A, Aguirre-Molina M, Molina CW. Latino health policy: Beyond demographic determinism. In: Aguirre-Molina M, Molina CW, Zambrana RE, eds. *Health Issues in the Latino Community.* San Francisco: Jossey-Bass; 2001:3–22.

10. Angel JL, Whitfield KE, eds. *The Health of Aging Hispanics: The Mexican-Origin Population.* New York: Springer Science+Business Media, LLC; 2007.

11. Aguirre-Molina M, Molina CW, Zambrana RE, eds. *Health Issues in the Latino Community.* San Francisco: Jossey-Bass; 2001.

12. Markides KS, Coreil J. The health of Hispanics in the Southwestern United States: An epidemiologic paradox. *Public Health Rep.* 1986;101(3):253–265.

13. Escobar JI. Immigration and mental health: Why are immigrants better off? *Arch Gen Psych.* 1998;55:781–782.

14. Lara M, Gamboa C, Kahramanian MI, et al. Acculturation and Latino Health in the United States: A review of the literature and its sociopolitical context. *Ann Rev Public Health.* 2005;26:367–397.

15. Centers for Disease Control and Prevention. *Fact Sheet: Hispanic Health Disparities, 2004.* http://www.cdc.gov/od/oc/Media. Accessed October 3, 2007.

16. Centers for Disease Control and Prevention. *National Immunization Survey 2005.* Atlanta: U.S. Department of Health and Human Services, Centers for Disease Control and Prevention; 2005.

17. Ogden CL, Carroll MD, Curtin LR, et al. Prevalence of overweight and obesity in the United States, 1999-2004. *JAMA.* 2006;295(13):1549–1555.

18. Johnson LD, O'Malley PM, Bachman JG, et al. *Monitoring the Future National Survey Results on Drug Use, 1975-2006: Volume I, Secondary School Students* (NIH Publication No. 07-6205). Bethesda, MD: National Institute on Drug Abuse; 2007.

19. U.S. Bureau of Labor Statistics. Civilian Labor force participation rates by sex, age, race, and Hispanic origin, 2004. http://www.bls.gov. Accessed on December 7, 2005.

20. U.S. Bureau of the Census. Income, poverty, and health insurance coverage in the United States, 2005. *Current Population Reports.* Washington DC: U.S. Government Printing Office; 2006.

21. Bastida E, Brown HS, Pagan JA. Health insurance coverage and health care utilization along the U.S.-Mexico border: Evidence from the border epidemiologic study of aging. In: Angel JL, Whitfield KE, eds. *The Health of Aging Hispanics: The Mexican-Origin Population.* New York: Springer Science+Business Media, LLC; 2007:222–234.

22. Kaiser Family Foundation. *Medicare and Minorities.* Menlo Park, CA: Author; 1999.

23. Carrillo JE, Trevino F, Betancourt JR, et al. Latino access to health care: The role of insurance, Medicaid managed care, and institutional barriers. In: Aguirre-Molina M, Molina CW, Zambrana RE, eds. *Health Issues in the Latino Community.* San Francisco: Jossey-Bass; 2001:55-106.

24. Bierman AS, Magari ES, Jette AM, et al. Assessing access as a first step toward improving the quality of care for very old adults. *J Ambul Care Man.* 1998;21(3):17–26.

25. Quinn K. *Working without Benefits: The Health Insurance Crisis Confronting Hispanic-Americans.* New York: Commonwealth Fund, 2000.

26. Cooper-Patrick L, et al. Race, gender, and partnership in the patient-physician relationship. *JAMA*. 1999;282(6):583–589.

27. Hornberger J, Itakura, H, Wilson SR. Bridging language and cultural barriers between physicians and patients. *Pub Health Rep*. 1997;112(5):410–417.

28. National Hispanic/Latino Health Initiative. *Pub Health Rep*. 1993;108:534–558.

29. David RA, Rhee M. The impact of language as a barrier to effective health care in an underserved urban Latino community. *Mount Sinai J Med*. 1998;65(5-6): 393–397.

30. Erzinger S. Communication between Spanish-speaking patients and their doctors in medical encounters. *Culture Med Psych*. 1991;15:91

31. Kirkman-Liff B, Mondragon D. Language of interview: Relevance for research of Southwest Hispanics. *Am J Public Health*. 1991;81(11):1399–1404.

32. Perez-Stable EJ, Napoles-Springer A, Miramontes JM. The effects of ethnicity and language on medical outcomes of patients with hypertension or diabetes. *Med Care*. 1997;35(12):1212–1219.

33. Solis JM, Marks G, Garcia M, et al. Acculturation, access to care, and use of preventive services by Hispanics; findings from HHANES 1982-84. *Am J. Public Health*. 1990;80(Suppl);11–19.

34. Manson A. Language concordance as a determinant of patient compliance and emergency room use in-patients with asthma. *Med Care*. 1988;26(12):1119–1128.

35. Stanton AL. Determinants of adherence to medical regimens by hypertensive patients. *J Behav Med*. 1987;10(4):377–394.

36. Chapa J, Saenz R, Rochin RI, McConnell ED. Latinos and the changing demographic fabric of the rural Midwest. In: Millard AV, Chapa J, with Burillo C, et al. *Apple Pie and Enchiladas: Latino Newcomers in the Rural Midwest*. Austin: University of Texas Press; 2004:47–73.

37. Millard AV, Chapa J. Ten myths about Latinos. In: Millard AV, Chapa J, with Burillo C, et al. *Apple Pie and Enchiladas: Latino Newcomers in the Rural Midwest*. Austin: University of Texas Press; 2004:22.

38. McConnell ED. Latinos in the rural Midwest: The twentieth-century historical context leading to contemporary challenges. In: Millard AV, Chapa J, with Burillo C, et al. *Apple Pie and Enchiladas: Latino Newcomers in the Rural Midwest*. Austin: University of Texas Press; 2004:26–40.

39. Portes A, Rumbaut RG. *Legacies: The Story of the Immigrant Second Generation*. Berkeley: University of California Press; 2001.

40. Ryder AG, Alden LE, Paulhus DL. Is acculturation unidimensional or bidimensional? A head-to-head comparison in the prediction of personality, self-identity, and adjustment. *J Personal Soc Psychol*. 2000;79(1):49–65.

41. Magana JR, de la Rocha OL, Amsel J, et al. Revisiting the dimensions of acculturation: cultural theory and psychometric practice. *Hisp J Behav Sci*. 1996;18(4): 444–468.

42. Marin G, Gamba RJ. A new measure of acculturation for Hispanics: The Bidimensional Scale for Hispanics. *Hisp J Behav Sci*. 1996;18(3):297–316.

43. Cuellar I, Arnold B, Maldonado R. Acculturation rating scale for Mexican Americans-II: a revision of the original ARSMA Scale. *Hisp J Behav Sci*. 1995;17(3): 275–304.

44. Deyo RA, Diehl AK, Hazuda H, et al. A simple language-based acculturation scale for Mexican-Americans: validation and application to healthcare research *Am J Public Health*. 1985;75(1):51–55.

45. Zea MC, Asner-Self KK, Birman D, et al. The abbreviated multidimensional acculturation scale: empirical validation with two Latino/Latina samples. *Cult Divers Ethn Minor Psychol*. 2003;9(2):107–126.
46. Marin G. Issues in the measurement of acculturation among Hispanics. In: Geisinger KF, ed. *Psychological Testing of Hispanics*. Washington DC: American Psychological Association; 1992:23–51.
47. Hu, DJ, Covell, RM. Health care usage by Hispanic outpatients as function of primary language. *West J Med*. 1986;144(4):490–493.
48. Marks G, Garica M, Solis JM. Health risk behaviors of Hispanics in the United States: findings from HHANES, 1982-84. *Am J Public Health*. 1990;80(Suppl.): 20–26.
49. Marin G, Posner SF. The role of gender and acculturation on determining the consumption of alcoholic beverages among Mexican-Americans and Central Americans in the United States. *Int J Addict*. 1995;30(7):779–794.
50. Vega WA, Aldrete E, Kolody B, et al. Illicit drug use among Mexicans and Mexican Americans in California: the effects of gender and acculturation. *Addiction*. 1998;93(12):1839–1850.
51. Velez CN, Ungemack, JA. Drug use among Puerto Rican youth; and exploration of generational status differences. *Soc Sci Med*. 1989;29(6):779–789.
52. Vega WA, Kolody B, Aguilar-Gaxiola S, et al. Lifetime Prevalence of *DSM-III-R* Psychiatric disorders among urban and rural Mexican Americans in California. *Arch Gen Psych*. 1998;55:771–778.
53. Zambrana RE, Scrimshaw S, Collins N, et al. Prenatal health behaviors and psychosocial risk factors in pregnant women of Mexican origin: The role of acculturation. *Am J Public Health*. 1997;87(6):1022–1026.
54. Findley SE, Irigoyen M, Schulman A. Children on the move and vaccination coverage in a low-income, urban Latino population. *Am J Public Health*. 1999;89(11): 1728–1731.
55. U.S. Bureau of the Census. Population projections of the United States by age, sex, race, and Latino origin: 1995 to 2050. *Current Population Reports*, Series P-25, No. 1130. Washington DC: U.S. Government Printing Office; 1999a.
56. Flores G, Zambrana RE. The early years: The health of children and youth. In: Aguirre-Molina M, Molina CW, Zambrana RE, eds. *Health Issues in the Latino Community*. San Francisco: Jossey-Bass; 2001:77–106.
57. Centers for Disease Control and Prevention. Update: Prevalence of overweight among children, adolescents, and adults—United States, 1988–1994. *MMWR*. 1997;46:198–202.
58. Carrillo-Zuniga G, Coutinho C, Shalat S, et al. Potential sources of childhood exposure to pesticides in an agricultural community. *J Children's Health*. 2004; 2(1):1–11.
59. Freeman N, Shalat S, Black K, et al. Seasonal pesticide use in a rural community on the U.S./Mexico border. *J Exposure Anal Environ Epidem*. 2004;14(6):473–478.
60. Shalat SL, Donnelly KC, Freeman NCG, et al. Non-dietary ingestion of pesticides by children in an agricultural community on the U.S./Mexico border: Preliminary results. *J Exposure Anal Environ Epidem*. 2002;12:42–48.
61. National Center for Health Statistics. *Health, United States, 2006, with Chartbook on Trends in the Health of Americans*. Hyattsville, MD: National Center for Health Statistics; 2006.

62. National Alliance for Hispanic Health. *A Manual for Providers*, 4th ed. Washington DC: Author; 2007.

63. Giachello, AL. The reproductive years: the health of Latinas. In: Aguirre-Molina M, Molina CW, Zambrana RE, eds. *Health Issues in the Latino Community*. San Francisco: Jossey-Bass; 2001:107–156.

64. Ventura SJ, Martin JA, Curtin SC, et al. Births: Final data for 1998. *National Vital Statistics Reports*, 48 (3). DHHS Publication No. [PHS] 00-1120, 0-0215. Hyattsville, MD: National Center for Health Statistics; 2000.

65. Abma J, Chandra A, Mosher W, et al. Fertility, family planning and women's health: New data from the 1995 National Survey of Family Growth. National Center for Health Statistics. *Vital Health Stat*. 1997;23:1.

66. Alan Guttmacher Institute. *Teenage Pregnancy: Overall Trends and State-by-state Information*. Washington DC: Author; 1999.

67. Giachello AL. Maternal/perinatal health issues. In: Molina CW, Aguirre-Molina M, eds. *Latino Health in the U.S.: A Growing Challenge*. Washington DC: American Public Health Association; 1994.

68. Giachello AL. Cultural diversity and institutional inequality. In: Adams DL, ed. *Health Issues for Women of Color: Cultural Diversity Perspective*. Thousand Oaks, CA: Sage; 1995.

69. American Diabetes Association. *Clinical Guidelines on Diabetes Care*. Washington DC: Author; 2000.

70. National Center for Health Statistics. *Natl Vital Stat Rep*. 2000;48(3):Table 25.

71. Guendelman S, Abrams B. Dietary, alcohol and tobacco intake among Mexican-American women of childbearing age. Results from NHANES data. *Am j Health Promotion*. 1994;8(5):363–372.

72. Villa VM, Torres-Gil FM. The later years: The health of elderly Latinos. In: Aguirre-Molina M, Molina CW, Zambrana RE, eds. *Health Issues in the Latino Community*. San Francisco: Jossey-Bass; 2001:157–178.

73. Cuellar J. Hispanic American aging: Geriatric educational curriculum for selected health professionals. In: Harper MS, ed. *Minority Aging: Essential Curricula Content for Selected Health and Allied Health Professions* (DHHS Publication No. HRS (P-DV-90-4). Washington DC: U.S. Government Printing Office; 1990:17–24.

74. Espino DV. Mexican-American elderly: Problems in evaluation, diagnosis, and treatment. In: Harper MS, ed. *Minority Aging: Essential Curricula Content for Selected Health and Allied Health Professions* (DHHS Publication No. HRS (P-DV-90-4). Washington DC: U.S. Government Printing Office; 1990:33–41.

75. Hazuda HP, Espino DV. Aging, chronic disease, and physical disability in Hispanic elderly. In: Markides KS, Miranda MR, eds. *Minorities, Aging and Health*. Thousand Oaks, CA: Sage Publications; 1997:127–148.

76. Markides K, Stroup-Benham C, Goodwin J, et al. The effect of medical conditions on the functional limitations of Mexican American elderly. *Ann Epidemiol*. 1996;6:386–391.

77. Wallace S, Lew-Ting C. Getting by at home—Community based long-term care of Latino elders. *West J Med*. 1992;157(3):337–344.

78. Carter-Pokras O, Zambrana R. Latino health status. In: Aguirre-Molina M, Molina CW, Zambrana RE, eds. *Health Issues in the Latino Community*. San Francisco: Jossey-Bass; 2001:23–54.

79. Hornick DB. Tuberculosis. In: Doebbeling BN, Wallace RB, eds. *Maxcy-Rosenau-Last Public Health and Preventive Medicine*, 14th ed. Stamford, CT: Appleton and Lange; 1988:208–217.

80. Bray GA, Bouchard C, James WPT. *Handbook of Obesity*. New York: Marcel Dekker; 1998.

81. Calle EE, Rodriguez C, Walker-Thurmond K, et al. Overweight, obesity, and mortality from cancer in a prospectively studied cohort of U.S. adults. *N Engl J Med*. 2003;348(17):1625–1638.

82. Must A, Spadano J, Coakley EH, et al. The disease burden associated with overweight and obesity. *JAMA*. 1999;282(16):1523–1529.

83. Paeratakul S, Lovejoy JC, Ryan DH, et al. The relation of gender, race and socioeconomic status to obesity and obesity comorbidities in a sample of U.S. adults. *Int J Obesity Related Metabol Disorder*. 2002;26(9):1205–1210.

84. Rawson ES, Freedson PS, Osganian SK, et al. Body mass index, but not physical activity, is associated with C-reactive protein. *Med Sci Sports Exer*. 2003;35(7):1160–1166.

85. Kuczmarski RJ, Flegal KM, Campbell SM, et al. Increasing prevalence of overweight among U.S. adults. The National Health and Nutrition Examination Surveys, 1960 to 1991. *JAMA*. 1994;272(3):205–211.

86. Baltrus PT, Lynch JW, Everson-Rose S, et al. Race/ethnicity, life-course socioeconomic position, and body weight trajectories over 34 years: the Alameda County Study. *Am J Public Health*. 2005;95(9):1595–1601.

87. Flegal KM, Ezzati TM, Harris MI, et al. Prevalence of diabetes in Mexican Americans, Cubans, and Puerto Ricans from the Hispanic Health and Nutrition Examination Survey, 1982–1984. *Diabetes Care*. 1991;14(7):628–638.

88. Hedley AA, Ogden CL, Johnson CL, et al. Prevalence of overweight and obesity among U.S. children, adolescents, and adults, 1999-2002. *JAMA*. 2004;291(23):2847–2850.

89. Seo DC, Torabi MR. Racial/ethnic differences in body mass index, morbidity and attitudes toward obesity among U.S. adults. *J Natl Med Assoc*. 2006;98(8):1300–1308.

90. Zhang Q, Wang Y. Socioeconomic inequality of obesity in the United States: Do gender, age, and ethnicity matter? *Soc Sci Med*. 2004;58(6):1171–1180.

91. Perez-Stable E, Juarbe T, Moreno-John G. Cardiovascular disease. In: Aguirre-Molina M, Molina CW, Zambrana RE, eds. *Health Issues in the Latino Community*. San Francisco: Jossey-Bass; 2001:245–276.

92. Rosenwaike I. Mortality differentials among persons born in Cuba, Mexico, and Puerto Rico residing in the United States. *Am J Public Health*. 1987;77(5):603–606.

93. Stern MP, Rosenthal M, Haffner SM, et al. Sex differences in the effects of sociocultural status on diabetes and cardiovascular risk factors in Mexican Americans: The San Antonio heart study. *Am J Epidemiol*. 1984;120(6):834–851.

94. Canto JG, et al. Presenting characteristics, treatment patterns, and clinical outcomes of non-black minorities in the National Registry of Myocardial Infarction 2. *Am J Cardiol*. 1998;82(9):1013–1018.

95. Cohen et al. Outcome of Hispanic patients treated with thrombolytic therapy for acute myocardial infarction: Results from the GUSTO I and III trials. Global utilization of streptokinase and TPA for occluded coronary arteries. *J Am Coll Cardiol*. 1999;34(6):1729–1737.

96. Madhavan S, Cohen H, Alderman MH. Angina pectoris by Rose Questionnaire does not predict cardiovascular disease in treated hypertensive patients. *J Hypertension*. 1995;13(11):1207–1212.

97. Centers for Disease Control and Prevention. *Web-based Injury Statistics Query and Reporting Systems (WISQARS)*, leading causes of death reports, 1999–2004 [2004 reports re Hispanic/Latinos]. http://webapp.cdc.gov/sasweb/ncipc/leadcaus 10.html. Accessed on September 20, 2007.

98. Mainous AG 3rd, Baker R, Koopman RJ, et al. Impact of the population at risk of diabetes on projections of diabetes burden in the United States: An epidemic on the way. *Diabetologia*. 2007;50(5):934–940.

99. Luchsinger JA. Diabetes. In: Aguirre-Molina M, Molina CW, Zambrana RE, eds. *Health Issues in the Latino Community*. San Francisco: Jossey-Bass; 2001:277–300.

100. Caballero AE. Diabetes in the Hispanic or Latino population: genes, environment, culture, and more. *Curr Diabetes Rep*. 2005;5(3):217–225.

101. Egede LE, Dagogo-Jack S. Epidemiology of type 2 diabetes: focus on ethnic minorities. *Med Clin North Am*. 2005;89(5):viii,949–975.

102. Flegal KM, Carroll MD, Ogden CL, et al. Prevalence and trends in obesity among U.S. adults, 1999-2000. *JAMA*. 2002;288(14):1723–1727.

103. Hanis CL, Hewett-Emmett D, Bertin TK, et al. Origins of U.S. Hispanics. Implications for diabetes. *Diabetes Care*. 1991;14(7):618–627.

104. Centers for Disease Control and Prevention. *Web-based Injury Statistics Query and Reporting Systems (WISQARS)*. http://www.cdc.gov/ncipc/wisqars. Accessed October 10, 2007.

105. Cowie CC, Rust KF, Byrd-Holt DD, et al. Prevalence of diabetes and impaired fasting glucose in adults in the U.S. population: National Health and Nutrition Examination Survey 1999-2002. *Diabetes Care*. 2006;29(6):1263-1268.

106. QuickStats: Diabetes death rate for Hispanics compared with non-Hispanic whites—United States versus counties along the U.S.-Mexico border, 2000–2002. *MMWR*. 2006;55:882.

107. Albertorio-Diaz J, Notzon F, Rodriguez-Lainz A. Diabetes hospitalization at the U.S.-Mexico border. *Prevent Chronic Dis*. 2007;4(2),1–15 [electronic resource]. http://www.cdc.gov/pcd/issues/2007/apr/06_0073.htm. Accessed September 4, 2007.

108. National Institute of Diabetes and Digestive and Kidney Diseases. *National Diabetes Statistics Fact Sheet: General Information and National Estimates on Diabetes in the United States, 2005*. NIH Publication No. 06–3892; 2005.

109. Lanting LC, Joung IM, Mackenbach JP, et al. Ethnic differences in mortality, end-stage complications, and quality of care among diabetic patients: a review. *Diabetes Care*. 2005;28(9):2280–2288.

110. Karter AJ, Ferrara A, Liu JY, et al. Ethnic disparities in diabetic complications in an insured population. *JAMA*. 2002;287(19):2519–2527.

111. Mitchell BD, Hazuda HP, Haffner SM, et al. Myocardial infarction in Mexican-Americans and non-Hispanic whites. The San Antonio Heart Study. *Circulation*. 1991;83(1):45–51.

112. Rewers M, Shetterly SM, Baxter J, et al. Prevalence of coronary heart disease in subjects with normal and impaired glucose tolerance and non-insulin-dependent diabetes mellitus in a biethnic Colorado population. The San Luis Valley Diabetes Study. *Am J Epidemiol*. 1992;135(12):1321–1330.

113. Cowie CC, Port FK, Wolfe RA, et al. Disparities in incidence of diabetic end-stage renal disease according to race and type of diabetes. *N Engl J Med.* 1989;321(16):1074–1079.

114. Pugh JA, Stern MP, Haffner SM, et al. Excess incidence of treatment of end-stage renal disease in Mexican Americans. *Am J Epidemiol.* 1998;127(1):135–144.

115. Hamman RF, Franklin GA, Mayer EJ, et al. Microvascular complications of NIDDM in Hispanics and non-Hispanic whites. San Luis Valley Diabetes Study. *Diabetes Care.* 1991;14(7):655–664.

116. Gregg EW, Sorlie P, Paulose-Ram R, et al. Prevalence of lower-extremity disease in the U.S. adult population >40 years of age with and without diabetes: 1999–2000 National Health and Nutrition Examination Survey. *Diabetes Care.* 2004;27(7):1591–597.

117. Ramirez AG, Suarez L. The impact of cancer on Latino populations. In: Aguirre-Molina M, Molina CW, Zambrana RE, eds. *Health Issues in the Latino Community.* San Francisco: Jossey-Bass; 2001:211–244.

118. American Cancer Society. *Cancer Facts & Figures for Hispanics/Latinos 2006-2008.* Atlanta: Author; 2006.

119. Heron MP, Smith BL. Deaths: Leading causes for 2003. *National Vital Statistics Reports*; 55(10). Hyattsville, MD: National Center for Health Statistics; 2007.

120. Miller BA, Hankey BF, Thomas TL. Impact of sociodemographic factors, hormone receptor status, and tumor grade on ethnic differences in tumor stage and size for breast cancer in U.S. women. *Am J Epidemiol.* 2002;155(6):534–545.

121. Jemal A, Clegg LX, Ward E, et al. Annual report to the nation on the status of cancer, 1975–2001, with a special feature regarding survival. *Cancer.* 2004;101(1):3–27.

122. Ries LAG, Harkins D, Krapcho M, et al. *SEER Cancer Statistics Review 1975–2003.* Bethesda, MD: National Cancer Institute; 2006.

123. Thomas DB, Karagas MR. Cancer in first and second generation Americans. *Cancer Res.* 1987;47(21):5771–5776.

124. Canto MT, Chu KC. Annual cancer incidence rates for Hispanics in the United States: Surveillance, epidemiology, and end results, 1992-1996. *Cancer.* 2000;88(11):2642–2652.

125. Wu ZH, Black SA, Markides KS. Prevalence and associated factors of cancer screening: Why are so many older Mexican American women never screened? *Prev Med.* 2001;33:268–273.

126. Fernandez LE, Morales A. Language and Use of Cancer Screening Services among Border and Non-Border Hispanic Texas Women. *Ethnic Health.* 2007;12(3):245–263.

127. Ramirez AG, Gallion KJ, Suarez L, et al. A national agenda for Latino cancer prevention and control. *Cancer.* 2005;103(11):2209–2215.

128. Vega WA, Alegría M. Latino Mental Health and Treatment in the United States. In: Aguirre-Molina M, Molina CW, Zambrana RE, eds. *Health Issues in the Latino Community.* San Francisco: Jossey-Bass; 2001:179–208.

129. Moscicki EK, Rae D, Regier DA, et al. The Hispanic health and nutrition examination survey: Depression among Mexican-Americans, Cuban-Americans and Puerto Ricans. In: Gaviria M, Arana JD, eds. *Health and Behavior: Research Agenda for Hispanics* [Simón Bolivar Research Monograph Series 1]. Chicago: University of Illinois at Chicago Press; 1987:145–159.

130. Vega WA, Warheit G, Buhl-Auth J, et al. The prevalence of depressive symptoms among Mexican Americans and Anglos. *Am J Epidemiol.* 1984;120:592–607.

131. Murray CJL, Lopez AD. *The Global Burden of Disease*. Cambridge: Harvard University Press; 1996.

132. Robins LN, Helzer JE, Croughan JL, et al. National Institute of Mental Health Diagnostic Interview Schedule: Its history, characteristics and validity. *Arch Gen Psych*. 1981;38:381–389.

133. Wittchen HU, Robins LN, Cottler LB, et al. Cross-cultural feasibility, reliability, and sources of variance of the Composite International Diagnostic Interview (CIDI). *Br J Psych*. 1991;159:645–653.

134. Narrow WE, Rae DS, Moscicki ED, et al. Depression among Cuban Americans: The Hispanic Health and Nutrition Examination Survey. *Soc Psychol Psych Epidemiol*. 1990;25:260–268.

135. Karno M, Hough RL, Burnam MA, et al. Lifetime prevalence of specific psychiatric disorders among Mexican Americans and non-Hispanic whites in Los Angeles. *Arch Gen Psych*. 1987;44:695–701.

136. Burnam A, Hough R, Karno M, et al. Acculturation and lifetime prevalence of psychiatric disorders among Mexican Americans in Los Angeles. *J Health Soc Behav*. 1987;28:89–102.

137. Canino GJ, Bird HR, Shrout PE, et al. The prevalence of specific psychiatric disorders in Puerto Rico. *Arch Gen Psych*. 1987;44:727–735.

138. Scribner R. Paradox as a paradigm: The health outcomes of Mexican Americans. *Am J Public Health*. 1996;86:303–305.

139. Grant BF, Stinson FS, Hasin DS, et al. Immigration and Lifetime Prevalence of *DSM-IV* Psychiatric Disorders Among Mexican Americans and Non-Hispanic whites in the United States: Results From the National Epidemiologic Survey on Alcohol and Related Conditions. *Arch Gen Psych*. 2004;61:1226–1233.

140. Escobar JI, Karno M, Burnam MA, et al. Distribution of major mental disorders in a U.S. metropolis. *Acta Psychiatrica Scandinavica*. 1988;78(344):45–54.

141. Alegría M, Mulvaney-Day N, Torres M, et al. Prevalence of Psychiatric Disorders Across Latino Subgroups in the United States. *Am J Public Health*. 2007;97(1):68–75.

142. Health Care Financing Administration. Medical recipients and vendor payments by race (Table 8); 1998. http://www.hcfa.gov/medicaid/2082-8htm.

143. Takeuchi DT, Sue S, Yeh M. Return rates and outcomes from ethnicity-specific mental health programs in Los Angeles. *Am J Public Health*. 1995;85(5): 638–643.

144. Saha S, Komaromy M, Koepsell TD, et al. Patient-physician concordance and the perceived quality and use of health care. *Arch Int Med*. 1999;159:991–1004.

145. Leigh WA, Lillie-Blanton M, Martinez RM, et al. Managed care in three states: Experiences of low-income African-Americans and Hispanics. *Inquiry*. 1999;36: 318–331.

146. Worby PA, Organista KC. Alcohol use and problem drinking among male Mexican and Central American immigrant laborers. *Hisp J Behav Sci*. 2007;29(4):413–455.

147. Gee GC, Ryan A, Laflamme DJ, et al. Self-reported discrimination and mental health status among African Descendants, Mexican Americans, and other Latinos in the New Hampshire REACH 2010 Initiative: The added dimension of immigration. *Am J Public Health*. 2006;96(10):1821–1828.

148. Hasin DS, Stinson FS, Ogburn E, et al. Prevalence, Correlates, Disability, and Comorbidity of *DSM-IV* Alcohol Abuse and Dependence in the United States.

Results From the National Epidemiologic Survey on Alcohol and Related Conditions. *Arch Gen Psych.* 2007;64:830–842.

149. Azevedo K, Ochoa-Bogue H. Health and occupational risks of Latinos living in rural America. In Aguirre-Molina M, Molina CW, Zambrana RE, eds. *Health Issues in the Latino Community.* San Francisco: Jossey-Bass; 2001:359–380.

150. Barr D, Thomas K, Curwin B, et al. Biomonitoring of exposure in farmworker studies. *Environ Health Perspect.* 2006;114:936–942.

151. National Association of Community Health Centers. *Access to Community Health Care: A National and State Data Bank.* Washington DC: Author; 1997.

152. National Migrant Resource Program. Proceedings of the 1992 migrant stream forums. Comprehensive program to improve the supply of rural family physicians. *Fam Med.* 1992;32(1):17–21.

153. Warrick LH, Wood A, Meister J, et al. Evaluation of a peer health worker prenatal outreach and education program for Hispanic farmworker families. *J Community Health.* 1992;17(1):13–26.

154. National Institute for Occupational Safety and Health. *Worker Health Chartbook: Census of Fatal Occupational Injuries.* Washington DC: U.S. Department of Labor, Bureau of Labor Statistics, Safety and Health Statistics Program. 2004; Publication No. 2004-146. www.bls.gov/iif/oshcfoi1.htm. Accessed October 11, 2007.

155. Arias E (2004). United States life tables, 2001. *Natl Vital Stat Rep.* 2004;52 (14).

156. Molla MT, Madans JH, Wagener DK, et al. *Summary Measures of Population Health: Report of Findings on Methodologic and Data Issues.* Hyattsville, MD: National Center for Health Statistics; 2003.

157. National Institute for Occupational Safety and Health. *Tracking Occupational Injuries, Illnesses, and Hazards: The NIOSH Surveillance Strategic Plan.* Cincinnati, OH: U.S. Department of Health and Human Services, Public Health Service, Centers for Disease Control and Prevention, National Institute for Occupational Safety and Health. DHHS (NIOSH) Publication No. 2001-118; 2001. www.cdc.gov/niosh/2001-118.html.

158. LaDou J. The Practice of Occupational Medicine. In: LaDou J., *Occupational Medicine.* Stamford, CT: Appleton and Lange; 1999.

159. U.S. Immigration and Naturalization Service. Illegal alien resident population. http://uscis.gov/graphics/shared/statistics/archives/illegal.pdf. Accessed September 10, 2007.

160. Cromartie SP. Labor force status of families: a visual essay. *Monthly Labor Rev.* 2007;130:7-8. http://www.bls.gov/opub/mlr/2007/07/ressum.pdf. Accessed September 25, 2007.

161. Rakesh K. *Latino Labor Report.* Washington DC: Pew Hispanic Center; 2006.

162. U.S. Bureau of Labor Statistics. *Census of Fatal Occupational Injuries, 2003.* Washington DC. http://www.bls.gov. Accessed October 10, 2007.

163. Greenhouse S. Government asked to act on teenager's job safety. *New York Times;* 2002. http://nytimes.com. Accessed September 30, 2007.

164. U.S. Bureau of Labor Statistics. *Current Population Survey, 2001.* Washington DC: U.S. Department of Labor, Bureau of Labor Statistics. http//www.bls.gov/cps. Accessed September 25, 2007.

165. Brunette MJ. Development of educational and training materials in safety and health: targeting Hispanic workers in the construction industry. *Fam Community Health.* 2005;28(3):253–266.

166. Public Citizen's Global Trade Watch. NAFTA's Broken Promises: Failure to Create U.S. Jobs. *Global Trade Watch*. 1997;(1);http://www.citizen.org/trade/nafta/jobs/articles.cfm. Accessed September 30, 2007.

167. Sawicki S. The maquiladoras: Back door pollution. *Norwalk: the environmental magazine*. 1998;9(4).

168. SafeKids Worldwide. Childhood unintentionally injury worldwide meeting the challenge. 2002;(10). Children's National Medical Center. http://www.safekids.org. Accessed October 8, 2007.

169. Hendrickson SG. Reaching an underserved population with a randomly assigned home safety intervention. *Injury Prevent*. 2005;11:313–317.

170. Miller TR, Romano EO, Spicer RS. The Future of Children (2000). The cost of childhood unintentional injuries and the value of prevention. *Unintentional Injuries Childhood*. 2000;10(1):137–163.

171. National Vital Statistics System, *2004 Mortality Data*. Hyattsville MD: National Center for Health Statistics; 2007.

172. Ignarro LJ, Balestrieri ML, Napoli C (2007). Nutrition, physical activity, and cardiovascular disease: an update. *Cardiovas Res*. 2007;73(2):326–340.

173. Kanaya AM, Narayan KM. Prevention of type 2 diabetes: Data from recent trials. *Primary Care*. 2003;30(3):511–526.

174. Kriska AM, Delahanty LM, Pettee KK. Lifestyle intervention for the prevention of type 2 diabetes: translation and future recommendations. *Current Diabetes Rep*. 1999;4(2):113–118.

175. World Health Organization. (2007) Diet and physical activity: A public health priority. http://www.who.int/dietphysicalactivity/en. Accessed February 28, 2007.

176. Ma GX, Shive SE, Tan Y, et al. Development of a culturally appropriate smoking cessation program for Chinese-American youth. *J Adolesc Health*. 2004;35(3):206–216.

177. Crespo CJ, Smit E, Andersen RE, et al. Race/ethnicity, social class and their relation to physical inactivity during leisure time: results from the Third National Health and Nutrition Examination Survey, 1988-1994. *Am J Prevent Med*. 2000;18(1):46–53.

178. Adams J (2006). Trends in physical activity and inactivity amongst U.S. 14–18 year olds by gender, school grade and race, 1993–2003: Evidence from the youth risk behavior survey. *BMC Public Health*, 2006;6,57.

179. National Cancer Institute. 5 A Day for Better Health Program Evaluation Report: Executive Summary; 2006. http://www.cancercontrol.cancer.gov/5ad_exec.html. Accessed September 21, 2007.

180. Thompson FE, Midthune D, Subar AF, et al. Dietary intake estimates in the National Health Interview Survey, 2000: Methodology, results, and interpretation. *J Am Dietetic Assoc*. 2005;105(3):352–363; quiz 487.

181. Prevalence of fruit and vegetable consumption and physical activity by race/ethnicity—United States, 2005. *MMWR*. 2007;56(13):301–304.

182. Thompson B, Demark-Wahnefried W, Taylor G, et al. Baseline fruit and vegetable intake among adults in seven 5 a day study centers located in diverse geographic areas. *J Am Dietetic Assoc*. 1999;99(10):1241–1248.

183. Briefel R, Ziegler P, Novak T, et al. Feeding infants and toddlers study: Characteristics and usual nutrient intake of Hispanic and non-Hispanic infants and toddlers. *J Am Dietetic Assoc*. 2006;106(1),Suppl 1:S84–S95.

184. Newell GR, Borrud LG, McPherson RS, et al. Nutrient intakes of whites, blacks, and Mexican Americans in southeast Texas. *Prevent Med*. 1988;17(5):622–633.

185. Zive MM, Berry CC, Sallis JF, et al. Tracking dietary intake in white and Mexican-American children from age 4 to 12 years. *J Am Dietetic Assoc.* 2002;102(5):683–689.

186. Lopez TK, Marshall JA, Shetterly SM, et al. Ethnic differences in micronutrient intake in a rural biethnic population. *Am J Prevent Med.* 1995;11(5):301–305.

187. Yang QH, Carter HK, Mulinare J, et al. Race-ethnicity differences in folic acid intake in women of childbearing age in the United States after folic acid fortification: Findings from the National Health and Nutrition Examination Survey, 2001–2002. *Am J Clin Nutr.* 2007;85(5):1409–1416.

188. Abraído-Lanza AF, Chao MT, Flórez KR. Do healthy behaviors decline with greater acculturation? Implications for the Latino mortality paradox. *Soc Sci Med.* 2005;61:1243–1255.

189. Ahmed NU, Smith GL, Flores AM, et al. Racial/ethnic disparity and predictors of leisure-time physical activity among U.S. men. *Ethnic Disparities.* 2005;15: 40–52.

190. Berrigan D, Dodd K, Troiano RP, et al. Physical activity and acculturation among adult Hispanics in the United States. *Res Qtrly Exercise Sport.* 2006;77(2): 147–157.

191. Crespo CJ, Smit E, Carter-Pokras O, et al. Acculturation and leisure-time physical inactivity in Mexican American adults: Results from NHANES III, 1988-1994. *Am J Public Health.* 2001;91(8):1254–1257.

192. Gordon-Larsen P, Harris KM, Ward DS, et al. Acculturation and overweight-related behaviors among Hispanic immigrants to the US: The National Longitudinal Study of Adolescent Health. *Soc Sci Med.* 2003;57(11):2023–2034.

193. Masel MC, Rudkin LL, Peek MK. Examining the role of acculturation in health behaviors of older Mexican Americans. *Am J Health Behav.* 2006;30(6):684–699.

194. Mazur RE, Marquis GS, Jensen HH. Diet and food insufficiency among Hispanic youths: acculturation and socioeconomic factors in the third National Health and Nutrition Examination Survey. *Am J Clin Nutr.* 2003;78(6):1120–1127.

195. Mier N, Ory MG, Zhan D, et al. Levels and correlates of exercise in a border Mexican American population. *Am J Health Behav.* 2007;31(2):159–169.

196. Neuhouser ML, Thompson B, Coronado GD, et al. Higher fat intake and lower fruit and vegetables intakes are associated with greater acculturation among Mexicans living in Washington State. *J Am Dietetic Assoc.* 2004;104(1):51–57.

197. Wilbur J, Chandler PJ, Dancy B, et al. Correlates of physical activity in urban Midwestern Latinas. *Am J Prevent Med.* 2003;25(3 Suppl 1):69–76.

198. Centers for Disease Control and Prevention. HIV/AIDS Surveillance Report, 2005. Vol. 17. Rev. ed. Atlanta: U.S. Department of Health and Human Services, Centers for Disease Control and Prevention. http://www.cdc.gov/hiv/topics/surveillance/resources/reports. Accessed September 4, 2007.

199. Anderson LM, Scrimshaw SC, Fullilove MT, et al. Culturally competent healthcare systems. A systematic review. *Am J Prevent Med.* 2003;24(Suppl):68–79.

200. Campo RE, Alvarez D, Santos G, et al. Antiretroviral treatment considerations in Latino patients. *AIDS Patient Care STDS.* 2005;19(6):366–374.

201. Centers for Disease Control and Prevention. Trends in reportable sexually transmitted diseases in the United States, 2005. National surveillance data for chlamydia, gonorrhea, and syphilis; 2006. Atlanta: U.S. Department of Health and Human Services, Centers for Disease Control and Prevention. http://www.cdc.gov/hiv/topics/surveillance/resources/reports. Accessed May 8, 2008.

202. McGrath C, René A, Jones B, et al. Descriptive study of sexually transmitted diseases in Tarrant County, Texas, from 1998 through 2000. *Texas Med.* 2003;99(2):48–53.

203. Mertz KJ, McQuillan GM, Levine WC, et al. A pilot study of the prevalence of chlamydial infection in a national household survey. *Sexually Transmitted Dis.* 1998;25(5):225–228.

204. Hallfors DD, Iritani BJ, Miller WC, et al. Sexual and drug behavior patterns and HIV and STD racial disparities: the need for new directions. *Am J Public Health.* 2007;97(1):125–132.

205. Harwood A. *Ethnicity and Medical Care.* Cambridge, MA: Harvard University Press; 1981.

206. Berlin EA, Fowkes WC Jr. A teaching framework for cross-cultural health care. Application in family practice. *West J Med.*; 1983:139(6):934–938.

207. Bernal G, Bonilla J, Bellido C. Ecological validity and cultural sensitivity for outcome research: issues for the cultural adaptation and development of psychosocial treatments with Hispanics. *J Abnormal Child Psychol.* 1995;23(1):67–82.

208. Cooper LA, Hill MN, Powe NR. Designing and evaluating interventions to eliminate racial and ethnic disparities in health care. *J Gen Intern Med.* 2002;17(6):477–486.

209. Mier N, Ory MG, Medina AA. Anatomy of culturally sensitive interventions promoting nutrition and exercise in Hispanics: A critical examination of existing literature. Manuscript submitted for publication; 2007.

210. Marin G, Marin BV. *Research with Hispanic Populations.* Newbury Park, CA: Sage; 1991.

Chapter 12

Health Disparities among Native American People of the United States

Adeola O. Jaiyeola, MD, DOHS, MHSc
Wehnona Stabler, MPH

The term *Native American* refers to the indigenous people of North, South, and Central America and includes American Indians and Alaska Natives (AI/AN). According to the 2000 U.S. Census, 4.3 million people, or 1.5 percent of the total U.S. population, reported that they were AI/AN. This included 2.4 million, or approximately 0.9%, who reported AI/AN only and 1.6 million or approximately 0.6% who reported AI/AN and one or more other races.[1]

Native Americans are a diverse group that includes members of 569 federally recognized tribes and an unknown number of tribes that are not federally recognized. Each tribe has its own culture, beliefs, practices, history, and language—all of which influence their health and well-being. While Native Americans reside throughout the United States, the greatest concentrations of AI/AN populations are in the West, Southwest, and Midwest, in particular in Alaska, Arizona, Montana, New Mexico, Oklahoma, and South Dakota.[2] Up to 60% of Native Americans live in urban areas. The health status of Native Americans may vary according to geographic location. The health disparities described in this chapter will focus mainly on individuals who identify as AI/AN only and who maintain tribal affiliation or community attachment, because data on their health status are more readily available. However, where available, national data on all Native Americans in the United States will be presented.

Historical Origin of Health Disparities in Native Americans

Health disparities in Native Americans can be traced back to the arrival of the first settlers and the diseases that accompanied them, to which Natives had little or no immunity. However, archaeological remains show that native groups were not living in a pristine, disease-free environment before European contact.[3] Archaeologists and physical anthropologists have identified the diseases present in the Americas prior to European contact by analyzing ancient skeletal remains.[4] The presence of numerous diseases in the New World have also been documented throughout history.[4] Such diseases included "common bacterial infections, salmonella and other food poisonings, dysentery, tuberculosis, viral influenzas and pneumonias, South American trypanosomiasis (African 'sleeping sickness'), viral and rickettsial fevers, typhus, American leishmaniasis (transmitted by kissing bugs), intestinal worms and other intestinal parasites, non-venereal syphilis, nutritional deficiency states (such as goiter), and various forms of arthritis."[4] However, these diseases were probably of low prevalence among Native Americans in the New World,[5] and there were several established indigenous or traditional healthcare systems effective in mitigating these diseases.[4]

There is documentation of a wide range of Native American collections of medicinal herbs traditionally used to treat New World diseases that are now known to be effective pharmaceuticals. Examples of such are "anesthetics, astringents, antiseptics, antibiotics, cathartics, anti-malarials, vermifuges (to kill intestinal parasites), and obstetric-gynecologic preparations." A communal approach to providing care when needed in harmony with nature and sustaining the environment were important aspects of maintaining health status in the New World.[4]

The arrival of Europeans brought Native Americans in contact with new diseases as well as lifestyle and social changes that were extremely different from their previous way of life. The collapse of the previous social system is partly responsible for the emerging epidemic of chronic debilitating diseases. Prevalence of diseases such as tuberculosis increased among Native Americans after European contact. The spread of tuberculosis was aided by malnutrition, overcrowding, war, social upheaval, poverty, alcoholism, and smoking, particularly from older adults to adolescents. Because of the chronicity of tuberculosis, there was a great toll on the childbearing population, thus affecting reproductive capacity. Old World diseases that were not present in the Americas until contact with Europeans include bubonic plague, measles, smallpox, mumps, chickenpox, influenza, cholera, diphtheria, typhus, malaria, leprosy, and yellow fever.[6] Native Americans had no acquired immunity to these diseases, which caused *virgin soil epidemics* and which occur in populations with no prior contact with an infectious agent and are, therefore, immunologically defenseless. All members of the population are infected simultaneously, and sometimes entire communities are decimated by infections with severe consequences, such as small pox.[7] The disruption of the social structures and cultures of Native Americans through war, famine, and deliberate acculturation and expulsion from their ancestral lands is key to understanding the spread of disease and current health disparities.

Federal Trust Relationship with Native American Tribes

The United States has a unique legal relationship with Indian tribal governments based on the U.S. Constitution, treaties, statutes, executive orders and court decisions beginning with the 1830s.[8,9] There is an established legal obligation requiring the U.S. government to provide economic and social programs to the Native people necessary to raise the standard of living and social well-being to a level comparable to non-Native society. The obligation to provide "social programs" encompasses the federal responsibility for health care for Native Americans. The federal government's obligations stem from Native Americans ceding more than 400 million acres of tribal land to the United States pursuant to promises and agreements.

Subsequent to the birth of the United States, the federal government became concerned about the health status of Native Americans and assigned responsibility for Native American health care to the Office of Indian Affairs in the War Department in 1803. The healthcare duties were subsequently transferred to the newly formed Department of Interior in 1849, where the responsible office was eventually named the Bureau of Indian Affairs (BIA).[10] Beginning in the 1920s, the inadequacy of the government healthcare programs for Native Americans became obvious, and this resulted in the formation of the Meriam Commission, which was mandated to inspect reservations, schools, and hospital settings. The Commission issued a report in 1928 that documented the substandard health conditions of reservations stemming from inefficient government programs and inadequate funding, and recommended increased funding.[11] In 1955, the division responsible for Native health was transferred to the Department of Health, Education, and Welfare (which later became the Department of Health and Human Services [DHHS]). Within DHHS, the Indian Health Service (IHS) is the main federal agency providing health care to Native Americans. The stated goal of IHS is to raise the health status of Native Americans "to the highest possible level."

Over the years, several laws have been enacted that codify the federal government's responsibility to Native Americans and that allocate funds for healthcare services. The first of these was the Snyder Act of 1921, which provides for the relief of distress and conservation of health and for employment of physicians for Indian tribes.[12] This act allowed Congress to authorize funding for the provision of healthcare services to tribes. In 1976, Congress enacted legislation to define further the Indian heathcare delivery system through the Indian Health Care Improvement Act (IHCIA). IHCIA established the basic structure for the delivery of health services to Native Americans and authorized the construction and maintenance of healthcare and sanitation facilities on reservations.[13] The IHCIA has been amended and reauthorized several times, but it expired in 2001. Currently (at the time of this writing, December 2007), a proposal for reauthorization is pending in House of Representatives and Senate Committees. Even though the federal government continues to fulfill its obligations without the reauthorization, not having the act in place leaves room for the federal government to renege on its responsibilities. Another piece of legislation that has a great potential to alter health delivery to the Native Americans, and thus affect health status, is Public Law 93-638 enacted in 1975. This is the Indian Self-Determination and Education Assistance Act. This law enables tribal governments to take over their health care from IHS.

Population and Socioeconomic Characteristics

According to Census data, the Native American population is relatively younger than the total U.S. population.[14] In 2000, about 33% of Native Americans were under age 18 compared with 26% of the total U.S. population, and only 5.6% of Native Americans were 65 and older compared with 12.4% of the total U.S. population.[14] The median age for Native Americans was 29 years—6 years below that of the total U.S. population median age of 35.[14] The younger age distribution of Native American population compared with the total U.S. population results from shorter life expectancies and higher birth rates; both factors have implications for patterns of mortality and disease prevalence.

Education levels of Native Americans were below those of the total U.S. population in 2000.[14] Seventy-one percent of Native Americans ages 25 and older had at least a high school education compared with 80% of the total U.S. population, and only 11% had a bachelor's degree compared with 24% of the total U.S. population. Educational attainment also varied among the tribal groupings. The Creek, Choctaw, Iroquois, and Tlingit-Haida tribes had educational attainment comparable to the total U.S. population, while others fared worse.[14] Educational attainment is related to employability and economic power, which in turn may affect health status and healthcare access.

The labor force participation for Native American men (66%) was lower than all men (71%), but for women, labor force participation (57%) was comparable to the total U.S. population (58%).[14] The majority of Native Americans in the labor force (75.7%) are employed in service; sales and office; farming, fishing, and forestry; construction, extraction, and maintenance; and production, transportation, and material moving services compared with 66.4% of all workers who were employed in these sectors. A lower percentage of Native Americans are employed in managerial, professional, or related positions when compared with the total U.S. population. The unemployment rate of Native Americans ages 16 years and older (12.3%) was twice that of the general population (5.7%). The percentage of Native American children who were members of a single-parent family household (43.5%) was substantially higher that of the general population (29.2%).[14]

The annual, median earnings of Native American men ($28,900) and women ($22,800) were substantially below those of all U.S. men ($37,100) and U.S. women ($27,200). In 1999, the percentage of Native Americans living below poverty level (25.7%) was more than twice that of the total population (12.4%). The percentage of Native Americans living below poverty level varies according to tribe. Roughly 18% or less of Creek, Cherokee, Lumbee, Aleut, and Tlingit-Haida live below the poverty level compared with 32% of Sioux, Navajo, and Apache.

Geographic Isolation and Cultural Barriers to Health Care

Geographic isolation is a major barrier to accessing health care by Native Americans. The majority of tribal reservations are located in remote rural areas that lack adequate transportation. Even within each reservation, tribal communities are far apart, and people have to travel miles to access available health care. The geographic isolation is a barrier to attracting competent healthcare professionals to remote communities. There is also a high turnover of healthcare staff, which affects continuity of care for the Natives.

Lack of cultural understanding and language barriers as well as healthcare providers' bias and stereotyping have also been recognized as contributing to health disparities among Native Americans.[15] Many of the current disparities are rooted in past segregationist practices, resulting in inferior housing, education, and physical environments. Along with these are a history of disenfranchisement; extermination of tradition, language, and land rights; broken treaties; sterilization of Native women; placement of Indian children in boarding schools; and other experiences of oppression, which have established deep-rooted intergenerational anger and grief as well as mistrust of government.[15] Healthcare providers' lack of cultural sensitivity and recognition of traditional healing practices and medicine are also barriers to receiving adequate health care.[10] Treatments provided in a culturally insensitive manner are ineffective, and they continue to propagate persisting disparities in health. Health care must recognize and comply with Natives' values, beliefs, and traditions in order to provide acceptable services.

Mortality

The following mortality data was obtained from the National Center for Health Statistics (NCHS) and the Indian Health Service (IHS). The population segments included in the data sources differ. While the NCHS data cover all AI/AN deaths in the United States reported by each state, the IHS data cover AI/AN in the IHS service delivery areas, which make up about 55% of all AI/AN.

The age-adjusted mortality rate for U.S. AI/AN in 2004 was 650 per 100,000 persons, lower than that of whites (786.3 per 100,000 persons).[16] These data are drawn from state vital registry systems and may not represent true mortality rates for the AI/AN population due to racial misclassification.[17] Racial misclassification occurs when there is misreporting of race/ethnicity in death certificates or other health reports. After adjusting for race misreporting, the 2000–2002 IHS report that the mortality rate was 1,039 per 100,000 for all areas, which is significantly higher than the 2001 figure of 854.5 per 100,000 for all races.[18]

Table 12–1 lists the 10 leading causes of mortality for the U.S. American Indians and Alaska Natives compared with the U.S. white and all races populations for 1980 and 2004. These comparisons demonstrate that in addition to the disparity in age-adjusted mortality rates, the causes of mortality differ for the AI/AN population, further demonstrating a need for unique health programming and intervention. In 2004, the leading causes of U.S. AI/AN mortality were diseases of the heart; malignant neoplasms; unintentional injuries; diabetes mellitus; cerebrovascular diseases; chronic liver diseases and cirrhosis; chronic lower respiratory diseases; suicide; influenza and pneumonia; and nephritis, nephritic syndrome, and nephrosis (Table 12–1). This reflects a change from 1980 when unintentional injuries followed diseases of the heart as the two leading causes of death. Homicide and certain conditions originating

Table 12–1 *Leading Causes of Death among Native Americans, Whites, and All U.S. Populations, 2004 versus 1980*

Native American

	2004		1980	
Ranking	*Cause of Death*	*# Deaths*	*Cause of Death*	*# Deaths*
	All causes	13,124	All causes	6,923
1	Diseases of the heart	2,598	Diseases of the heart	1,494
2	Malignant neoplasms	2,392	Unintentional injuries	1,290
3	Unintentional injuries	1,520	Malignant neoplasms	770
4	Diabetes mellitus	746	Chronic live disease and cirrhosis	410
5	Cerebrovascular diseases	581	Cerebrovascular diseases	322
6	Chronic liver disease and cirrhosis	577	Pneumonia and influenza	257
7	Chronic lower respiratory diseases	486	Homicide	217
8	Suicide	404	Diabetes mellitus	210
9	Influenza and pneumonia	291	Certain conditions originating in the perinatal period	199
10	Nephritis, nephritic syndrome, and nephrosis	247	Suicide	181

Whites

	2004		1980	
Ranking	*Cause of Death*	*# Deaths*	*Cause of Death*	*# Deaths*
	All causes	2,056,643	All causes	1,738,607
1	Diseases of the heart	565,703	Diseases of the heart	683,347
2	Malignant neoplasms	478,134	Malignant neoplasms	368,162
3	Cerebrovascular diseases	127,868	Cerebrovascular diseases	148.734
4	Chronic lower respiratory diseases	112,914	Unintentional injuries	90,122
5	Unintentional injuries	95,890	Chronic obstructive pulmonary diseases	52,375
6	Alzheimer's disease	61,087	Pneumonia and influenza	48,369

continues

Table 12–1 *Leading Causes of Death among Native Americans, Whites, and All U.S. Populations, 2004 versus 1980 (Continued)*

	2004		1980	
Ranking	*Cause of Death*	*# Deaths*	*Cause of Death*	*# Deaths*
7	Diabetes mellitus	58,078	Diabetes mellitus	28,868
8	Influenza and pneumonia	52,430	Atherosclerosis	27,069
9	Nephritis, nephritic syndrome, and nephrosis	33,691	Chronic live disease and cirrhosis	25,240
10	Suicide	29,251	Suicide	24,829

All United States

	2004		1980	
Ranking	*Cause of Death*	*# Deaths*	*Cause of Death*	*# Deaths*
	All causes	2,397,615	All causes	1,989,841
1	Diseases of the heart	652,486	Diseases of the heart	761,085
2	Malignant neoplasms	553,888	Malignant neoplasms	416.509
3	Cerebrovascular diseases	150,074	Cerebrovascular diseases	170,225
4	Chronic lower respiratory diseases	121,987	Unintentional injuries	105,718
5	Unintentional injuries	112,012	Chronic obstructive pulmonary diseases	52,375
6	Diabetes Mellitus	73,138	Pneumonia and influenza	48,369
7	Alzheimer's disease	65,965	Diabetes mellitus	28,868
8	Influenza and pneumonia	59,664	Chronic live disease and cirrhosis	30,583
9	Nephritis, nephritic syndrome, and nephrosis	42,480	Atherosclerosis	29,449
10	Septicemia	33,373	Suicide	26,869

Source: National Center for Health Statistics. *Health, United States, 2006. With Chartbook on Trends in the Health of Americans* Hyattsville, MD: Author; 2006

in the perinatal period were also included in the ten leading causes of deaths for U.S. AI/AN in 1980 but not in 2004. The leading cause of mortality among the AI/AN in 2004 was different from that of whites. For U.S. white and all races populations, cerebrovascular diseases and chronic lower respiratory disease replaced unintentional injuries and diabetes mellitus as the third and fourth leading causes of death. Alzheimer's disease, the sixth leading cause for U.S. white and all races does not rank among the ten leading causes of death for AI/AN. Unintentional injuries, the third leading cause of death for AI/AN, ranks fifth for U.S. white and all races populations. Diabetes and suicide, the fourth and sixth leading causes of death for AI/AN, rank seventh and tenth, respectively, for U.S. white and all races populations. Chronic liver diseases and cirrhosis, which rank as the sixth leading cause of death for AI/AN, does not rank for U.S. white and all races as one of the ten leading causes of death.

The 1999–2001 life expectancy for AI/AN residing in the IHS service area is 2.4 years less than the U.S. all races population (74.5 years versus 76.9 years, respectively). The 2000–2002 Native American infant mortality rate was 8.5 per 1000 live births compared with 6.8 for the U.S all races population.[18] A closer look at each of the causes of mortality will shed more light on health disparities that exists among the Native Americans and the general U.S. population.

Cardiovascular Diseases

Heart disease and strokes, which were very rare diseases among AI/AN population in the past, have recently risen to become the first and the fifth leading causes of death. Even though the overall number of AI/AN developing cardiovascular diseases appears to be increasing, their overall age-adjusted cardiovascular disease death rate decreased from 240.6 per 100,000 persons in 1980 to 148 in 2004. This decreasing trend is consistent with the overall national trend among all races. However, as is the case with overall mortality, IHS reported that heart disease mortality for individuals residing in IHS service areas, after adjusting for racial misreporting, is higher than the nationally reported rates for the U.S. AI/AN population. From 2000–2001, the IHS reported a heart disease mortality rate of 236.2 for AI/AN compared with 247.8 in 2001 for U.S. all races.[18] The reason for the low mortality rate for heart disease may be that Native Americans are a relatively young population and have not caught up with the rest of the population in prevalence of heart diseases.

Malignant Neoplasms

Cancer is a growing concern among Native Americans, particularly for Native women.[19] Although U.S. AI/AN statistics indicate lower incidence and mortality rates than for the U.S. white population, cancer became the second leading cause of death in 2004, surpassing unintentional injuries.[16] Cancer is the leading cause of death for Alaska Native women and the second leading cause for American Indian women.[18] Native women have the lowest all-sites-combined cancer incidence rates, but the third highest cancer death rates.[20] American Indians and Alaska Natives have the poorest survival rate from all cancers than any other racial group,[21] which may indicate disparities in healthcare access and utilization related to cancer screening and treatment.

In the past, health professionals have also noticed important regional and cancer-specific differences in mortality that would have been masked by the low overall incidence and mortality. From 1994 to 1998, higher rates of cancer mortality appeared in Alaska and the Northern Plains with rates of 217.9 and 238.6 deaths per 100,000, respectively, while the overall cancer mortality for the United States in this period was 164.2.[22] These high cancer mortality rates are attributed to disparities in specific cancer sites, such as colorectal, gallbladder, kidney, liver, lung, and stomach.[22,23] Similarly, cervical cancer mortality rates were higher among Native women than all racial and ethnic populations (3.7 versus 2.6, respectively).[24]

Unintentional Injuries

Death and disabilities from unintentional injuries are major public health concerns affecting all Americans, but they are of particular concern for Native people and are an area of great health disparity. The most recent national, age-adjusted AI/AN unintentional injury death rate was 53.1 per 100,000 compared with 37.7 for the U.S. all races population.[16] The IHS all areas unintentional injury death rate after adjustment for racial misclassification was 90.1 per 100,000 in 2000–2002, more than twice the rate of 35.7 for U.S. all races in 2001.[18]

Although unintentional injuries ranks third as the leading cause of death among all Native people,[16] it ranks as the leading cause of death for Native Americans below the age of 44.[25] In fact, injuries account for 75% of all deaths among Native American children and youth.[26] Native Americans suffer injuries rates 1.5 to 5 times the rates for other Americans.[25] Injuries result in 46% of all years of potential life lost (YPLL) for Native Americans, which is five times greater than the YPLL of 8% due to heart disease, the next highest cause.[27] Motor vehicle crashes were the leading cause of unintentional injury-related death, followed by firearms events, pedestrian events, drownings, and fires.[28] A recent IHS report highlighted the following disparity between IHS all areas and the U.S. white populations[29,15]:

- American Indian children died in motor vehicle crashes at about twice the rate for white children.
- American Indian children died in pedestrian-related motor vehicle crashes at about three times the rate for white children.

- American Indian children died from drowning at about twice the rate for white children.
- Native American Children died from fire-related injuries at about three times the rate for white children.

Diabetes Mellitus

Type 2 diabetes is one of the most serious health challenges facing Native Americans. Compared with other racial/ethnic populations in the United States, diabetes affects Native Americans disproportionately,[30,31] and the prevalence continues to increase.[31,32] **Figure 12–1** shows an increasing trend in the prevalence of diabetes and a continued widening of gap between the overall U.S. adult population and AI/AN adults. In 2002, the age-adjusted prevalence of diabetes among Native Americans was 15.3% compared with 7.3% for total U.S. adults.[32] The difference was distributed across all ages and genders.

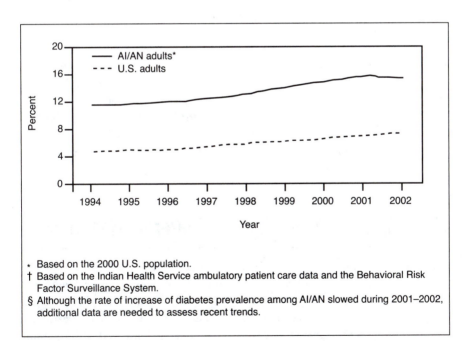

* Based on the 2000 U.S. population.
† Based on the Indian Health Service ambulatory patient care data and the Behavioral Risk Factor Surveillance System.
§ Although the rate of increase of diabetes prevalence among AI/AN slowed during 2001–2002, additional data are needed to assess recent trends.

Figure 12–1   *Age-Adjusted Prevalance of Diagnosed Diabetes among American Indian/Alaska Native (AI/AN) and U.S. Adults Aged ≥ 20 years, 1994–2002*
Source: Acton KJ, Burrows NR, Geiss LS, Thompson T. Diabetes prevalence among American Indians and Alaska Natives and the overall population—United States, 1994–2002. *MMWR.* 2003;52(30):702–704. http://www.cdc.gov/mmwr/preview/mmwrhtml/mm5230a3.htm#fig.

Type 2 diabetes has become a significant threat to the health of young Native Americans. In a study examining the user population of IHS facilities between 1990 and 1998, the number of Native Americans younger than 35 years with diagnosed diabetes increased by 71%, and the crude prevalence of diabetes increased by 46% from 6.4 to 9.3 per 1000.[33] In contrast, diabetes prevalence among the U.S. general population younger than 45 years increased by 14% between 1990 and 1994.[34] In a more recent study, the AI/AN population aged 35 or younger using the IHS system doubled their prevalence rate of diabetes from 8.5 to 17.1 per 1000 between 1994 and 2004.[35]

Type 2 diabetes accounts for major morbidities among Native Americans, including blindness, kidney failure, lower-extremity amputations, cardiovascular diseases, disability, decreased quality of life, and premature mortality[36]; it is also a major cause of congenital anomalies, malformations, and perinatal deaths.[37] Early onset of diabetes is an even greater concern because it increases the lifetime duration of disease with increased risk of disabling complications.[38] The high prevalence of diabetes in Native American females (and the behavior associated with it) also has implications for the next generation because it may set up a cycle of diabetes during pregnancy, diabetes onset at a young age in offspring, and diabetes during pregnancy in the subsequent generations.[33]

Although diabetes ranked as the fourth leading cause of death for Native Americans in 2004, the true extent of deaths from diabetes is grossly underestimated because a large proportion of deaths from heart disease, the leading cause of death among Native Americans, is associated with diabetes.[39,40] In 2004, the reported age-adjusted death rate for diabetes of 39.2 per 100,000 in Native Americans was higher than that of the 24.5 per 100,000 for U.S. all races population. The 2000–2002 IHS all areas diabetes mortality rates, after adjusting for racial misclassification, was 73.2 per 100,000 compared with 25.3 for U.S. all races in 2001.[17]

Natality, Infant Mortality, and Maternal Health

The infant mortality rate is generally accepted as an important indicator of the health status and social well-being of a nation. Historically, Native Americans have had high infant mortality rates, especially during the post-neonatal period.[41] Although improvements have been made that have drastically reduced infant mortality rates for Native Americans, compared with the total U.S. population, disparities still persist—and it is evident that more needs to be done to decrease the disparity.

Recent IHS data show that the total AI/AN area birthrate is 24.0 per 1000, nearly 1.7 times the rate of the total U.S. population (14.5).[31] In 2000–2002, infant deaths among Native Americans were 1.3 times those of U.S. all races (8.5 per 1000 versus 6.8 per 1000). Infant mortality rates continue to decline compared with the 1996–1998 rate of 8.9 per 1000 for Native American and the 1997 rate of 7.2 per 1000 for all of the U.S population.[17] The death rate in the neonatal period for Native Americans does not differ from whites (4.8 per 1000 live births), but the post-neonatal period shows a significant disparity (4.4 versus 2.5 per 1000 live births).[31]

In 1998–2000, the leading causes of infant death in Native Americans were congenital anomalies, sudden infant death syndrome (SIDS), disorders relating to short gestation and unspecified low birth weight, accidents, influenza, and pneumonia. This differs somewhat from that of white infants in which SIDS ranks third and respiratory distress syndrome ranks fifth. A greater proportion of Native American infant deaths than white infant deaths is attributable to SIDS (16.8% versus 11.0%, respectively).[42]

Important health disparities have also been identified between Native American mothers and U.S. mothers of all races in certain maternal characteristics and behaviors that affect birth outcomes. Specifically, 68.5% of Native mothers accessed prenatal care in the first trimester of pregnancy compared with 82.5% for U.S. all races mothers. Native mothers were more likely than U.S. mothers of all races to have diabetes during pregnancy (50.2% versus 32.8%), drink alcohol during pregnancy (3.6% versus 1.1%), and smoke tobacco during pregnancy (20.2% versus 13.2%).[31]

Suicide

The 2000–2002 IHS reported suicide rate of 17.3 per 100,000 for Native Americans, after adjustment for racial misclassification, was 190% higher than that of all U.S. races (10.7 per 100,000) for 2001. There was no significant difference in the rates for both groups compared with a previous year (1996–1998 for AI/AN and 1997 for all U.S. races).[17] While the highest suicide rate was for persons 74 and older in the U.S. population, the highest rate in Native Americans was for ages 15 to 34. The death rate from suicide in this age range was more than double that of the general population.[31] Suicide is the second leading cause of death following unintentional injuries in Native Americans ages 15 to 34 years and the third leading cause of death in 5 to 14 year olds.[31]

Suicide is a fatal symptom of depression: the most common mental health problem facing Americans today. Depression, untreated or inadequately treated, may lead to suicide. Depression in Native Americans is attributable to several factors, including isolation on distant reservations, pervasive poverty, hopelessness, and intergenerational trauma.[15] Underlying mental health and behavioral health problems may be related to colonization, historical trauma, and adverse past U.S. policies.[15]

Substance Abuse

Alcohol abuse is rampant in Native American communities. Native Americans use and abuse alcohol and other drugs at a younger age and at a higher rate than the general U.S. population. The latest age-adjusted alcohol-induced death mortality rate, after adjusting for racial misclassification, was 7.3 times that of the U.S. population.[17] Chronic liver disease and liver cirrhosis, a severe consequence of alcohol abuse, is the sixth leading cause of death among Native Americans with death rate about five times that of the U.S. general population.[31]

Sexually Transmitted Disease/HIV

In 2004, reported rates of chlamydia, gonorrhea, and primary and secondary syphilis were two to six times those of whites.[43] Similar to the overall pattern in the United States, chlamydia remains the most commonly reported infectious disease among the Native Americans. In 2004, the total chlamydia rate for Native Americans was twice that of the U.S. population: 705.8 cases per 100,000 AI/AN population compared with 319.6 per 100,000 U. S. population.[43] The total incidence of gonorrhea for AI/AN in 2004 is comparable to that of U.S. total (117 per 100,000 versus 113.5 per 100,000, respectively). The rate for primary and secondary syphilis in Native Americans was comparable to that of U.S. total. However, certain areas have higher rates of chlamydia, gonorrhea, and primary and secondary syphilis than the national average for American Indians.[43]

HIV/AIDS is a growing problem among Native Americans.[44] In 2005, HIV/AIDS was diagnosed for an estimated 195 AI/AN (adults, adolescents, and children). Furthermore, AI/AN with HIV/AIDS had shorter survival rates than Asians and Pacific Islanders, whites, or Hispanics.[44] After 9 years, 67% of AI/AN were alive, compared with 66% of blacks, 74% of Hispanics, 75% of whites, and 81% of Asians and Pacific Islanders.[44] Even though the HIV/AIDS rates in Native American communities are currently low, the existence of high rates of *Chlamydia trachomatis* infection, gonorrhea, and syphilis suggests that the sexual behaviors that facilitate the spread of HIV are relatively common.

Behavioral Health Risk Characteristics

The results of the Behavioral Risk Factor Surveillance System (BRFSS) survey conducted from 1997 to 2000 revealed several disparities in the self-reported health risks of Native American adults and the U.S. population.[45] Compared with the general population, Native American respondents were more likely to report "fair" or "poor" health status (23.8% versus14.6%); more likely to be obese based on body mass index (BMI), calculated from height and weight (23.9% versus 18.7%); more likely to have been told by a healthcare professional that they have diabetes (9.7% versus 5.7%); more likely to smoke (32.2% versus 22.3%); and less likely to engage in leisure physical activity (32.5% versus 27.5%).[45] Surprisingly, binge drinking and drinking and driving by Native American men were comparable to other racial/ethnic groups.[45]

Native American women with an intact uterine cervix were more likely to never have had a Pap test than other racial/ethnic groups (10.3% versus 6.1%) or to have had their last Pap test more that 3 years ago (21.3% versus 15.3%).[45]

Oral Health

Dental caries is the most common form of chronic disease in childhood. Dental caries disproportionately affects the AI/AN population.[46] The AI/AN population has the highest tooth decay rate of any cohort in the United States, five times the U.S. average for children 2 to 4 years of age. Of AI/AN children aged 2 to 5 years, 79% have tooth decay, with 60% of these having severe early childhood caries (baby bottle tooth decay). Of AI/AN children aged 6 to 14 years, 87% have a history of decay and have dental caries twice that of the general population. Of AI/AN young people aged 15 to19 years, 91% have caries. In total, 68% of AI/AN children have untreated dental caries. One-third of AI/AN schoolchildren report missing school because of dental pain, and 25% report avoiding laughing or smiling because of the way their teeth look.[46] The observed oral health disparities are due to little or no access to dental care for the AI/AN population, which results from geographic isolation and difficulties in attracting dentists to rural dental facilities that serve Native people.[47]

Other Areas of Health Disparities

Although the prevalence of tuberculosis (TB) is declining among Native Americans, it continues to affect them disproportionately.[48] In 2002, TB incidence among Native Americans was approximately double the incidence for U.S. all races population at 7 cases per 100,000. Furthermore, the age adjusted TB mortality rate reported by IHS from 2000–2002 for AI/AN was seven times that of the U.S. all races population (2.1 versus 0.3 per 100,000).[17]

Pneumonia and influenza also disproportionately affect Native Americans, with an age-adjusted mortality rate of 31.1 per 100,000, after adjusting for racial misclassification, compared with 22.0 per 100,000 for the U.S population.[17]

Population to Health Professionals Ratio

There is documentation of a low healthcare professional/population ratio throughout the Indian healthcare system.[49]

- In 1998, there were 74 physicians per 100,000 AI/AN beneficiaries, compared with 242 per 100,000 in the overall U.S. population.
- In 1998, there were 232 registered nurses per 100,000 AI/AN beneficiaries, compared with 876.2 per 100,000 in the overall U.S. population.
- In 1998, there were 289 public health nurses in the IHS. This represents a ratio of 19.8 per 100,000 AI/AN beneficiaries.
- In 2000–2001, there were 21 IHS psychiatrists, 63 IHS psychologists, and 19 podiatrists to treat the more than 60,000 AI/AN diagnosed with diabetes.
- In 2001, there were 11 vacancies for optometrists.
- In fiscal year 1998, the dentist to AI/AN beneficiary ratio was 1:2793 compared with 1:1743 for the overall U.S. population.

Indian Healthcare System

Since 1955, the Indian Health Service has been the agency within the department of Health and Human Services responsible for the delivery of health care to federally recognized American Indian tribes and Alaska Native villages and corporations. The current system serves 1.8 million Native Americans with 48 hospitals, 268 health centers, 135 health stations, 11 school health stations, 162 Alaska village clinics, 34 urban Indian health programs, and 11 tribal epidemiology centers. The mission of IHS is to raise the physical, mental, social, and spiritual health of AI/AN to the highest level. Since the inception of the IHS, the health status of Native Americans has improved significantly due to access to health care and public health efforts to reduce the effects of infectious disease. However, despite these improvements, there is persistent disparity in the health of Native Americans compared with the overall population, and several researchers have alluded to the fact that IHS is not adequately funded to meet the healthcare needs of American Indians.[50]

In 2003, the federal funding per capita for Indian health was only $1914, an amount that is below mainstream health plans and other federal government plans. **Figure 12–2** illustrates the disparity between per capita IHS spending and federal health expenditures for other groups.

Addressing Health Disparities in American Indians

Eliminating persistent health disparities between the Native American population and the general U.S. population is a challenge. Any lasting solution has to take into consideration the multiple factors that have contributed to the current state of affairs. Healthcare solutions for Native Americans must take a holistic approach that includes education, housing, economic opportunities,

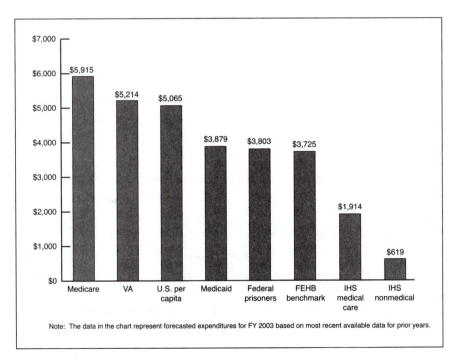

Figure 12–2 *Comparison between IHS Appropriations per Capita and Other Federal Health Expenditures in 2003*
Source: Commission on Civil Rights, July, 2003. *A Quiet Crisis: Federal Funding and Unmet Needs in Indian Country.* http://www.usccr.gov/pubs/na0703/na0204.pdf.

culture, and spirituality, as well as empowerment through self-determination and self-governance. The system must take into consideration the physical, mental, emotional, and spiritual health of the Native American.

There is need for more federal funding to increase the numbers of health-care professionals—Native American healthcare professionals in particular—to serve Native American communities. Services provided to Native communities need to be expanded to offer more preventive services. The reauthorization of Indian Health Care Act that is currently (December 2007) being considered in the House of Representatives holds some hope for increased federal government funding as well as expansion of IHS mandate to provide more preventive services. The services provided by IHS or any other entity must be culturally appropriate for acceptability and effectiveness among Native Americans. Prevention and health education should be framed in the context of cultural values.

The federal government is increasingly employing extensive tribal consultation prior to making decisions affecting the Native American communities; this trend must continue to ensure proper decisions. Also the trend toward empowerment and self-determination will enable Native Americans to take over their health care, and education will enable them to create a healthcare system that is culturally appropriate. New and innovative ways of delivering IHS health care, such as tele-medicine and tele-pharmacy to diminish geographic barriers, are also being initiated. However, for the system to be most effective, it has to be adequately funded.

Public health services are grossly inadequate in tribal communities. Although, IHS is responsible for public health activities as well as healthcare service delivery, it is not adequately funded or structured to conduct the 10 essential services of public health:

1. Monitor health status to identify community health problems.
2. Diagnose and investigate health problems and health hazards in the community.
3. Inform, educate, and empower people about health issues.
4. Mobilize community partnerships to identify and solve health problems.
5. Develop policies and plans that support individual and community health efforts.
6. Enforce laws and regulations that protect health and ensure safety.
7. (a) Link people to needed personal health services and (b) ensure the provision of health care when otherwise unavailable.
8. Ensure a competent public health and personal healthcare work force.

9. Evaluate effectiveness, accessibility, and quality of personal and population-based health services.

10. Research for new insights and innovative solutions to health problems.

Many state systems do not provide these services within tribal jurisdictions, and no parallel funding systems support public health infrastructure within tribal jurisdictions. However, IHS has recently started funding regional tribal epidemiology centers with the mission of providing leadership, technical assistance, and epidemiological support to tribes for public health programming. Twelve have been established across the country. There is also a lack of mental health services to address the high rates of depression and suicide among Native Americans. Increasing federal funding may help to reduce suicides. Along with funding, there is also a need to train healthcare providers to be culturally competent and respectful of Native American culture.

Because health is not an isolated issue, any attempts to improve the health status of Native Americans must also attempt to improve their economic well-being. Opportunities for economic development should be provided to Native communities as well as support for economic and transportation infrastructures, housing, and other key factors that are both determinants and indicators of social well-being that influence health.

The school system needs to provide an adequate, well-rounded education for Native American children that will give them a solid basis to compete with the general U.S. population. Education should be tailored toward their physical, mental, emotional, and spiritual well-being.

Finally, there needs to be more timely research and data on Native Americans. The paucity of timely data is due to many factors, including inadequate data infrastructure, cultural barriers, and researchers' lack of knowledge of Native cultures. As more Native researchers are trained, knowledge of Native cultures and spirituality is increasing, and researchers are learning how best to conduct research by honoring and respecting Native culture, values, beliefs, and traditions. Community-based participatory research (CBPR) is a way of conducting research that is evolving from experiences in the Native communities. CPBR involves a partnership between researchers and the community whereby community members have input into a research study— from the inception of formulating the research question to conducting the research and disseminating the results. This approach to research is improving the availability of more timely and accurate data for monitoring health status, planning health programs, and supporting health policy changes. The National Institutes of Health (NIH) have also begun to fund the Native American Research Center for Health (NARCH) through the IHS as a way to increase research conducted in Native communities.

SUMMARY

Although the health status of Native Americans has improved remarkably over the years, disparities in health continue to exist. To make any further inroads into improving the health of Native Americans, several factors have to be taken into consideration from a holistic perspective: providing adequate funding for health services, expanding the scope of services provided to include preventive and public health services, allowing integration of culture and spirituality into health services, providing opportunities for economic development, improving education, promoting self-governance and self-determination, and conducting research in a culturally appropriate way.

REFERENCES

1. U.S. Census Bureau. *Census 2000: Brief Overview of Race and Hispanic Origin*. Census Bureau, Census 2000.
2. Martin DL, Goodman AH. Health conditions before Columbus: Paleopathology of native North Americans. *West J Med*. 2002;176(1):65–68.
3. Micozzi MS. Health and disease in the New World. *Encounters*. 1992;5–6:42–43.
4. Ortner DJ, Putschar WGJ. *Identification of Pathological Conditions in Human Skeletal Remains*. Washington, DC: Smithsonian Institution Press; 1981
5. Larsen CS. In the wake of Columbus: Native population biology in the postcontact Americas. *Yearbook Phys Anthropol*. 1994;37:109–115.
6. Crosby AW Jr. Virgin soil epidemics as a factor in the aboriginal depopulation in America. *William Mary Q*. 1976;33:289–299.
7. Executive Order No. 13084, 63 *Federal Register* 27655 (1998).
8. Executive Order No. 13175, 65 *Federal Register* 67249-67252 (2000).
9. Kuschell-Haworth, HT. Traditional healers and the Indian Health Care Improvement Act, citing *American Indian Policy Review Commission Report on Indian Health: Task Force Six*; 1976.
10. Meriam Commission, *The Problem of Indian Administration* (Report of a survey made at the request of the Honorable Hubert Work, Secretary of Interior, and submitted to him, February 21, 1928), Chapter I. http://www.alaskool.org/native_ed/research_reports/IndianAdmin/Chapter1.html#chap1. Last accessed February 3, 2004.
11. Snyder Act of 1921 Chapter. 115, 42 Stat 208, 25 USC 13(1921).
12. Indian Health Care Improvement Act, Pub. L. No. 94-437, 90 Stat. 1402 (codified as amended in scattered sections of 25 U.S.C.).
13. Ogunwole SU. *We the People: American Indians and Alaska Natives in United States: 2000*. Washington, DC: U.S. Census Bureau; February 2006.
14. U.S. Commission on Civil Rights. *Broken Promises: Evaluating the Native American Health Care System*. Washington, DC: U.S. Commission Civil Rights; September 2004.
15. National Center for Health Statistics. *Health, United States, 2006*. With Chartbook on Trends in the Health of Americans. Hyattsville, MD: Author; 2006.
16. Indian Health Service. *Adjusting for Miscoding of Indian Race on State Death Certificates*. Rockville, MD: U.S. Public Health Service; 1996.

17. Indian Health Services. *United States, Facts on Indian Health Disparities*. Washington, DC: U.S. Department of Health and Human Services; January 2006.

18. Native American Research Corporation. *Native Americans and Cancer*. http://members.aol.com/natamcan/nativeca.htm. Accessed July 5, 2007.

19. U.S. Cancer Statistics Working Group. *United States Cancer Statistics: 1999–2002 Incidence and Mortality Web-based Report*. Atlanta, GA: U.S. Department of Health and Human Services, Centers for Disease Control and Prevention and National Cancer Institute; 2005.

20. Haynes MA, Smedley BD, Institute of Medicine. *The Unequal Burden of Cancer. An Assessment of NIH Research and Programs for Ethnic Minorities and the Medically Underserved*. Washington, DC: National Academy Press; 1999.

21. Espey D. *Regional Patterns of Cancer Mortality in American Indians and Alaskan Natives in the U.S. 1994–1998*. Washington, DC: American Public Health Association;

22. Espey D, Paisano R, Cobb N. Regional patterns of cancer mortality in American Indians and Alaskan Natives, 1990–2001. *Cancer* 2005;103(5):1045–1053.

23. Centers for Disease Control. Cancer mortality among American Indians and Alaska Natives—United States, 1994–1998, *MMWR* 2003;52(30):704–707.

24. Indian Health Services. Injuries. *IHS Health and Heritage Brochure—Health Disparities*. http://www.info.ihs.gov.

25. Wallace LJD. *Injuries among American Indian and Alaska Children, 1985–1996*. Atlanta, GA: Centers for Disease Control and Prevention; 2000.

26. U.S Department of Health and Human Services, Centers for Disease Control and Preventions. *Healthy People 2010*, Chapter 15: Injury and Violence Prevention; Washington, DC: Author; 2008.

27. Centers for Disease Control. Injury mortality among American Indian and Alaska Native children and youth—United States 1989–1998. *MMWR*. 2003;52(30): 697–701.

28. Broderick EB. Quantifying the unmet need in IHS/Tribal EMS. A project funded by the Office of Program Planning and Evaluation, Office of Public Health, IHS Headquarters, 1999-2001:9–10.

29. Valway S, Freeman W, Kaufman S, Welty T, Helgerson SD, Gohdes D. Prevalence of diagnosed diabetes among American Indians and Alaska Natives, 1987. *Diabetes Care* 1993;16(suppl 1):271–276.

30. *Trends in Indian Health*. Rockville, MD: Indian Health Services; 2000–2001.

31. Centers for Disease Control. Diabetes prevalence among American Indians and Alaska Natives and the overall population—United States 1994–2002. *MMWR*. 2003;52(30):702–704.

32. Acton KJ, Burrows NR, Moore K, Querec L, Geiss LS, Engelgau MM. Trends in diabetes prevalence among American Indian and Alaskan Native children, adolescents, and young adults. *AJPH*. 2002;92(9):1485–1490.

33. Centers for Diseases Control and Prevention diabetes surveillance, 1999.

34. Centers for Disease Control, Diagnosed diabetes among American Indians and Alaska Natives Aged <35 years—United States 1994–2004. *MMWR*. 2006;55(44): 1201–1203.

35. Ghodes D. Diabetes in American Indians: A growing problem. *Diabetes Care*. 1986;9:609–613.

36. Aberg A, Westbom L, Kallen B. Congenital malformations among infants whose mother had gestational diabetes or pre-existing diabetes. *Early Hum Dev*. 2001;61: 85–95.

37. Harris MI. Chapter 1: Summary. In: Harris MI, Cowie CC, Stern MP, Boyko EJ, Reibe GE, Bennett PH, eds. *Diabetes in America*, 2nd ed. DHHS publication no. NIH 95-1468. Washington, DC: U.S. Department of Health and Human Services; 1995:1–13.

38. *National Health Care Disparities Report*. Washington, DC: U.S. Department of Health and Human Services, Agency for Healthcare Research and Quality; December 2003.

39. Bild D, Stevenson, J. Frequency of recording of diabetes on U.S. death certificates: Analysis of the 1986 National Mortality Follow Back Survey. *J Clin Epidemiol*. 1992;454:275–281.

40. Nakamura RM, King R, Kimball EH, Oye RK, Helgerson SD. Excess infant mortality in an American Indian population, 1940 to 1990. *JAMA*. 1991:266:2244–2248.

41. Tomashek KM, Qin C, Hsia J, Iyasu S, Barfield WD, Flowers LM. Infant mortality trend and differences between American Indian/Alaska Native infant and white infants in the United States, 1989–1991 and 1998–2000. *AJPH*. 2006;96(12): 2222–2227.

42. Centers for Disease Control and Prevention. *Indian Health Surveillance Report: Sexually Transmitted Diseases*, Atlanta, GA: Author: 2004.

43. Centers for Disease Control and Prevention. *HIV/AIDS Surveillance Report, 2005*. Vol. 17. Rev ed. Atlanta, GA: Author; 2007:1–46.

44. Centers for Disease Control and Prevention. Surveillance for health behaviors of American Indians and Alaska Natives: Findings from the Behavioral Risk Factor Surveillance System, 1997–2000. *MMWR*. 2003:52(SS07):1–13.

45. *The 1999 Oral Health Survey of American Indian and Alaska Native Dental Patients*. Rockville, MD: Indian Health Service, Division of Dental Services; 2002:106.

46. Nash DA, Nagel RJ. Confronting oral health disparities among American Indian/Alaska native children: the pediatric oral health therapist. *Am J Public Health*. 2005;95:1325–1329.

47. Butler JC, et al. Emerging infectious diseases among indigenous peoples. *Emerging Infectious Diseases*. 2001;7(3suppl.):55–54.

48. Reauthorization of the Indian Health Care Improvement Act. Testimony of Michael Bird, MSW, MPH Senate Indian Affairs Committee On Behalf of the Friends of Indian Health; July 31, 2001. http://www.apha.org/advocacy/priorities/comments/legislativetestcommindianhealth.htm. Accessed July 22, 2007.

49. Level of Need Funded Workgroup. *Final Report: Level of Need Funded Cost Model—Indian Health Services*; 2005.

Chapter 13

Addressing Health Disparities in Immigrant Populations in the United States

Patti Patterson, MD, MPH
Gordon Gong, MD

The United States is a nation of immigrants from all over the world with vastly different cultures, who have had a tremendous impact on the population growth, economic development, cultural enrichment and political structure of the United States. Low-skilled laborers, educators, scientists, as well as elite immigrants such as Albert Einstein and Enrico Fermi have contributed to every aspect of life in this country. According to the U.S. Census Bureau, foreign-born persons accounted for more than 11% (31 million) of the United States population in 2000.[1] The foreign-born population grew to 35.7 million in 2004, according to a recent estimate.[2] Nearly one-third (11 million) of foreign-born persons were undocumented immigrants.[3] Sixteen percent of the U.S. nonelderly population (18–65 years of age) was foreign-born.[4] These newcomers often face legal and structural barriers in the new environment because of culture shock, prejudice, language barriers, unemployment, low income, and lack of education, among others. As a result, many have no health insurance and have limited access to preventive, primary, and nonemergent health care, and they tend to have disproportionately high rates of health problems, the nature of which varies with the country origin.

The causes of health disparities in immigrant populations are varied and multifactorial. Immigrants' health issues have implications for the health of the community and nation as well as being of critical importance for the appropriate delivery of quality care to the individuals themselves. The region of origin; history of travel to the native country; length of time since immigration; and cultural, social, and nutritional practices all affect the diagnoses of various health conditions. It is critical for policy makers as well as health-care organizations and professionals to understand and address health issues particular to immigrant populations in order to reduce health disparities in the United States.

Immigration reform has become a major national issue and a subject of hot debate. Conflicting opinions about the economic benefits and societal implications of national immigration policy have come to the forefront, particularly the potential impacts on health care, public education, and businesses such as agriculture, construction, and service industries. Whatever policies the U.S. government adopts, healthcare professionals, hospitals, and public health institutions will be caring for people with serious illnesses and untreated preventable conditions. These challenges must be addressed to preserve the health and well-being of immigrants and the U.S. population as a whole.

Definitions of Immigrants, Foreign-Born Persons, Refugees, and Naturalized Citizens

The terms *immigrants*, *foreign-born persons*, *naturalized citizens*, *non-citizens*, *permanent residents*, *illegal* (or *undocumented* or *unauthorized*) *aliens*, *refugees*, and others are frequently encountered in medical, public health, and social sciences literature, as well as in laws, rules, and regulations. It is essential to clarify these terms and their relationships.

Immigrants

While it is often said that the United States is a nation of immigrants, in the sense that 99.3% of the population is immigrants or descendants of immigrants,[5] precise definitions of the various terms are necessary to discuss health disparities. The Kaiser Family Foundation and many authors refer to those in the United States who were born in foreign countries as immigrants, including legal permanent residents, refugees, temporary immigrants, undocumented (or illegal) immigrants, and naturalized citizens.[4-7] Some refer to their children and grandchildren as "the second- and third-generation-immigrants" although they are born in the United States and are U.S. citizens.[7] However, according to U.S. Citizenship and Immigration Services (USCIS), an *immigrant* is "an alien admitted to the United States as a lawful permanent resident. Permanent residents are also commonly referred to as immigrants; however, the Immigration and Nationality Act (INA) broadly defines an immigrant as any alien in the United States, except one legally admitted under specific nonimmigrant categories (INA) section 101(a(15). An illegal alien who entered the United States without inspection, for example, would be strictly defined as an immigrant under the INA" (last amendment of INA in 1996).[8] In this chapter, we use USCIS's definition of immigrant unless specified. Thus, those who came to the United States as immigrants and subsequently became U.S. citizens (naturalized citizens) are no longer considered to be immigrants.[8]

Foreign-Born Persons

After becoming U.S. citizens, former immigrants will often maintain many aspects of their foreign culture, language, and foreign accents. These characteristics along with their low socioeconomic status (SES) and prejudices against them may contribute to health disparities. For many purposes (social, political, medical), there has been a need for a category of *foreign-born*, which refers to "anyone who is not a U.S. citizen at birth. This includes naturalized U.S. citizens, Lawful Permanent Residents (immigrants), temporary migrants (such as students), humanitarian migrants (such as refugees), and persons illegally present in the United States."[9] This chapter covers both immigrants and foreign-born persons in addressing health disparities and cultural proficiency. The impact of legal status on health disparity among immigrants and cultural proficiency will also be discussed.

The Numbers of Immigrants and Foreign-Born Persons in the United States

To understand the magnitude of health disparities and the importance of cultural proficiency in dealing with immigrant populations, it is crucial to know the numbers of immigrants and foreign-born persons.

Permanent Residents

In the 1990s, the United States experienced the largest immigration surge in terms of the absolute number of legal immigrants in history, far exceeding the numbers in the three previous great waves (1815–1860, 1865–1890, and

1890–1914) (see **Figure 13–1**).[10, 11] From 2004 to 2006, more than 3 million persons immigrated legally into the United States (see **Table 13–1**).[12] Unlike immigrants in the previous waves, who came mainly from Europe, immigrants in the recent wave were mainly from Latin America and Asia. European immigrants from 2004 to 2006 accounted for only 13% to 17% of the legal immigrant population in the United States (Table 13–1).[12] The largest numbers are coming from Mexico, China, Philippines, India, Cuba, and Colombia. Although immigrants from Africa account for only 7% to 9.3% of all legal immigrants in the United States, their share increased compared with previous years.[12]

Foreign-Born Persons

More than 35 million of the U.S. population were foreign-born in 2004.[2] California, Florida, New York, New Jersey, and Nevada have the highest proportions of foreign-born persons, accounting for 17.2% to 27.2% of their populations **(Figure 13–2)**.[13] One in nine residents, one in seven workers, and one in five low-wage workers are foreign born, while one in five children under 18 years of age has a foreign-born parent.[14–17] More than

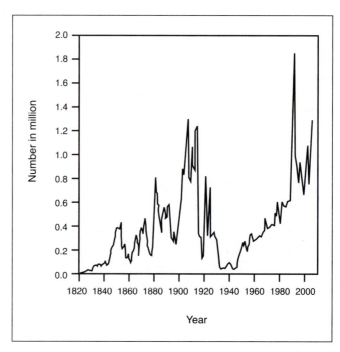

Figure 13–1 *Legal Permanent Residents in the United States, 1820–2006*
Source: U.S. Department of Homeland Security. *2006 Yearbook of Immigration Statistics.*
http://www.dhs.gov/ximgtn/statistics/publications/yearbook.shtm. Accessed September 27, 2007.

Table 13–1 *Legal Permanent Residents by Region and Country of Birth: Fiscal Years 2004–2006*

	2006		2005		2004	
	Number	**Percent**	**Number**	**Percent**	**Number**	**Percent**
Total	1,266,264	100	1,122,373	100	957,883	100
Region						
Africa	117,430	9.3	85,102	7.6	66,422	6.9
Asia	422,333	33.4	400,135	35.7	334,540	34.9
Europe	164,285	13	176,569	15.7	133,181	13.9
North America	414,096	32.7	345,575	30.8	342,468	35.8
Carribbean	146,771	11.6	108,598	9.7	89,144	9.3
Central America	75,030	5.9	53,470	4.8	62,287	6.5
Other North America	192,295	15.2	183,507	16.4	191,037	19.9
Oceania	7,385	0.6	6,546	0.6	5,985	0.6
South America	138,001	10.9	103,143	9.2	72,060	7.5
Unknown	2,734	0.2	5,303	0.5	3,227	0.3
Country						
Mexico	173,753	13.7	161,445	14.4	175,411	18.3
China, People's Republic	87,345	6.9	69,967	6.2	55,494	5.8
Philippines	74,607	5.9	60,748	5.4	57,846	6
India	61,369	4.8	84,681	7.5	70,151	7.3
Cuba	45,614	3.6	36,261	3.2	20,488	2.1
Colombia	43,151	3.4	25,571	2.3	18,846	2
Dominican Republic	38,069	3	27,504	2.5	30,506	3.2
El Salvador	31,783	2.5	21,359	1.9	29,807	3.1
Vietnam	30,695	2.4	32,784	2.9	31,524	3.3
Jamaica	24,976	2	18,346	1.6	14,430	1.5
Korea	24,386	1.9	26,562	2.4	19,766	2.1

continues

Table 13–1 *Legal Permanent Residents by Region and Country of Birth: Fiscal Years 2004–2006 (Continued)*

	2006		2005		2004	
	Number	*Percent*	*Number*	*Percent*	*Number*	*Percent*
Guatemala	24,146	1.9	16,825	1.5	18,920	2
Haiti	22,228	1.8	14,529	1.3	14,191	1.5
Peru	21,718	1.7	15,676	1.4	11,794	1.2
Canada	18,207	1.4	21,878	2	15,569	1.6
Brazil	17,910	1.4	16,664	1.5	10,556	1.1
Ecuador	17,490	1.4	11,608	1	8,626	0.9
Pakistan	17,418	1.4	14,926	1.3	12,086	1.3
United Kingdom	17,207	1.4	19,800	1.8	14,915	1.6
Ukraine	17,142	1.4	22,761	2	14,156	1.5
Other countries	457,050	36.1	402,478	35.9	312,801	32.7

Source: U.S. Department of Homeland Security. *2006 Yearbook of Immigration Statistics.*
http://www.dhs.gov/ximgtn/statistics/publications/yearbook.shtm. Accessed September 27, 2007.

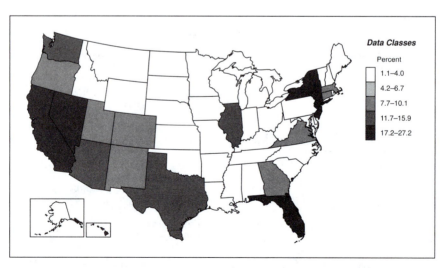

Figure 13–2 *Percentage of Foreign-Born Persons in the United States by States*
Source: U.S. Census Bureau. Percent of people who are foreign born: 2005. http://factfinder.census
.gov/servlet/ThematicMapFramesetServlet?_bm=y&-geo_id=01000US&-tm_name=ACS_2005_EST_
G00_M00615&-ds_name=ACS_2005_EST_G00_&-_MapEvent=displayBy&-_dBy=040. Accessed
September 27, 2007.

50% of foreign-born individuals have limited English proficiency, and 18% of foreign-born individuals live below the poverty line compared with 12% of native-born persons. The poverty rate was the highest (23%) among noncitizens **(Table 13–2)**.

First-generation immigrant children under 18 are twice as likely to be poor compared to children of later generations (35% and 17%, respectively).

Table 13–2 *Foreign-Born Residents, 2000*

Percent Size and Growth	
Total U.S. population, 2000	281,421,906
Foreign-born population, 2000	31,107,889
Percent who were foreign-born, 2000	11
Percent of foreign-born population who arrived 1990–2000	43
Countries and Regions of Origin	
Percent of foreign-born population in 2000 from top five countries of origin	
Mexico	30
China	5
Philippines	4
India	3
Vietnam	3
Percent of foreign-born in 2000, by regions of origin	
Latin America	52
Asia	26
Europe	16
Africa	3
North America	3
English Proficiency	
Percent of the total U.S. population ages 5 or older with limited English proficiency	8
Percent of foreign-born population ages 5 or older with limited English proficiency	51

continues

Table 13–2 *Foreign-Born Residents, 2000 (Continued)*

Poverty	
Percent of residents living at or below the federal poverty level in 2000	
Foreign-born	18
Native-born	12
Naturalized citizens	11
Noncitizens	23
Naturalized Citizens	
Percent naturalized, by period of entry	
Before 1970	82
1970–1979	66
1980–1989	45
1990–2000	13
Legal permanent resident (LPR population in 2002)	11.4 million
Population eligible to naturalize in 2002	7.8 million
Number of persons naturalized in fiscal year 2002	573,708

Source: U.S. Department of Homeland Security, U.S. Citizenship and Immigration Services, Office of Citizenship, *Helping Immigrants Become New Americans: Communities Discuss the Issues.* Washington, DC, 2004. http://www.uscis.gov. Also see U.S. Census Bureau. http://quickfacts.census.gov/qfd/states/00000.html.

About half of immigrant children are living with families with an annual income below 200% of the poverty level compared with 34% among U.S.-born children.[18] Foreign-born children are twice as likely to have no health insurance, and four times as likely to live in crowded housing than U.S.-born children.[19] Immigrant children are more likely to be exposed to developmental risk factors, which include a mother without a high school diploma, poverty, living in a linguistically isolated household, and living in a single-parent family. More children (67%) of immigrant parents had at least one of these risk factors and 17% had three, compared with 45% and 4%, respectively, of children of U.S.-born parents.[20]

The fastest growing foreign-born populations are Hispanics/Latinos and Asians. The Hispanic/Latino population increased 58% from 22.4 million in 1990 to 35.3 million (58.5% were Mexican descendants in 2000),[21] and Asians increased 48% from 6.9 to 10.2 million during the same period.[22] Immigration of Hispanics/Latinos is a major contributor to demographic shifts in the U.S. population. Half of all Hispanics/Latinos live in two states: California and Texas.[21]

Undocumented Immigrants

In the 1990s, an estimated 350,000 *undocumented immigrants* entered the United States each year.[23] Among the 11 million undocumented immigrants in the United States in 2004,[3,15] 81% were from Latin America, 9% from China, 6% from Europe and Canada, and 4% from Africa and other countries. Children under 18 years of age (1.7 million) accounted for 17% of the undocumented population in 2004.[3]

Refugees

According to the United Nations, a *refugee* is a person who, "owing to a well-founded fear of being persecuted for reasons of race, religion, nationality, membership in a particular social group, or political opinion, is outside the country of his nationality, and is unable to or, owing to such fear, is unwilling to avail himself of the protection of that country."[24] More than 2 million refugees were admitted to the United States between 1975 and 2000 **(Table 13–3)**.[25]

Table 13–3 *Number of Refugees in the United States*

Area	*Period*	*Number*
Africa	1980–2000	Total >85,000. >30,000 Ethiopian; ~25,000 Somali; the remainder Sudanese, Liberian, Zairian, Rwandan, Ugandan, and Angolans
Southeast Asia	1975–2000	Total >1.4 million. ~ 900,000 Vietnamese; the remainder Laotians, Cambodian, and Burmese
Near East, South Asia	1980–2000	Total 112,500. ~47,000 Iranian, ~31,200 Iraqi, ~28,000 Afghan
New Independent States and the Baltic	1989–2000	Total >378,000
Former Soviet Union	1989–2000	Total 546,516
Yugoslavia	1992–2000	Total ~107,000
Latin America	1975–2000	Total 79,634

Source: U.S. Department of State, Bureau of Population, Refugees, and Migration, January 18, 2000. http://www.state.gov/www/global/prm/admissions_resettle.html#fact; Refugee health—Immigrant health. Background on refugees. http://www3.baylor.edu/~Charles_Kemp/background_on_refugees.htm. Both accessed September 25, 2007.

Health Disparities in Immigrant and Foreign-Born Populations

Major Health Conditions with Health Disparities

Eliminating health disparities in minorities requires addressing health disparities in immigrant and foreign-born populations. In the United States, 45.6% (or 16.1/35.3 million) of all Latinos and 75% (or 7.6/10.2 million) of all Asians were foreign-born.[9,21,22] The range of health issues facing immigrants is complex and varied. Communicable diseases, health behaviors and lack of access to care all affect the health of these populations. Disparities of several major diseases and conditions such as stress are more often seen in immigrants. These include tuberculosis, HIV/AIDS, Hepatitis B, obesity, cancer, mental health, and mortality.

Tuberculosis

In 2005, there were 14,093 tuberculosis cases (4.8 cases per 100,000) reported in the United States. Between 1993 and 2005, the number of tuberculosis (TB) patients was steadily decreasing among U.S.-born citizens but was essentially unchanged in foreign-born populations **(Figure 13–3)**.[26] The prevalence of tuberculosis among the foreign-born was 8.7 times that of U.S. born persons in 2005 **(Figure 13–4)**.[26] More than one-fourth of the children in the United States 14 years of age or younger with TB are foreign-born.[27] The number of multi-drug-resistant (MDR, defined as resistance to at least isoniazid and rifampin) TB cases increased by 13.3% in the United States from 1993 to 2005.[26] The rate of MDR TB cases increased significantly in foreign-born persons from 26% (105 of 410) in 1993 to 80% (76 of 95) in 2005.[26] Although the total number of MDR TB cases is relatively small, these cases present a significant public health threat due to the transmission potential and the cost and difficulty of treatment. People infected with human immunodeficiency virus (HIV) are more susceptible to TB infection because of reduced immunity. As a result, the percentage of TB cases with HIV infection is high (12.4% in 2006), and HIV infection is contributing to global resurgence of TB.[28] Although the total number of TB cases had decreased among foreign-born persons, the rate of decrease was slower than in U.S.-born persons in 2006. A majority of Asians (95.6% or 3,126/3,269) and Hispanics/Latinos (74.7% or 3,024/4,050) with TB were foreign-born, while only 29.9% (1,110/3,712) of blacks and 17.8% (427 of 2,404) of whites with TB were foreign-born.[28]

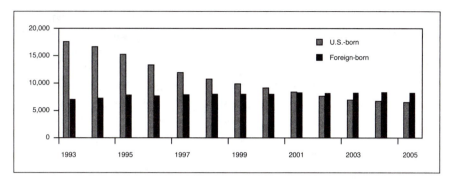

Figure 13–3   *Tuberculosis Cases in U.S.-Born versus Foreign-Born Persons in the United States*
Source: Centers for Disease Control and Prevention. *Reported Tuberculosis in the United States,*
2005. Atlanta, GA: U.S. Department of Health and Human Services; September 2006.
http://www.cdc.gov/tb/surv/surv2005/PDF/TBSurvFULLReport.pdf. September 25, 2007.

Because many immigrants come from countries with inadequate resources
for appropriate surveillance and treatment of TB, a global approach is essential to TB control. To prevent the spread of TB from other countries, the Centers for Disease Control and Prevention (CDC) requires that all applicants for
an immigrant visa 2 years of age or older receive tuberculin skin testing. For

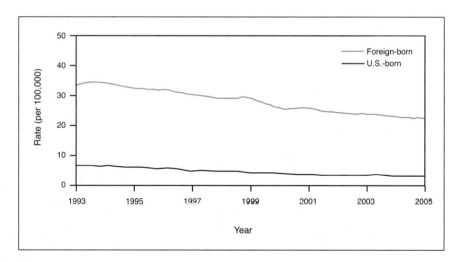

Figure 13–4   *U.S. Tuberculosis Rates by Country of Birth*
Source: Centers for Disease Control and Prevention. *Reported Tuberculosis in the United States,*
2005. Atlanta, GA: U.S. Department of Health and Human Services; September 2006.
http://www.cdc.gov/tb/surv/surv2005/PDF/TBSurvFULLReport.pdf. September 25, 2007.

those with a skin test reaction of 5 mm, a chest radiograph is required.[29] **Table 13–4** shows that tuberculosis is more prevalent among persons in the United States who were born in Asia and Latin Americas.[26] Currently, the CDC is helping these countries improve their surveillance and treatment of TB cases.[28] In addition, the CDC recommended in 2006 that in the United States, "all patients initiating treatment for TB be screened routinely for HIV infection." CDC strategies for TB control also include increasing awareness of healthcare providers regarding TB/HIV co-infection and developing new drugs for drug-resistant TB.[28]

TB screening of immigrants, which might be an attractive strategy, has been criticized for discrimination and stigmatization.[30] However, when immigrants in London were offered screening for tuberculosis, most recipients val-

Table 13–4 *Tuberculosis Cases and Rates in Foreign-Born Persons in Top 14 Countries of Origin of Birth, 2005*

	Number	*Percent*
Mexico	1,942	25
Philippines	829	11
Vietnam	577	8
India	567	7
China	392	5
Haiti	238	3
Guatemala	209	3
Korea	173	2
Honduras	165	2
Ecuador	155	2
Peru	154	2
Ethiopia	154	2
Somalia	147	2
El Salvador	142	2

Source: Centers for Disease Control and Prevention. *Reported Tuberculosis in the United States, 2005.* Atlanta, GA: U.S. Department of Health and Human Services; September 2006. http://www.cdc.gov/tb/surv/surv2005/PDF/TBSurvFULLReport.pdf. September 25, 2007.

ued the offer with few mentioning potential discrimination.[31] The screening acceptance rate was 77% in Canada,[32] but only 33% (213/649) undocumented immigrants accepted TB screening in Italy.[33] There is a lack of such data for the United States. This important public health issue deserves further study to determine appropriate ways to improve disease surveillance, treatment of cases and identification of contacts for screening, diagnosis, and treatment with respect to undocumented immigrants.

Hepatitis B Virus Infection

Hepatitis B Virus (HBV) infection is transmitted through blood and sexual intercourse. Chronic HBV is the most common cause of liver cirrhosis and liver cancer and results in 1 million deaths each year worldwide.[34] Approximately 2 billion people have been infected with HBV worldwide, of whom 350 million people have lifelong (chronic) infection.[34] In the United States, 1 million people have chronic HBV infection, and half of them are Asians/Pacific Islanders.[35] They likely acquired the infection before coming to the United States but were unaware of their status.[35] The HBV-related death rate among Asians/Pacific Islanders is seven times that of whites.[36] A recent study by the Asian American Hepatitis B Program showed that the prevalence of chronic HBV infection among foreign-born Asians is approximately 15% in New York City, which is 35 times the overall rate in the U.S. population.[37] The prevalence is particularly high among those born in China: about one in five newly tested Chinese Americans was infected **(Table 13–5)**.[37] Screening programs in Atlanta, Chicago, Philadelphia, and California have reported similarly high prevalence of chronic HBV infection (10%–15%) among Asian immigrants.[38] The high prevalence among China-

Table 13–5 *Country of Birth and Prevalence of HBV Infection among Newly Tested Individuals More Than 20 Years Old, in New York City, January 22–June 30, 2005*

	Total Number	*Number of Infected*	*Percent of Infected*	*95% Confidence Interval*
China	566	121	21.4	18.0–24.8
South Korea	280	13	4.6	2.2–7.1
Other Asian countries*	69	3	4.3	0.5–9.1
United States	10	0	—	—

Source: Centers for Disease Control and Prevention. Screening for Chronic Hepatitis B among Asian/Pacific Islander Populations—New York City, 2005. *MMWR*. 2006;55(18):505–528 May, 2006. http://www.cdc.gov/mmwr/preview/mmwrhtml/mm5518a2.htm.

born Americans is related to the fact that about 60% of China's population has a history of HBV infection, and close to 10% remains chronically infected.[39] Vertical transmission from mother to child is common.[35,40]

The 2004 National Health Interview survey in the United States showed that more than half of adults aged 18 to 49 years at high risk for HBV infection were not vaccinated.[38] Although the rate of HBV vaccination among high-risk adults increased significantly between 2000 and 2004 (from 30% to 45%) in the United States, it remains lower than other age groups: 92% for children and 86% for adolescents. Recently, China implemented universal hepatitis B vaccination for infants, with the goal to reduce HBV infection to below 1% among young children by 2010.[39] Such a measure will be beneficial in reducing the prevalence of HBV in future immigrants from China to the United States. In 1996, USCIS began requiring that all people, including children, from areas with endemic HBV infection seeking an immigrant visa provide proof of immunization with at least the first dose of all recommended vaccines. An exception is internationally adopted children younger than 10 years of age; these children must be vaccinated after arrival in the United States.[41]

AIDS/HIV

It was estimated that in 2005, 33.4 to 46.0 million people worldwide were living with HIV, 3.4 to 6.2 million became newly infected with HIV, and 2.4 to 3.3 million died of AIDS.[42] The prevalence of HIV peaked and reached a plateau in late 2000. Close to three-quarters (21.8 to 27.7 million) of the world's HIV carriers are in sub-Saharan Africa. Deaths due to AIDS in sub-Saharan Africa (1.8 to 2.4 million) accounted for 72% of the global total. HIV carriers in a single country, South Africa, accounted for 32% of all people living with HIV in the world.[43] Approximately 7% of all sub-Saharan Africans and 15% of young women (15–24 years) in South Africa and Zimbabwe are living with HIV. Although the rates of HIV infection are stabilizing in certain parts of the African continent, they are on the rise in most parts of the south.[44]

In the United States, it was estimated that more than a million persons had HIV/AIDS in 2003. Among them, 417,000 persons were diagnosed with HIV infection, 415,000 were diagnosed with AIDS, and 252,000 to 312,000 (24% to 27%) carried HIV but were undiagnosed.[45] The CDC estimated that there are 40,000 new cases infected with HIV each year in the United States.[46] Under U.S. immigration laws, persons with AIDS/HIV and other communicable diseases of public health significance are not admissible to the United States and are not eligible for adjustment to lawful permanent resident status under "medical grounds of inadmissibility" with certain exceptions (e.g., humanitarian reasons, to assure family unity). For example, a refugee will not be denied adjustment to lawful permanent resident because of HIV infection, but he or she is required to identify a healthcare provider in the United States. HIV-positive children or a spouse of a U.S. citizen can file a request for waiver of the inadmissibility.[46] Although there is a lack of data on the number and percentage of immigrants with HIV/AIDS, certain states are concerned about HIV/AIDS among immigrants from Sudan, Ethiopia, and Laos, and among migrant workers.[47]

Obesity

The prevalence of obesity in the United States has increased dramatically in the past 20 years. In 1985, only 8 out of 20 states surveyed had obesity prevalence of 10% to 15%, the remaining 12 states had obesity prevalence below 10%, and no states had prevalence >15%. In 1995, no states had rates >20%, although most states had obesity prevalence at 15% to 19%. By 2005, however, all but 4 of the 50 states had obesity prevalence >20%, and 17 had a 25% prevalence and 3 states had a 30% prevalence.[48] These factors affect the health of immigrants as they become integrated into American society and have both additional health risks and advantages associated with their home countries.

The longer immigrants stay in the United States, the more likely they are to become obese.[49] The Sample Adult Module of the 2000 National Health Interview Survey showed that only 8% of immigrants living in the United States for less than 1 year were obese, but 19% of those living in the United States for 15 years or more were obese, approximating the rate of U.S.-born persons (22%).[49] Such a trend was not observed in immigrants of African origin,[49] although a recent study showed that body mass index (BMI) derived by actually measuring body weight and height (rather than by surveying) in African immigrants was positively correlated with their length of stay in the United States.[50] The prevalence of obesity among U.S.-born Asian Americans and Hispanic adolescents is more than twice that of those who came to the United States as immigrants.[51,52] Children from higher-income countries who arrived in the United States at 12 years of age or older tend to gain more weight than children of similar age from lower-income countries. Also, among children with lower SES from low-income countries, those who came to the United States at 12 years of age or older tend to gain more weight than those who came to the United States at 11 years of age or younger.[53] These facts suggest that environmental factors play an important role in the etiology of obesity.

Once obese, immigrants from countries of low obesity prevalence may be more vulnerable because of lack of awareness of the risks of diseases associated with obesity and lack of knowledge of preventive measures in a new environment. It has been shown that immigrants and foreign-born persons are less likely than U.S.-born persons to discuss diet and exercise with clinicians.[54] Lack of health insurance, inadequate language skills, lack of knowledge of U.S. healthcare and social services, and passive attitudes toward illness and treatment often make immigrants even more vulnerable to chronic diseases.[55] The longer they stay in the United States, the higher the risk for heart disease.[56] It is reported that Asian immigrants' life expectancy is lower than that of white American citizens, although life expectancy of immigrants from all countries is 3 to 4 years longer than white citizens.[57]

Cancer

2007 Cancer Statistics shows that cancer causes more deaths than heart disease in persons fewer than 85 years of age, despite recent progress in cancer control.[58] Stomach, liver, and cervical cancer mortality in Asian immigrants is significantly higher than in U.S.-born citizens. Asian immigrants tend to have lower mortality rates from lung, colorectal, breast, prostate, and esophageal cancers. However, as with obesity, the rate of cancer is positively correlated with length of stay in the United States such that the prevalence of many types of cancer increase similar to that for U.S.-born person within a generation among immigrants from Asia or Africa where incidence of some cancers is typically low.[59]

Early detection through appropriate screening and early intervention are critical to cancer control. Thus, it is important to reduce health disparities in screening and treatment rates between immigrants/foreign-born and U.S.-born populations. However, cancer screening is less likely to be sought by Asian Americans who immigrated to the United States more recently.[60] Compared with U.S.-born whites, foreign-born Hispanic and Asian Americans or Pacific Islanders are less likely to have Pap-smear examinations, fecal occult blood testing, or sigmoidoscopy. Foreign-born Asian Americans or Pacific Islanders are less likely to have been recommended mammography screening. The difference between U.S.-born and foreign-born persons' compliance with cancer screening measures is partially attributed to the difference in access to health care.[61]

The rate of compliance with cancer screening recommendations is also related to citizenship status. Noncitizen women are less likely to have a mammogram than U.S.-born women. Noncitizen Latinas are less likely to have Pap smears than U.S.-born Latinas.[60] Lack of acculturation is partly responsible for the differences because immigrants are more likely than nonimmigrants to deem Pap smears a private and invasive procedure and to prefer female gynecologists for medical care.[62] Outreach efforts should focus on helping immigrants understand the importance of cancer screening and ensuring access to follow-up diagnosis and treatment for positive tests. Family-centered approaches with qualified translators is very important to increase cancer screening among immigrants.[60]

Mental Health

Recent immigrants often have mental distress related to leaving their homes, difficulties adjusting to new environments, coping with traumatic experiences in their native countries, overcoming cultural and language barriers, and encountering discrimination.[63] Immigrants often are separated from family and support systems, including traditional community and religious supports. They may also face loss of income, traditions, values, and property. These difficulties are more prominent among immigrant children, women, the disabled, and the poor.[63]

Before coming to the United States, immigrants may have experienced extreme poverty, human trafficking, war, torture, and natural disasters. Some immigrant women and children have been exposed to rape, HIV/AIDS, and other sexually transmitted and infectious diseases. As a result, many suffer from depression, anxiety, and posttraumatic stress disorder.[63] The risk of suicide is high among immigrants.[63] Despite the hardships they face, immigrants are less likely to receive quality mental health care. More than 50% of immigrants and ethnic minorities in the United States with clinical depression received no diagnosis or treatment because of lack of health insurance or misdiagnosis resulting from culture and language problems or mistrust of health providers in the United States. Immigrant children and adolescents often leave school to work to support their families, resulting in limited educational attainment and emotional and behavioral problems.[63]

The prevalence of mental disorders among immigrants/foreign-born persons varies with ethnicity and country of origin. For example, foreign-born non-Hispanic black and Hispanic immigrant adults experience fewer symptoms of serious psychological distress than U.S.-born non-Hispanic black and Hispanics, respectively.[64] The prevalence of anxiety and depression is also lower in recent Russian immigrants than in the general U.S. population.[65] The prevalence of mental disorders is greater in descendants of immigrants than in the immigrants themselves. In the United States, the first-generation Caribbean black immigrants have a lower rate of psychiatric disorders than their U.S.-born children and grandchildren.[66] This might be related to increased exposure to minority status of later generations in the United States.[66]

Mortality and Life Expectancy among Immigrants

Singh and Siahpush showed that mortality was 18% and 13% lower among immigrant men and women, respectively, than U.S.-born men and women of similar ethnic backgrounds after adjusting for age between 1979 and 1989.[67] The lower mortality rates were more pronounced among younger and black and Hispanic immigrants.[67] Also, life expectancy of female and male immigrants was 3.4 and 2.5 years longer, respectively, than U.S.-born populations of similar ethnic composition.[57] The greater life expectancy was especially prominent in black immigrant men and women: 9.4 and 7.8 years longer, respectively, than U.S.-born black men and women.[57] However, Chinese, Japanese, and Filipino immigrants had lower life expectancies than the respective U.S.-born populations. Compared with U.S.-born Asians, Asian immigrants had higher stomach, liver, and cervical cancer mortality rates.[57] Another study showed that foreign-born blacks, Hispanics, Asians/Pacific Islanders, and whites had lower mortality risks when compared with U.S.-born whites of equivalent socioeconomic and demographic background.[68]

Infant Mortality

Despite the disadvantages of low socioeconomic status, less education, and language barriers, infant mortality and low-birth-weight rates are lower among Mexican and Cuban Americans than Whites.[69–71] This phenomenon is termed the *epidemiological paradox*[70,72,73] or *Latina paradox*.[74,75] When compared with Asian Indian immigrants, Hispanic/Latino immigrants also have lower rates in infant mortality and low birth weight, although they tend to have lower maternal education and access to prenatal care with private insurance than Asian Indians,[76] while there were no differences between foreign-born and U.S.-born Asian Indian mothers.[77] The Latina paradox is more pronounced among Mexico-born women than U.S.-born Mexican American women.[74] However, this "paradox" is not limited to Latinos. Infants of foreign-born black and Chinese mothers also have lower rates of mortality and/or low birth weight than those of native-born black and Chinese mothers, respectively, after controlling for potential confounders.[78–82] It should be noted that U.S.-born blacks and foreign-born blacks may or may not be of the same ethnicity because they are ethnically diverse.[83]

How do we explain the Latina paradox? Some attribute better birth outcomes in Latina immigrants to their unique social support systems of family, friends, community members, and lay health workers, which U.S.-born Latinos tended to lose.[74] Others propose "migrant selection" as an explanation, noting that the infant mortality rate is lower in recent migrant Puerto Rican families than families in Puerto Rico[84] and that the incidence of low birth weights in Latinas in the United States (6.5%) is much lower than in Mexico, Peru, Guatemala, Nicaragua, and El Salvador (9% to 13%).[74]

The advantage of foreign-born Hispanics/Latinos is observed not only in obesity and mortality rates but also in other disorders. A recent study of blood pressure and metabolic and inflammatory risk profiles of 4,206 adults aged 40 years and older found that U.S.-born Mexican Americans had higher biological risk scores than whites (all U.S.-born) and foreign-born Mexican Americans after controlling for SES. These findings suggest the role of health behaviors conditional on environment in the etiology and pathogenesis of many diseases.[85]

Access to Health Care among Immigrants

The rates of the uninsured among naturalized citizens, foreign-born persons, and noncitizens were 17.9% (2.5 million), 33.6%, and 43.6% (9.5 million), respectively, in 2005, much higher than the 13.4% uninsured rate among the U.S.-born population.[86] The high rate of uninsured persons among foreign-born persons and noncitizens was paralleled by the high poverty rate: 16.5% (5.9 million) of foreign-born population, compared with the poverty rate of 12.1% (31.1 million) among the U.S.-born population in 2005.[86] Poverty rates were 10.4% for naturalized citizens and 20.4% for noncitizens in 2005.[87] Approximately 73% of uninsured noncitizen adults are below 200% of the federal poverty level (FPL).[4]

In 1996, Congress passed the federal Welfare Reform Act that excluded immigrants from eligibility for Medicaid except for emergency care.[88] This law not only restricts Medicaid for undocumented immigrants but also for legal immigrants who arrived in the United States after August 1996 during the first five years of their residency. As a result, the percentage of low-income noncitizens enrolled in Medicaid declined from 19% in 1996 to 13% in 1998.[88] One in three foreign-born persons in the United States has no health insurance.[89] Nearly a third (6.7 of the 22.3 million) of foreign-born persons with health insurance are covered by government programs such as Medicaid and Medicare.[89]

Currently, emergency medical care is the only service universally covered in the United States regardless of immigration status. In North Carolina, 99% of patients who received emergency care reimbursed under Emergency Medicaid were undocumented; a majority were Hispanic women in labor or with complications of pregnancy. The remaining cases were related to injuries, severe acute complications of chronic diseases, and other acute emergencies.[90] In addition, low-income noncitizens were less likely to use emergency services than low-income citizens, regardless of health insurance coverage. Noncitizens with health insurance were less likely to use emergency services than insured citizens. Uninsured people receive less care and have worse outcomes of emergency care or newly diagnosed chronic diseases than the insured.[4]

The disparity in health insurance between foreign-born and native-born persons is more strongly correlated with differences in socioeconomic factors than country of birth. However, noncitizens, especially undocumented immigrants and their children, have reduced access to private and public nonemergency health care even when covered by health insurance, after adjusting for confounding factors such as socioeconomic status. This suggests that other factors, such as immigration status, racial/ethnic origin, and cultural factors may also play a role.[91]

Policies and Practices Intended to Eliminate Health Disparities among Immigrants

In response to the 1996 federal law that excludes immigrants from eligibility for Medicaid benefits, some states have used state funds to cover recent legal immigrants and undocumented children and pregnant women. As of 2004, 25 states had offered such coverage to provide essential services for immigrants.[92] A June 2007 report shows that 17 states have used state funds to cover some nonpregnant adult immigrants not eligible for Medicaid.[4]

Over a period of 10 years (1998–2007), there has been a significant reduction in the number of uninsured children in the United States because of the State Children's Health Insurance Program (SCHIP).[93] As of 2006, seven states (Vermont, New Jersey, Connecticut, Maryland, New Hampshire, West Virginia, and Massachusetts) had expanded their SCHIP eligibility to families at or below 300% of the FPL, covering almost all uninsured U.S. *citizen* children in these states.[94] Although the number of uninsured citizen children dropped, the percentage of low-income *immigrant* children increased since the enforcement of restriction of the eligibility of legal immigrants for Medicaid and CHIP by federal law. Approximately half of low-income immigrant children are uninsured.[93]

It was believed that reauthorization of SCHIP in 2008 would allow states to expand insurance coverage by public funds to legal immigrant children living in the United States less than 5 years and to women for their prenatal, delivery, and postpartum care, which may bring us closer to universal coverage for America's children.[94] This debate has become a focal point for philosophical differences in government's role in healthcare financing. Recently, Congress voted to expand the SCHIP by $35 billion over the next 5 years, covering 4 million children in addition to the 6.6 million who are already enrolled.[95] President Bush vetoed the bill, and opponents argue that the bill goes beyond the original intent of helping low-income children.[96]

Because the United States will continue to absorb a large number of immigrants, reducing health disparities between immigrant/foreign-born and U.S.-born populations is important to ensure the health and economic viability of society as a whole. The recent surge in legal and undocumented immigrants from developing countries makes the issue more pressing. Some believe that health disparities originate from social, political, and economic inequality, and it is critical to transform institutions, policies, and practices that cause health disparities.[97] These reforms may include substantial government investments in housing, child care, education, employment, medical care, and food access.[97] While economic justice might be a long-term goal, universal access to health care is considered more urgent and more realistic to reduce health disparities.[98,99] Providing an appropriate range of healthcare services for immigrants and other vulnerable populations remains a major challenge for the 21st century.

Cultural Proficiency among Healthcare Providers and Researchers

Language Services

According to the U.S. Census Bureau, 18% of the U.S. population speaks a language other than English at home.[100] Most immigrants have limited English proficiency. According to the 2000 Census, 21.3 million of the 31 million foreign-born persons speak English "less than very well," up from 13.9 million in 1990.[101] Language barriers in immigrants may result in incomplete or inaccurate information necessary for diagnosis and treatment. The federal government requires that providers offer all non-English-speaking patients free language assistance to ensure quality services. Federal funds from Medicaid and the SCHIP matching funds are used for oral and written translation services, which have improved the health of many immigrant families. However, some clinics and hospitals use unqualified interpreters, such as minor children, for translation. This may compromise accuracy of translation and should be avoided.[101]

A recent study found that pediatricians most frequently used patients' family members (70%) as interpreters.[102] Those in regions where persons with limited English proficiency are highly concentrated are even less likely to have trained interpreters for language services.[102] The U.S. federal government spent $267.6 million for interpretation services in 2002.[101] However, there are no data about the portion of the budget allocated to rural areas that serve large populations of immigrants. Health providers proficient in English and other languages, modern technologies, and qualified interpreters are needed in such areas to ensure quality health care to immigrants and foreign-born persons in general.

Cultures of Immigrants

Health providers in the United States often find themselves unable to gain cooperation from immigrants in medical treatment because of differences in language and culture. Newcomers are often suspicious of unfamiliar therapies. Understanding immigrant patients' cultures and respect for their beliefs is required for better outcomes.[103]

Culture is the "customary beliefs, social forms, and material traits of a racial, religious, or social group,"[104] which are typically passed on from one generation to another.[105] There is no unique immigrant culture; there are different cultural factors deriving from country of origin and/or race/ethnicity. The racial/ethnical classification by the Office of Management and Budget (OMB) has been said to "represent a political-social construct."[106] Because it is neither anthropologically nor scientifically based,[106] this classification has been controversial.[107] For example, Asian Indians and Chinese are different in history, culture, and physical appearances, and Latinos are of different racial/ethnic groups **(Table 13–6)**.[108]

Table 13–6 *Percentage of Ethnic Groups in Latin America*

Ethnic groups	Mestizo	Mulatto	Mixed	Amerindian	White	Black	Other
Mexico	60			30	9		1
Cuba		51			37	11	1*
Colombia	58	14			20	4	
Dominican Republic			73		16	11	
El Salvador	90			1	9		
Brazil	53.7	38.5				6.2	1.6
Peru	37			45	15		3‡
Guatemala	59.4**			40.6†			

*Chinese; ‡Blacks, Japanese, Chinese, and other; **Mestizo and European; †Indigenous peoples (Mayans) including K'iche (9.1%), Kaqchikel (8.4%), Mam (7.9%), Q'eqchi (6.3%), other Mayan (8.6%), others (0.3%).

Source: Central Intelligence Agency. *The World Factbook.* https://www.cia.gov/library/publications/the-world-factbook/docs/profileguide.html. Accessed September 30, 2007.

Cultures of Hispanics/Latinos[109,110]

More than 90% of Hispanics define themselves as being Roman Catholic, and the church has great influence on their daily lives and community affairs. *Family* usually refers to extended family that may include grandparents and grandchildren. Family ties and sense of community are usually strong and are believed to be an important factor in the better health outcomes among Hispanic immigrants, partially accounting for the Latina paradox.[74] The father or oldest male is generally in charge, although some cultures of Hispanics/Latinos are more matriarchal. Women are expected to respect their husbands, at least publicly. Family members have a moral responsibility to help each other deal with financial, health, and other problems. Healthcare providers should understand family dynamics and encourage family involvement in healthcare planning.

Recently, community-based medical practices and health-literacy education and research have become important approaches to health care. These approaches may better serve immigrant communities and other populations. Involvement of Hispanic community leaders in the planning, delivery, and evaluation can facilitate these efforts. It is often desirable to hold educational programs in churches, local libraries, and recreational centers.

Direct disagreement or confrontation is uncommon, and silence in a healthcare context is usually an expression of disagreement with a healthcare provider. As a result, healthcare providers may not accurately discern complaints or problems. Hispanics/Latinos often perceive failure in communication as prejudice and may not return. Clinicians should be aware that although most Hispanics are Catholic, many Latinas use contraception with or without their husbands' knowledge.[109]

Many health problems are considered as "hot" and "cold" conditions. Menstrual cramps, rhinitis, pneumonia, and colic are "cold" conditions, while pregnancy, hypertension, diabetes, acid indigestion are considered as "hot" problems. It is believed that "cold" conditions can be balanced by hot medications and vice versa.[109] While Hispanics may seek folk medication, most will not reject modern medications, such as antibiotics and high blood pressure medications. When sick, Hispanics tend to try home remedies (with herbs, spices, or fruits) first, followed by seeking help from herbalists, massage therapists, and midwives if home remedies do not work. Such practices may be more common among immigrants.

Among Latinas, breastfeeding is common among immigrants and for two generations of descendants. Many Mexican Americans believe that type 2 diabetes is caused by *susto* (fright), unhealthy lifestyle, and heredity. Some see diabetes as controlled by God, "while others believe that God gave them strength to cope with their illness."[111] Knowledge of various religious traditions and beliefs is important for physicians to understand the health-seeking behaviors of different groups.

The Chinese Cultures

Health providers should understand the culture and belief systems of immigrant or foreign-born Chinese patients in order to provide appropriate care. A psychiatrist may miss the diagnosis of depression when a Chinese immigrant's main complaints are discomfort, dizziness, or fatigue instead of sadness.[112] Chinese immigrants may find a diagnosis of depression unacceptable.[112] An obstetrician's recommendation to a Chinese woman to get outdoor exercise less than a month after giving birth may be met with resistance and disbelief because, after giving birth, the mother is supposed to stay home for a month ("sitting for the month"), according to Chinese belief.[113,114] Some would attribute subsequent illnesses to their failure to follow the postpartum rules.

There are 56 major ethnic groups in China, including Han (92%), Zhuang, Uygur, Hui, Yi, Tibetan, Miao, Manchu, Mongol, Buyi, Korean, and others.[115,116] Buddhism, Islam, and Christianity have been among the main religions, with Buddhism being the most ancient (more than 2,000 years old) and popular. Although most Chinese consider themselves as nonreligious,[117] believers and nonbelievers tend to share some Buddhist beliefs: reward for benevolence, punishment for malevolence; do not kill any form of life; vegetables are good and meats are bad for health.

However, Confucianism has been the predominant belief system since its founding by Qiu Kong (551–479 B.C.) also known as Kong Fuzi (Master Kong or Confucius).[118] Confucianism set a certain moral, social, and political standard for conduct. Accordingly, respect to elders and superiors and obedience to parents have been the norm in Chinese daily life. As a result, family ties are strong, and taking care of the elderly is an important moral responsibility among Chinese people. After coming to the United States, strong family ties are still observed. For example, in a recent study, older Chinese (most of them first-generation immigrants) in nursing homes in New York were found to be less likely to have lived alone and were more likely to depend on family members for decision making when compared with whites.[119]

The Chinese have a long history of traditional medicine that is very effective in treating many diseases. For example, they have used the antibiotic Berberine[120] since the Han dynasty (206 B.C.–220 A.D.). As a result, the theory and practice of traditional Chinese medicine have a great influence in Chinese health beliefs. Herbal medication and acupuncture are popular among Chinese immigrants in the United States. A recent study[120] showed that almost all Chinese patients in the United States had used traditional Chinese medicine for musculoskeletal or abdominal pain, fatigue, and health maintenance during the year prior to the study. Self-medication with herbal products was most common. However, few physicians had asked whether they had taken Chinese medicines. A large proportion of Chinese, including immigrants, believe that Western medicine is more efficient for treating acute conditions, while traditional Chinese medicine is superior in treating chronic illnesses.[121] Familiarity with health beliefs among Chinese immigrants is useful for health providers.

Common Traits among Immigrants

Immigrants, though of different cultures, have some things in common. As newcomers, immigrants and foreign-born persons are more likely to have limited English proficiency, different degrees of acculturation, and retain the strong influences of their original cultures. Undocumented immigrants may be reluctant to tell details of their personal profile for fear of deportation of themselves or their families. Sensitivity in dealing with immigrants and foreign-born persons is essential and requires special attention from health professionals.

Ethical, Legal and Social Implications of Research with Immigrants as Subjects

Many diseases are caused by genetic predispositions interacting with environmental factors. Certain diseases may occur in one environment but not in another.[122] For example, bone mineral density in Sudanese immigrants is positively correlated to their length of residence in the United States,[50] and life expectancy is generally higher in immigrants than in U.S.-born persons.[56] There is a growing interest among researchers in studying gene–environment interactions in immigrants. However, most immigrants are unfamiliar with American culture and the U.S. legal system. Many are economically and educationally disadvantaged, and might not be able to understand the complex scientific concepts in research projects and the potential risks and benefits involved. Some may have participated in research simply for the stipends, without adequately considering potential harms such as stigmatization. For example, researchers may attribute lower cognitive ability test scores in minorities to "biological inferiority" rather than educational or other environmental factors.[123] The Tuskegee experiment (1932–1972), sponsored by the U.S. Public Health Service, investigated the natural history of untreated syphilis using illiterate black men living in a poor rural Alabama town without their knowledge of the diagnosis or that there were effective treatments (no U.S. government officials apologized to the volunteers and their families for the unethical conducts until President Bill Clinton did so in 1997).[124]

Research on immigrants who do not fully understand the risks involved can be compared to the Tuskegee example, even though the immigrants may have signed a consent form. A recent study found that 35% of the 1,789 non-immigrant participants in a clinical trial could not recall the purpose of the trial, and close to 70% could not recall the main side-effect although they had signed the consent form.[125] It is alarming that participants of ethnic minority were more than two and half times more likely than whites to incorrectly tell the purposes of the trial.[125] Another study showed that those with less education had the poorest knowledge about the information conveyed in the consent form.[126] It would be more difficult for educationally disadvantaged immigrant participants to understand the purposes and risks involved in genetic research because even highly educated professionals such as physicians are not well informed about genetics and are often even misinformed.[127] Thus, genetic researchers should be extremely cautious in the process of obtaining informed consent from immigrant populations with low literacy rates, such as those from south Sudan where 90% of women are illiterate, a rate consistent with our impression from our recent studies.[50,128] It is essential to determine whether immigrants are fully informed when they sign consent forms to participate in research.

For several reasons, the Agency for Healthcare Research and Quality, Department of Health and Human Services, classifies immigrants as a vulnerable population[129] and the ethical, legal, and social implications of genetic studies with immigrants as subjects are under investigation.[130] Attention should also be given to the ethical, legal, and social implications in other medical research with immigrants as subjects. In the process of recruiting immigrants and obtaining their consent, it is very important for researchers to pay attention to cultural and language issues. It is advisable to work with immigrant community leaders in planning, design, and budgeting. In genetic research, education using lay language with the aid of graphic illustration such as video tapes should be a routine before obtaining consent from educationally disadvantaged immigrant participants.

SUMMARY

It is very important for policy makers, healthcare organizations, and professionals to address health disparities among immigrant populations in the United States. Immigrants represent a substantial portion of the population. Their health status significantly impacts the health status of the nation as a whole. Certain health conditions including transmissible diseases such as tuberculosis and hepatitis B are more prevalent among immigrants of certain ethnic groups. In the new environment of the United States, immigrants tend to lose their advantage such as healthier diet adopted in their original countries and tend to become obese, while the "Latina paradox" of lower infant mortality rate among Latino immigrants tends to disappear over time. Most immigrants have limited English proficiency which may result in incomplete or inaccurate information necessary for diagnosis and treatment. Immigrants are more likely to be uninsured and less likely to access primary and preventative health care. Cultural, language, and socioeconomic barriers often contribute to limited knowledge about prevention of diseases such as cancer screening and preventive measures for cardiovascular diseases. Providing effective, high-quality health care for immigrant populations requires using trained interpreters, developing cultural proficiency of healthcare personnel in addressing health disparities, understanding family dynamics, and encouraging family involvement in healthcare delivery. Involvement of community leaders is recommended in the planning, delivery, and evaluation of medical care delivery and health education and research.

REFERENCES

1. U.S. Department of Homeland Security, U.S. Citizenship and Immigration Services, Office of Citizenship, *Helping Immigrants Become New Americans: Communities Discuss the Issues*. Washington, DC, 2004. http://www.uscis.gov. Also see U.S. Census Bureau. http://quickfacts.census.gov/qfd/states/00000.html.
2. Passel JS. Background briefing prepared for task force on immigration and America's future. http://pewhispanic.org/files/reports/46.pdf. Accessed September 25, 2007.
3. Pew Hispanic Center. Estimates of the Unauthorized Migrant Population for States based on the March 2005 CPS. http://pewhispanic.org/files/factsheets/17.pdf. Accessed September 25, 2007.
4. Schwartz K, Artiga S. Health insurance coverage and access to care for low-income non-citizen adults. http://www.kff.org/uninsured/upload/7651.pdf. Accessed September 25, 2007.
5. Walker PF, Jaranson J. Refugee and immigrant health care. *Med Clin North Am.* 1999;83(4):1103–1120.
6. Velie EM, Shaw GM, Malcoe LH, et al. Understanding the increased risk of neural tube defect–affected pregnancies among Mexico-born women in California: Immigration and anthropometric factors. *Paediatr Perinat Epidemiol.* 2006;20(3):219–230.
7. Allen ML, Elliott MN, Morales LS, Diamant AL, Hambarsoomian K, Schuster MA. Adolescent participation in preventive health behaviors, physical activity, and nutrition: Differences across immigrant generations for Asians and Latinos compared with Whites. *Am J Public Health.* 2007;97(2):337–343.
8. U.S. Citizenship and Immigration Services. Glossary. http://www.uscis.gov/. Accessed September 27, 2007.
9. U.S. Census Bureau. http://www.census.gov/population/www/socdemo/immigration.html. Accessed September 27, 2007.

10. Schultz SK, Tishler WP. Foreign immigrants in industrial America. *American History 102: Civil War to the Present*. http://us.history.wisc.edu/hist102/lectures/lecture08.html. Accessed September 27, 2007.

11. Jefferys K. U.S. legal permanent residents: 2006. http://www.dhs.gov/xlibrary/assets/statistics/publications/IS-4496_LPRFlowReport_04vaccessible.pdf. Accessed September 27, 2007.

12. U.S. Department of Homeland Security. *2006 Yearbook of Immigration Statistics*. http://www.dhs.gov/ximgtn/statistics/publications/yearbook.shtm. Accessed September 27, 2007.

13. U.S. Census Bureau. Percent of people who are foreign born: 2005. http://factfinder.census.gov/servlet/ThematicMapFramesetServlet?_bm=y&-geo_id=01000US&-tm_name=ACS_2005_EST_G00_M00615&-ds_name=ACS_2005_EST_G00_&-_MapEvent=displayBy&-_dBy=040. Accessed September 27, 2007.

14. Capps R. Fix M, Passel, Ost J, Perez-Lopez D. A profile of the low-wage immigrant workforce.http://www.urban.org/UploadedPDF/310880_lowwage_immig_wkfc.pdf. Accessed September 25, 2007.

15. Immigration Studies. A program of the Urban Institute. http://www.urban.org/toolkit/issues/immigration.cfm#about#about. Accessed September 25, 2007.

16. Elmelech Y, McCaskie K, Lennon MC, Lu HH. Children of immigrants: A statistical profile. http://www.nccp.org/publications/pub_475.html. Accessed September 25, 2007.

17. Federation for American Immigration Reform. Immigration and poverty. http://www.fairus.org/site/PageServer?pagename=iic_immigrationissuecenters93c3. Accessed June 20, 2008.

18. Capps R, Fix M, Ost J, Reardon-Anderson J, Passel JS. The health and well-being of young children of immigrants. http://www.urban.org/UploadedPDF/311182_immigrant_families_5.pdf. Accessed September 25, 2007.

19. Capps R. Hardship among children of immigrants: Findings from the 1999 National Survey of America's Families. http://www.urban.org/UploadedPDF/anf_b29.pdf. Accessed September 25, 2007.

20. Haskins R. Federal policy for immigrant children: Room for common ground? *Future of Children Policy Brief*. Summer 2004. http://www.brookings.edu/es/research/projects/wrb/publications/pb/foc_14_2.htm. Accessed June 20, 2008.

21. U.S. Census Bureau. The Hispanic population. *Census Brief: 2000*. http://www.census.gov/prod/2001pubs/c2kbr01-3.pdf. Accessed September 25, 2007.

22. U.S. Census Bureau. The Asian population. *Census Brief: 2000*. http://www.census.gov/prod/2002pubs/c2kbr01-16.pdf. Accessed September 25, 2007.

23. Migration Policy Institute. Unauthorized immigration to the United States. http://www.migrationpolicy.org/pubs/two_unauthorized_immigration_us.pdf. Accessed September 25, 2007.

24. United Nations. Definition of the UNHCR, United Nations High Commissioner for Refugees. http://www.lnf.org.lb/migrationnetwork/definition.html#unrwa. Accessed June 20, 2008.

25. U.S. Department of State, Bureau of Population, Refugees, and Migration, January 18, 2000. http://www.state.gov/www/global/prm/admissions_resettle.html#fact; Refugee health—Immigrant health. Background on refugees. http://www3.baylor.edu/~Charles_Kemp/background_on_refugees.htm. Both accessed September 25, 2007.

26. Centers for Disease Control and Prevention. *Reported Tuberculosis in the United States, 2005*. Atlanta, GA: U.S. Department of Health and Human Services; Sep-

tember 2006. http://www.cdc.gov/tb/surv/surv2005/PDF/TBSurvFULLReport.pdf. Accessed September 25, 2007.

27. American Academy of Pediatrics. In: Pickering LK, Baker CJ, Long SS, McMillan JA, eds. *Red Book: 2006 Report of the Committee on Infectious Diseases.* 27th ed. Elk Grove Village, IL: American Academy of Pediatrics; 2006:679.

28. Centers for Disease Control and Prevention. Trends in tuberculosis incidence—United States, 2006. *MMWR.* 2007;56(11);245–250.

29. Centers for Disease Control and Prevention. Updates on the medical examination of aliens (refugees and immigrants). Required evaluation by civil surgeons for tuberculosis (TB). http://0-www.cdc.gov.mill1.sjlibrary.org/ncidod/dq/updates .htm. Accessed September 25, 2007.

30. Paterson R. Screening immigrants for infectious diseases. *Lancet Infect Dis.* 2003;3(11):681.

31. Brewin P, Jones A, Kelly M, et al. Is screening for tuberculosis acceptable to immigrants? A qualitative study. *J Public Health (Oxf).* 2006;28(3):253–260.

32. Levesque JF, Dongier P, Brassard P, Allard R. Acceptance of screening and completion of treatment for latent tuberculosis infection among refugee claimants in Canada. *Int J Tuberc Lung Dis.* 2004;8(6):711–717.

33. Carvalho AC, Saleri N, El-Hamad I, et al. Completion of screening for latent tuberculosis infection among immigrants. *Epidemiol Infect.* 2005;133(1):179–185.

34. World Health Organization. Hepatitis B. hhttp://www.who.int/mediacentre/ factsheets/fs204/en/. Accessed September 25, 2007.

35. Centers for Disease Control and Prevention. Screening for chronic hepatitis B among Asian/Pacific Islander populations—New York City, 2005. *MMWR.* 2006;55:505–509.

36. Centers for Disease Control and Prevention. Characteristics of persons with chronic hepatitis B—San Francisco, California, 2006. *MMWR.* 2007;56(18):446–448.

37. Centers for Disease Control and Prevention. Screening for Chronic Hepatitis B among Asian/Pacific Islander Populations—New York City, 2005. *MMWR.* 2006; 55(18):505–528. http://www.cdc.gov/mmwr/preview/mmwrhtml/mm5518a2.htm.

38. Waknine Y. Highlights from *MMWR*: Asian Immigrants at high risk for HBV infection and more. http://www.medscape.com/viewarticle/532289. Accessed May 29, 2007.

39. Centers for Disease Control and Prevention. Progress in Hepatitis B prevention through universal infant vaccination—China, 1997–2006, *MMWR.* 2—7;56(18): 441–445.

40. Wikipedia. Hepatitis B. http://en.wikipedia.org/wiki/Hepatitis_B. Accessed September 30, 2007.

41. American Academy of Pediatrics. Immunization in special clinical circumstances. In Pickering LK, Baker CJ, Long SS, McMillan JA ed. *Red Book: 2006 Report of the Committee on Infectious Diseases* 27th ed. Elk Grove Village, IL: American Academy of Pediatrics; 2006:96.

42. World Health Organization. HIV/AIDS. http://www.who.int/hiv/mediacentre/news60/ en/index.html. Accessed September 30, 2007.

43. United Nations. Sub-Saharan Africa, 2006 AIDS epidemic update. http://data .unaids.org/pub/EpiReport/2006/04-Sub_Saharan_Africa_2006_EpiUpdate _eng.pdf. Accessed September 30, 2007.

44. Ruben M. Scourge of a continent: The devastation of AIDS, HIV prevention policies, and the relief effort in Sub-Saharan Africa. http://www.csa.com/ discoveryguides/afraid/review.php#n2.

45. Glynn M, Rhodes P. Estimated HIV prevalence in the United States at the end of 2003. National HIV Prevention Conference; June 2005; Atlanta. Abstract T1-B1101. http://www.aegis.com/conferences/NHIVPC/2005/T1-B1101.html. Accessed May 30, 2007.

46. Centers for Disease Control and Prevention. Guidelines for national human immunodeficiency virus case surveillance, including monitoring for human immunodeficiency virus infection and Acquired Immunodeficiency Syndrome. *MMWR Recomm Rep.* 1999;48(RR-13):1–28.

47. Centers for Disease Control and Prevention. Immigrant, refugee and migrant health. http://www.cdc.gov/ncidod/dq/refugee/. Accessed September 30, 2007.

48. Centers for Disease Control and Prevention. U.S. obesity trends 1985–2005. http://www.cdc.gov/nccdphp/dnpa/obesity/trend/maps/. Accessed September 30, 2007.

49. Goel MS, McCarthy EP, Phillips RS, Wee CC. Obesity among US immigrant subgroups by duration of residence. *JAMA.* 2004;292(23):2860–2867.

50. Gong G, Haynatzki G, Haynatzka V, et al. Bone mineral density of recent African immigrants in the United States. *J Natl Med Assoc.* 2006;98(7):746–752.

51. Popkin BM, Udry JR. Adolescent obesity increases significantly in second and third generation U.S. immigrants: The national longitudinal study of adolescent health. *J Nutr.* 1998;128(4):701–706.

52. Cho J, Juon H-S. Assessing overweight and obesity risk among Korean Americans in California using world health organization body mass index criteria for Asians. *Prev Chronic Dis.* 2006;3(3):A79.

53. Van Hook J, Balistreri KS. Immigrant generation, socioeconomic status, and economic development of countries of origin: a longitudinal study of body mass index among children. *Soc Sci Med.* 2007;65(5):976–989.

54. Goel MS, McCarthy EP, Phillips RS, Wee CC. Obesity among US immigrant subgroups by duration of residence. *JAMA.* 2004;292(23):2860–2867.

55. Flaskerud JH, Kim S. Health problems of Asian and Latino immigrants. *Nurs Clin North Am.* 1999;34(2):359-380.

56. Mooteri SN, Petersen F, Dagubati R, Pai RG. Duration of residence in the United States as a new risk factor for coronary artery disease (The Konkani Heart Study). *Am J Cardiol.* 2004;93(3):359–361.

57. Singh GK, Miller BA. Health, life expectancy, and mortality patterns among immigrant populations in the United States. *Can J Public Health.* 2004;95(3):I14–I21.

58. Jemal A, Siegel R, Ward E, Murray T, Xu J, Thun MJ. Cancer statistics, 2007. *CA Cancer J Clin.* 2007;57(1):43–66.

59. Sandler RS. Epidemiology and risk factors for colorectal cancer. *Gastroenterol Clin North Am.* 1996;25(4):717–735.

60. Wong ST, Gildengorin G, Nguyen T, Mock J. Disparities in colorectal cancer screening rates among Asian Americans and non-Latino whites. *Cancer.* 2005;104(12 Suppl):2940–2947.

61. Goel MS, Wee CC, McCarthy EP, Davis RB, Ngo-Metzger Q, Phillips RS. Racial and ethnic disparities in cancer screening: the importance of foreign birth as a barrier to care. *J Gen Intern Med.* 2003;18(12):1028–1035.

62. Echeverria SE, Carrasquillo O. The roles of citizenship status, acculturation, and health insurance in breast and cervical cancer screening among immigrant women. *Med Care.* 2006;44(8):788-792.

63. American Psychological Association. The mental health needs of immigrants. http://www.apa.org/ppo/ethnic/immigranthealth.html. Accessed September 30, 2007.

64. Dey AN, Lucas JW. Physical and mental health characteristics of U.S.- and foreign-born adults: United States, 1998–2003. *Adv Data.* 2006;369:1–19.
65. Hoffmann C, McFarland BH, Kinzie JD, et al. Psychological distress among recent Russian immigrants in the United States. *Int J Soc Psychiatry.* 2006;52(1):29–40.
66. Williams DR, Haile R, González HM, Neighbors H, Baser R, Jackson JS. The mental health of Black Caribbean immigrants: results from the National Survey of American Life. *Am J Public Health.* 2007;97(1):52–59.
67. Singh GK, Siahpush M. All-cause and cause-specific mortality of immigrants and native born in the United States. *Am J Public Health.* 2001;91(3):392–399.
68. Singh GK, Siahpush M. Ethnic-immigrant differentials in health behaviors, morbidity, and cause-specific mortality in the United States: An analysis of two national databases. *Hum Biol.* 2002;74(1):83–109.
69. Becerra JE, Hogue CJ, Atrash HK, Pérez N. Infant mortality among Hispanics. A portrait of heterogeneity. *JAMA.* 1991;265(16):2065–2066.
70. Scribner RA. Infant mortality among Hispanics: the epidemiological paradox. *JAMA.* 1991;265(2):217–221.
71. James SA. Racial and ethnic differences in infant mortality and low birthweight. A psychosocial critique. *Ann Epidemiol.* 1993;3(2):130–136.
72. Fuentes-Afflick E, Lurie P. Low birthweight and Latino ethnicity. Examining the epidemiologic paradox. *Arch Pediatr Adolesc Med.* 1997;151(7):665–674.
73. Fuentes-Afflick E, Hessol NA, Perez-Stable EJ. Testing the epidemiologic paradox of low birthweight in Latinos. *Arch Pediatr Adolesc Med.* 1999;153(2):147–153.
74. McGlade MS, Saha S, Dahlstrom ME. The Latina paradox: an opportunity for restructuring prenatal care delivery. *Am J Public Health.* 2004;94(12):2062–2065.
75. Hessol NA, Fuentes-Afflick E. The perinatal advantage of Mexican-origin Latina women. *Ann Epidemiol.* 2000;10:516–523.
76. Gould JB, Madan A, Qin C, Chavez G. Perinatal outcomes in two dissimilar immigrant populations in the United States: a dual epidemiologic paradox. *Pediatrics.* 2003;111(6 Pt 1):e676–e682.
77. Palaniappan L, Urizar G, Wang Y, Fortmann SP, Gould JB. Sociocultural factors that affect pregnancy outcomes in two dissimilar immigrant groups in the United States. *J Pediatr.* 2006;148(3):341–346.
78. Rosenberg KD, Desai RA, Kan J. Why do foreign-born blacks have lower infant mortality than native-born blacks? New directions in African-American infant mortality research. *J Natl Med Assoc.* 2002;94(9):770–778.
79. Singh GK, Yu SM. Adverse pregnancy outcomes: differences between US- and foreign-born women in major US racial and ethnic groups. *Am J Public Health.* 1996;86(6):837–843.
80. Liu KL, Laraque F. Higher mortality rate among infants of US-born mothers compared to foreign-born mothers in New York City. *J Immigr Minor Health.* 2006;8 (3):281–289.
81. Salihu HM, Mardenbrough-Gumbs WS, Aliyu MH, et al. Influence of nativity on neonatal survival of Black twins in the United States. *Ethn Dis.* 2005;15 (2):276–282.
82. Forna F, Jamieson DJ, Sanders D, Lindsay MK. Pregnancy outcomes in foreign-born and US-born women. *Int J Gynaecol Obstet.* 2003;83(3):257–265.
83. Kosoko-Lasaki O, Gong G, Haynatzki G, Wilson MR. Race, ethnicity and prevalence of primary open angle glaucoma. *J Natl Med Assoc.* 2006;98:1626–1629.

84. Landale NS, Oropesa RS, Gorman BK. Migration and infant death: assimilation or selective migration among Puerto Ricans? *Am Soc Rev*. 2000;65(6):888–909.

85. Crimmins EM, Kim JK, Alley DE, Karlamangla A, Seeman T. Hispanic paradox in biological risk profiles. *Am J Public Health*. 2007;97:1305–1310.

86. DeNavas-Walt C, Proctor BD, Lee CH. Income, poverty, and health insurance coverage in the United States: 2005. http://www.census.gov/prod/2006pubs/p60-231.pdf. Accessed September 30, 2007.

87. U.S. Census Bureau News. U.S. Department of Commerce. Income climbs, poverty stabilizes, uninsured rate increases. http://www.census.gov/Press-Release/www/releases/archives/income_wealth/007419.html. Accessed September 30, 2007.

88. Ku L. Matani S. Left out: Immigrants' access to health care and insurance. *Health Affairs (Millwood)*. 2001;20(1):247–256.

89. The Migration Policy Institute. Health insurance coverage of the foreign born in the United States: Numbers and trends. http://www.migrationpolicy.org/pubs/eight_health.pdf. Accessed September 30, 2007.

90. DuBard CA, Massing MW. Trends in emergency Medicaid expenditures for recent and undocumented immigrants. *JAMA*. 2007;297(10):1085–1092.

91. Goldman DP, Smith JP, Sood N. Legal status and health insurance among immigrants. *Health Affairs (Millwood)*. 2005;24(6):1640–1653.

92. Kaiser Family Foundation. Medicaid and the uninsured. http://www.kff.org/uninsured/upload/Health-Coverage-for-Immigrants-Fact-Sheet.pdf. Accessed September 30, 2007.

93. Ku L. Reducing disparities in health coverage for legal immigrant children and pregnant women. http://www.cbpp.org/4-20-07health2.pdf. Accessed August 30, 2007.

94. Berman S. State children's health insurance program reauthorization: Will it get us closer to universal coverage for America's children? *Pediatrics*. 2007;119(4):823–825.

95. Babington C. House votes to expand insurance for kids. *The Washington Post*. September 25, 2007. http://www.washingtonpost.com/wp-dyn/content/article/2007/09/25/AR2007092502287.html?tid=informbox. Accessed September 30, 2007.

96. Lee C, Weisman J. House passes children's health bill: Despite strong Republican support, threatened veto will probably stand. *Washington Post*. September 26, 2007:A04.

97. Plough A. Promoting social justice through public health policies, programs, and services. In: Richard Hofrichter ed. *Tackling Health Inequities Through Public Health Practice: A Handbook for Action*. 2006:77. http://www.naccho.org/topics/justice/documents/NACCHO_Handbook_hyperlinks_000.pdf. Accessed October 1, 2007.

98. Trotochaud K. Ethical issues and access to healthcare. *J Infusion Nurs*. 2006;29(3):165–170.

99. Daniels N. Rescuing universal health care. *Hastings Cent Rep*. 2007;37(2):3.

100. U.S. Census Bureau. *State & County QuickFacts*. http://quickfacts.census.gov/qfd/states/00000.html. Accessed September 30, 2007.

101. National Conference of State Legislatures. Immigrant Policy Project. Language access: Giving immigrants a hand in navigating the health care system. http://www.ncsl.org/programs/immig/SHNarticle.htm. Accessed September 30, 2007.

102. Kuo DZ, O'Connor KG, Flores G, Minkovitz CS. Pediatricians' use of language services for families with limited English proficiency. *Pediatrics*. 2007;119(4): e920–e927.

103. Kraut AM. Healers and strangers. Immigrant attitudes toward the physician in America—A relationship in historical perspective. *JAMA*. 1990;263(13): 1807–1811.

104. *Merriam-Webster Dictionary*, http://www.m-w.com/dictionary/culture.

105. Lipson JG. Culturally competent nursing care. In: Lipson JG, Dibble SL, Minarik PA, eds. *Culture & Nursing Care*. San Francisco: UCSF Nursing Press; 1996:1–6.

106. Office of Management and Budget, Office of Information and Regulatory Affairs. Recommendations from the interagency committee for the review of the racial and ethnic standards to the Office of Management and Budget concerning changes to the standards for the classification of federal data on race and ethnicity. http://www.census.gov/population/www/socdemo/race/Directive_15.html. Accessed June 20, 2008.

107. American Anthropological Association. Response to OMB Directive 15: Race and ethnic standards for federal statistics and administrative reporting. http://www.aaanet.org/gvt/ombdraft.htm. Accessed September 30, 2007.

108. Central Intelligence Agency. *The World Factbook*. https://www.cia.gov/library/publications/the-world-factbook/docs/profileguide.html. Accessed September 30, 2007.

109. Kemp C. Mexican & Mexican-Americans: Health beliefs and practices. http://www3.baylor.edu/~Charles_Kemp/hispanic_health.htm. Accessed June 20, 2008.

110. Ohio State University. Fact sheet, family and consumer sciences. http://ohioline.osu.edu/hyg-fact/5000/5237.html. Accessed September 30, 2007.

111. Caban A, Walker EA. A systemic review of research on culturally relevant issues for Hispanic with diabetes. *Diabetes Educator*. 2006;32(4):584–594.

112. Kleinman A. Culture and depression. *N Engl J Med*. 2004;351(10):951–952.

113. Chinese cultural beliefs related to pregnancy, birth and post partum care. http://www.hawcc.hawaii.edu/nursing/RNChinese02.html. Accessed September 30, 2007.

114. Wikipedia. Childbirth. http://en.wikipedia.org/wiki/Childbirth. Accessed September 30, 2007.

115. People's Daily Online. China's ethnic minorities. http://english.people.com.cn/data/minorities/ethnic_minorities.html. Accessed September 30, 2007.

116. Central Intelligence Agency. *The World Factbook*. https://www.cia.gov/library/publications/the-world-factbook/geos/ch.html#People. Accessed September 30, 2007.

117. Wikipedia. People's Republic of China. http://en.wikipedia.org/wiki/People's_Republic_of_China. Accessed September 30, 2007.

118. *Stanford Encyclopedia of Philosophy*. Confucius. http://plato.stanford.edu/entries/confucius/. Accessed September 30, 2007.

119. Huang ZB, Neufeld RR, Likourezos A, et al. Sociodemographic and health characteristics of older Chinese on admission to a nursing home: a cross-racial/ethnic study. *J Am Geriatr Soc*. 2003;51(3):404–409.

120. Shen Nong's Herbal (_____). http://bk.baidu.com/view/15091.htm. Accessed September 30, 2007.

121. Wu AP, Burke A, LeBaron S. Use of traditional medicine by immigrant Chinese patients. *Fam Med*. 2007;39(3):195-200.

122. González Burchard E, Borrell LN, Choudhry S, et al. Latino populations: A unique opportunity for the study of race, genetics, and social environment in epidemiological research. *Am J Public Health*. 2005;95(12):2161–2168.

123. Brown RP, Day EA. The difference isn't black and white: Stereotype threat and the race gap on Raven's Advanced Progressive Matrices. *J Appl Psychol*. 2006;91(4):979-985.

124. Public Broadcasting System. An apology 65 years late. http://www.pbs.org/newshour/bb/health/may97/tuskegee_5-16.html. Accessed September 30, 2007.

125. Griffin JM, Struve JK, Collins D, Liu A, Nelson DB, Bloomfield HE. Long term clinical trials: How much information do participants retain from the informed consent process? *Contemp Clin Trials*. 2006;27(5):441–448.

126. Kucia AM, Horowitz JD. Is informed consent to clinical trials an "upside selective" process in acute coronary syndromes? *Am Heart J*. 2000;140(1):94–97.

127. Kegley JA. An ethical imperative: Genetics education for physicians and patients. *Med Law*. 2003;22(2):275–283.

128. Gong G, Haynatzki G, Haynatzka V, et al. Bone mineral density–affecting genes in Africans. *J Natl Med Assoc*. 2006;98(7):1102–1108.

129. QualityTools. Glossary. Vulnerable populations. http://www.qualitytools.ahrq.gov/resources/glossary.aspx#tool. Accessed September 30, 2007.

130. U. S. Department of Health and Human Services. http://grants.nih.gov/grants/guide/pa-files/PA-07-277.html. Accessed September 30, 2007.

Chapter 14

Minority Attitudes and Perception of Health Care: A Comparison of Comments from a Cultural Competency Questionnaire and Focus Group Discussion

Cynthia T. Cook, PhD

Research documents the disparities that exist among ethnic and racial minorities in the United States.[1] Research also indicates that many Native Americans,[2-8] African Americans,[5,6,9-15] and Hispanic Americans[5,6,14,15] do not trust healthcare providers or the healthcare delivery system, do not have health insurance[1] and are reluctant to participate in health care research.[2,4,5,6,8,16] To better understand the healthcare concerns of Nebraska's minorities, a healthcare questionnaire was administered,[16] and focus groups were conducted in Omaha, Nebraska, during the summer and fall of 2003 as part of a cultural proficiency study supported by the Nebraska Tobacco Settlement funds.

The main purpose of the study was to give local residents the opportunity to express their concerns regarding health care in the Omaha community. A second objective was to build a bridge between the Creighton University Medical Center (CUMC) and local community organizations in order to increase the number of ethnic and racial minorities that participate in healthcare research. An unintended consequence of the research indicated that the *Hawthorne effect*[17] may have been operating: respondents were reluctant to express their bad experiences with health care on the questionnaire because the study personnel were directly or indirectly affiliated with those institutions. However, during the focus group discussion, the respondents indicated that they had had many unfavorable experiences with healthcare providers in the Omaha area, which included the institution conducting the study.

Research Design

Hypothesis

The design of the study and the results have been previously detailed.[16,18,19] In this paper we discuss the hypothesis that minority groups will be more willing to express their negative experiences with healthcare providers when among members of their own racial/ethic group. We compare the results of the administered questionnaire with the verbal comments from the focus group discussions that immediately followed the administration of the questionnaire.

Data Collection/Focus Group Recruitment

Key community organizations representing the Native American, Sudanese, Hispanic, Vietnamese, African American, and whites were contacted and asked to host a study session (see **Table 14–1** dates and size of focus groups). Hosting required the use of their neighborhood facility, provision of refreshments, and recruitment of 10 participants. To ensure 10 participants at each study session, we solicited confirmation from at least 12 potential participants. All participants who arrived at the designated site were included in the study. The only requirement for participation was that the participant had visited a healthcare provider in the Omaha area within 12 months preceding the session.

All members of the focus group were asked to complete a questionnaire before participating in the group discussion. The questionnaire asked about the cultural competency of their healthcare providers, use of folk or traditional medicine, need for interpreters, respondent's knowledge about the healthcare needs of his/her ethnic/racial group, and his or her willingness to participate in healthcare research.[16]

Table 14–1 *Administration of Focus Group by Race/Ethnicity, Number, and Date*

Racial/Ethnic	Number	Date
Native American	13	August 20, 2003
Sudanese men	10	September 10, 2003
Hispanic men	8	September 17, 2003
African American	12	September 22, 2003
Sudanese women	7	September 29, 2003
Hispanic women	12	October 1, 2003
Vietnamese	10	November 9, 2003
White	8	November 24, 2003
Total	**80**	

If the focus group's first language was not English, the host organization was responsible for providing interpreters. However, CUMC provided the interpreters for the Hispanic and Vietnamese groups; these persons were employed by the medical center. The interpreters stood next to the CU study presenter/organizer and focus group facilitator (an African American professor from University of Nebraska at Omaha) and translated every sentence to ensure consistency among all the study groups. Bilingual staff members affiliated with the host organization were also available to provide additional assistance to respondents. The Sudanese women's and men's groups presented the greatest challenge; interpreters were needed for the Nuer, Dinka, and Arabic languages.

At the beginning of each study session, respondents were given an overview regarding the purpose of the study and asked to sign a consent form. When all consent forms had been collected, the questionnaire was distributed. Respondents were given approximately 30 minutes to complete the questionnaire. After the questionnaires were collected, the facilitator began the focus group discussion.

There was no set format for the focus group discussion; the facilitator attempted to build rapport with the participants to enable them to speak more openly about their healthcare experiences. The discussion time was limited to approximately 1 hour because all focus groups were held in the late afternoon or early evening and their facilities were being kept open after normal hours. However, the Sudanese and white focus groups were held at CUMC. In addition, the women's Sudanese group had to be moved to another location because they exceeded the time limit for the use of the room, and two of the Arabic-speaking males were relocated to the cafeteria to complete the questionnaire while the male Sudanese discussion began.

The white group presenter was a white female, affiliated with CUMC. This is the only group in which consistency of presentation was not maintained. The original female presenter, a local African American, had moved out of state. The white group was added as a reference group for the study; they were not part of the original research design and will not be discussed in this paper.

Respondents were paid $50 for travel expenses. The host organization was compensated $250 for its assistance. Creighton University Institutional Review Board (IRB) approval was obtained for both the administration of the questionnaire and the focus group. No audio-video equipment was used; all focus groups were recorded and transcribed by the same transcriptionist.

Results

The demographic characteristics have been detailed in a previous publication.[16] In summary, the Hispanics and Sudanese had the largest groups because separate focus groups were convened for men and women, while the smallest was the white group. The total sample size was 80; 43.8% were men and 55% women. Fifty-one percent of the respondents were married, but none of the African Americans were. The data also indicated that more women were married than men.

The participants ranged in age from 18 to 80. However, more than 50% of the respondents were in their 30s or 40s, and 32% had no children living at home under age 19. With respect to education, five individuals did not answer this question or said "none." *None* is interpreted as "no formal education." One man had a doctorate, two respondents had master's degrees, and seven respondents had bachelor's degrees. The majority of the respondents had a high school education or more. All of the African Americans were high school graduates; more than half had some college or a college degree.

English was not the first language for the majority of the respondents. Non-English languages spoken included Arabic, Dinka, and Nuer (Sudanese languages); Dakotaxh (a Native American language); Spanish; and Vietnamese. Twenty-four, or 53%, of the non-English-speaking population had less than a high school education in comparison to only three, or 10%, of the English-speaking population.[16,19]

Although the study was conducted by personnel affiliated with Creighton University Medical Center, only 52 (65%) of the respondents had been treated by a CUMC provider. In addition, only 33 (43%) said the last visit to a healthcare provider was at a CUMC facility or provider. The results of these focus group discussions are not indicative of the care received at CUMC specifically, but the Omaha medical community generally.

Native Americans

The Native American group consisted of 13 respondents. Only three had not completed high school; the rest were high school graduates, and six had some college. Seven of the 13 said the last healthcare provider they visited was not affiliated with CUMC. Only four said they went to the emergency room on their last visit to a provider; all others went to the clinic or doctor's office. Twelve of the 13 rated the care they received from doctors as adequate or better. In fact, 9 said it was good or excellent, and 11 said if they got sick again they would visit the same healthcare provider. Based on the data collected on the questionnaire, the respondents were satisfied with healthcare providers within the Omaha community. However, during the focus group discussion when the facilitator asked about quality of care, one person said that the quality of care depended on what you were going for: "if you're dying maybe they will see you, but if you have a broken finger or broken arm you will have to wait a long time."

When asked about treatment by doctors, the comments included the following:

"Some doctors treat you professionally and do not talk down to you."

". . . doctors talk down to you . . . They do not communicate well with minorities. You are stereotyped if you are Black, Hispanic or Native American, it doesn't matter."

"Doctors blame you for the disease. They always ask if you have been drinking or how much do you drink before they ask you anything about what is wrong with you."

"If you don't have insurance you are treated badly."

"Doctors disrespect Indian men, it is like Cowboys and Indians, and we are the Indians. We are not treated like Americans."

"Indian healing ceremonies are warm and caring, everyone wants to help you get better, but the 'White Man's medicine' is very cold and insensitive."

"You go to the office, and they ask you what is wrong with you, but you don't know what is wrong with you. They have you drop your pants; they stick you in the butt and push you out the door. That's it! All our older people stay away from the doctor's office. They feel embarrassed. My father, for example would not go to the doctor's office, because every time he would go, they would embarrass him. We as Native Americans need the White man's medicine but they could be more respectful."

These comments indicated that our respondents have had negative experience with healthcare providers, but only one rated the care below adequate at last visit.

When we asked discussants about the cultural sensitivity of their healthcare providers, the comments were:

"Doctors don't recognize the value of Indian medicine."

"Older folks have their own ways of healing themselves. They (White man) took that knowledge away from us."

"Doctors feel that everything stems from alcohol. I don't like it when it is the first thing they ask you is 'Do you drink or when was the last time you had a drink or took some drugs.' They think that Native Americans just want drugs, that you are not really sick."

"They still don't tell you anything. My daughter had a broken leg and a young doctor told us it was just a sprain. We took her to an older doctor and he said that her leg was broken in two places."

"You just get a bunch of pills. But many people don't take them."

"I have been coming to this clinic for 27 years. They tell me that I have diabetes. So I asked the doctor 'Why am I diabetic?' After all this time, no one has explained it to me. He will not explain what caused it. He said that diet doesn't cause it; he said pancreas fails but he can't explain why the pancreas failed. I asked him why but I do not get any answers."

"Need to provide more education about illnesses. We need more information on how to treat ourselves."

These responses indicate that the discussants perceive healthcare providers as being culturally insensitive to the healthcare needs of the Native American population. However, only 2 of the 13 Native Americans said in the survey that they were not comfortable with the healthcare providers' medical knowledge of their illness; and only 4 said they did not think the healthcare provider was familiar enough with their cultural background to treat someone from their ethic/racial group. The survey data imply satisfaction with healthcare providers; but the focus group discussion indicates that Native Americans believe they do not get good health care, and that they are stereotyped (e.g., Native Americans have a drinking problem).

The discrepancy between the survey data and the focus group may be related to problems with doctor/patient communication. The Native Americans had this to say about communication:

"When I go to clinics out West and I know they do not see Native Americans very often, so I tell the doctors upfront what my health needs are. I speak up because I know they do not know. But I know a lot of people won't do that."

"You are misdiagnosed and given pills."

"I always ask the doctor to explain all new medication to me or I will not take them. She gives me an explanation."

"Every time I go to the doctor he wants me to restrict my coffee. He says drink decaffeinated. But then another doctor tells me that the chemicals they use to decaffeinate coffee are not good for you. So which is better? Why should I drink something that has chemicals in it?"

Only 1 of the 13 participants in our survey indicated that he required the use of an interpreter. This was an elderly man who was legally blind. The complaints regarding communication are not unique to Native Americans (as we will see later with our other focus groups), although they may have the perception that they are the only ones getting "bad medicine."

The majority of discussants answered yes when asked if they felt they had to assimilate into the American culture; however, on the survey 12 respondents answered no to feeling uncomfortable because they talked, dressed, or looked different, and all 13 answered no when asked if they felt pressured to behave or act different when visiting a healthcare provider. However, two Native Americans said they felt pressured to accept treatment or therapy that they did not want. The contradictory responses may have to do with the respondents getting their present health care at a Native American clinic. The survey data asked about treatment in the last 12 months, but our respondents discussed their overall experience with healthcare providers. Comments regarding assimilation include:

"Native American people are not asked to be a part of America. America looks at all Native Americans and lumps us all together. It's political. We are not considered a part of America so how can we assimilate."

"We as Native Americans are different from whites."

"A study says drink cow's milk, I drank cow's milk all my life, but it does not benefit the Native American. Maybe there are other things our bodies cannot tolerate. What are some other foods as a group that we should not eat because our diet has changed from traditional foods?"

"Treatment is not related to the Native American culture. Native American need to participate more in health care."

"Need more programs for Native Americans especially diabetes."

The purpose of our survey and focus group was to ascertain why Native Americans and other minorities did not participate in healthcare research that could be used to reduce health disparities. When our focus group was asked what type of health studies they would participate in, they said:

"Diabetes because it is the number one killer of Native Americans."

"It depends on the study . . . I know a friend who had to take some pills. They paid people $1000 for the study. The medication had adverse effects. The side effects were bad. I don't see any good in that."

"We need more educational programs on diabetes—basic education. . . ."

"I went to emergency room with bronchitis and a back problem. They did not care about my back problem. They said that I had to come back to get treated for that. I only go to the emergency room when something is real bad because I hate doctors . . . they don't treat what you need help for. They will only deal with one thing at a time."

"When you go the first thing they ask is do you have insurance? I don't have insurance so I go to the Native American hospital for medical needs every month. They give me a big bag of pills. Sometimes I don't take them."

"There is a difference between the ways that you are treated on the reservation versus the city. I had a 70% blockage in my neck. The doctor told me to have the nurse schedule me for some tests. The nurse asks me if I had insurance. I said no. So she said that they had to reschedule me for the tests. I never got a call. So I went to the reservation."

"Medicine is expensive so I always ask for supplements."

"When I go to the clinic, I get a different doctor each time, and a different diagnosis each time for the same thing. Then I get different drugs. I have gotten reactions to some of the medication."

"We get 'band-aid' services."

"You don't get help without insurance. You are sent back to the reservation."

"Reservation services are different from urban. You will not get 100% of the services if you are urban."

The survey did not ask if respondents received their health care on the reservation. When the facilitator asked where the discussants got their health care, one or two people said emergency room and the Fred LeRoy Indian

Health Center and Wellness Center operated by the Ponca Tribe of Nebraska. Perhaps this is the reason the majority of respondents said they were satisfied with their last visit to a healthcare provider but had had bad experiences with providers not affiliated with the reservation clinic.

When the facilitator asked if the participants would take medication that was offered by a Native American doctor, one respondent said "No, I would not . . . if the researcher would take the drugs also then maybe I would." On the survey, nine respondents said they would say yes if asked to participate in a healthcare study, only three said no, and one said he didn't know. One of the three who said no offered an explanation. He said he would not take the meds unless they had been approved by the FDA.

In summary, although our respondents indicated on the questionnaire that they were satisfied with health care, many of them have had negative experience with healthcare providers. We can assume that the Hawthorne effect was operating; respondents were reluctant to say anything negative on paper as a result of being asked to participate in the study, and perhaps the promise of $50. However, during the focus group, the Hawthorne effect had disappeared; respondents were candid about their negative experience with health care.

African Americans

Six men and five women were recruited to participate in the African American focus group. None of the subjects were married, although many were divorced or separated, and all were high school graduates. One respondent had a bachelor's degree, and a second a master's degree. All of the African Americans except one rated the doctor care at last visit as adequate or better. One person rated the nursing care as below adequate. All of the African Americans except one said they would want to see the same healthcare provider the next time they were ill. Overall, based on the survey, African Americans appear satisfied with the Omaha healthcare system. However, because the study was conducted by Creighton University Medical Center, they may have assumed that we wanted them to rate CUMC.

The facilitator asked the discussants about the quality of care they received at healthcare facilities. Their comments were:

"It depends on the hospital and where you are going. With St. Joe (Creighton University), it is terrible. You sit 1½ hours and more to wait to see someone."

"It is filling out lots of paperwork—that turns you off. You know what is going to happen."

"After many years of bad care, I now have a good private doctor. She takes time to answer all my questions. I do not have to wait a long time."

"A particular doctor at St. Joe is good. She diagrams and answers all your questions."

The respondents are discussing the care they received at Creighton Clinics and St. Joseph Hospital, the CUMC inpatient facility. When the participants were asked where they got their health care, many of them said Family Medicine, St. Joe's, University Hospital (University of Nebraska Medical Center or UNMC), and private doctors. It should be noted that the presenter knew many of the participants who participated in this focus group; one was her brother. The facilitator was also an African American political science professor at University of Nebraska at Omaha, with roots in the community. These participants were comfortable with one another, the presenter, and the facilitator.

The facilitator asked about written forms, and the discussants said:

"If you are seriously ill, things happen before you can be seen. While they are getting information, they should do something with you."

"Money is an issue—they want their money now. I had an appointment at Creighton; the lady treated me poorly. It (the bill) was even already paid for by my job. I had to tell her over and over that she had been notified."

"If you don't have insurance, you go to the end of the line. They don't treat you right."

"In 1999 at St. Joe I went in with pain. The doctor asked me what is wrong . . . I asked (him) to check for fibroids in the glands. I don't like needles. They did everything but what I asked them to do. I spend six hours in the ER and then I was asked to spend the night. I didn't have the money. Two years later I had fibroids and ended up having surgery. I still have a bill for $3,000 that has not been paid. If they would have listened at the beginning, this could have been avoided. I am the patient—you don't know my body like I do. You wait for hours in the first place, and then I had to pay for things I didn't need."

African Americans have the same complaints as Native Americans with respect to communication and care: healthcare professionals' failure to listen carefully to their complaints/symptoms, and quality of care is related to your ability to pay (i.e., insurance). When probed regarding patient/doctor communication, comments included:

"Consistency in receiving the same doctor is important. You see anyone in public clinics. If you have to see a new doctor every time, the information needs to be re-communicated to the new doctor. You repeat the same information to each new doctor."

"It helps to have a doctor who knows your history."

The facilitator asked the discussants about participating in their own health care. One person said, "We need to take care of ourselves in the first place. The doctor doesn't systematically deal with you on your level." Another person who was from the Caribbean added, "I have not had a problem with the university. Even going into emergency with chronic renal failure, there was not a problem. The doctors here are more up to date than the doctors in my country." A third person said: "University (UNMC) and Clarkson have better facilities than the others."

As indicated earlier, all of the African Americans were high school graduates and some had college. Based on their comments, they have learned how to work the system. They have also compared healthcare systems. The Native American compared the Omaha health community, including Creighton, with the health care received on the reservation. Our African American participants, aware that Creighton was sponsoring this study, were comparing CUMC with its competitors.

When the facilitator asked if the level of communication caused a problem, the comments were: "Many people do lots of comparing, maybe for the money" and "I am rushed through, and who cares?" When the facilitator asked if doctors listened to their comments and did they understand, one person revealed that she was a nurse and did not have problems communicating or understanding doctors. No other significant comments were made.

The issue of cultural sensitivity was addressed. Only 6 out of the 11 respondents in the survey said the healthcare provider was familiar enough with their cultural background to treat someone of their ethnic/racial group. Seven respondents said they were comfortable with the providers' medical knowledge, and three persons said some illnesses are better treated by someone of the same ethnic or racial group. The discussants' comments concerning cultural sensitivity were:

"There are a lot who do not understand. The first thing they ask is about insurance . . . They should already have this information. They want to make sure everything is current."

"I have seen signs in hospitals saying no discrimination."

"Patients should know their rights. They cannot turn you away . . . in an emergency situation."

"If you sit for 2 to 3 hours, you are going to leave."

"My sister had pain. One person was asking questions, and we waited for over an hour. By the time someone did come, we were ready to leave. The doctor said, 'we are not going to be responsible.' We waited for so long (pause). The pain goes away."

"I think we (African Americans) tend to be more agreeable in the beginning, whereas Caucasians are more interested in the results."

"Another thing is that as a group of people, we have faith in healing. We may not go see a doctor until the last minute. When asked to wait, it makes a bad situation worse."

Cultural sensitivity for African Americans is not about doctors understanding their culture but about having access to health care when you do not have health insurance. In addition, waiting hours for treatment is a complaint many people have who have had to use the emergency room. This group implied that the use of the emergency room is a last resort after alternative home remedies have failed. When probed further regarding alternative care, the participants said:

"I think it begins before we get to the hospital—in the community . . . We are scared of doctors. They (doctors) need to be brought into the community."

"By the time we get to the hospital, we are overly frustrated. The doctor needs to come to the community to talk with the people and the children."

The facilitator asked the discussants what they took before going to the doctor. They said,

"Drugs—something that takes your mind away—quick and strong."

"Home remedies, Amodium [sic] AD, because I haven't paid the first bill yet. They will turn you away if the bill is not paid."

"I make too much money with OPS (Omaha Public School). You don't want to keep adding on bills so you figure out what you could do at home."

These comments indicate that many do not have health insurance and that home remedies are being used to save money. However, there is no discussion of how effective home remedies are.

The assimilation question was raised. The respondents were asked how "we" are expected to act when we see a healthcare provider (a reminder that the presenter and facilitator are local African Americans; I, too, am African American). Some of the responses were:

". . . They expect you to be clinical like them."

"You talk differently to the doctor. I have had my doctor for years and call her by her first name."

"I have been going to Creighton with the same doctor for ten years. She is, in my book, 'the best of Omaha.' I go in and sit down and joke with them. The doctor is a professional, and I think you get better interaction that way."

"They must go to your level to understand patients."

"I think some doctors . . . our questions to them are burdening. . . . They want to move on to something else. How do we say we don't understand—they want to move on?' You need to find a doctor who will listen."

"If your income is limited, you don't have as many choices."

"When you go to hospitals with students, you have lots of people looking at you. You are a guinea pig. If you are sick, then you say I am the one having pain."

"Just because you have the paper (credentials), you do not always know what the problem is."

"If income is limited, your options are limited." [The response to this was: "There are places where they will work with you. If you have a good doctor, follow that doctor. If you know the system, there is a way to get to the doctor. Even within limits, explore the options."]

"The people do not interact with you when you go into a strange place. You are in their way. You go in and no one pays attention to you." [The response to this comment was: "The doctors have privileges at more than one facility. Find out where they have privileges."]

"If you are hurting now and don't have the money, your options are limited."

Assimilation is not an issue for African Americans. They are concerned with identifying and keeping a good doctor, and limiting their healthcare costs. The facilitator probed further the alternative medicine question. The respondents indicated that it was difficult to get information about their healthcare needs, but that people should do their research before going to the doctor:

"There is some information out there, but I do not think as much information gets out as it should."

"I had a bee sting. I needed to know if I am allergic. I went to several places. All I wanted was a question answered. I ended up incurring a doctor bill."

"Do your research yourself and take it with you to the doctor. Check the Internet. Or go to the library."

"For blacks, and the situation at Tech High School, the information is no longer available. It takes a village to raise a child. A community approach should be used to educate ourselves."

The last question presented to the focus group was about participation in healthcare studies. The survey indicated that most of our respondents were reluctant. The focus group discussion did not change their attitude. Comments included:

"I am willing to do another questionnaire."

"I would not be willing to take meds."

"After the study, is the system going to change? If I have to spend my time filling out forms and talking, it defeats the purpose, regardless of how much money we have."

"You must first make sure there is something wrong with you."

"Many kids are on drugs. Many of these are illegal for adults, but they are given to children."

"Don't do research on my baby. Don't put all those drugs in his body. As a result, we have ADHD. How much are we willing to do for money, because now they are adults and are crazy!"?

"Let's find the real reason about what the problem is."

Hispanic Americans

The Hispanic American focus group was divided into men and women and conducted on two separate days. The research team felt that women (or men) would express themselves more freely in a separate discussion group. There were 8 men and 12 women for a total of 20 people. Seven of the 20 Hispanic participants had a high school diploma or more. One man had a post-graduate degree. Fourteen of the 20 were married; the rest were single, divorced, or separated. The men were not asked where they received their health care, but the women were. They said the Chicano Center, Creighton, and/or University Hospital (UNMC).

The male discussants were asked about the quality of care. Only two men responded:

"I have had good and bad. Very good over at St. Joe Dental School and at Creighton. I have had a bad experience with a private clinic. I took my little boy in with a fractured tendon. Doctor charged $160 for an x-ray and sent the child to school. Nothing happened. That was my bad experience. Another good experience was over at Chicano Indian Clinic."

"I have had a good experience with a doctor . . . and nurses."

When the women were asked the same question about quality of care, most said the care was excellent, but others said,

"Receptionists are very rude and critical . . . When we call them, they take forever to answer."

"They chat with others in the background."

"The front office personnel need to be nicer."

"I have paid my bills but continue to get charged over and over."

"I went to emergency; I got a bill that cost $600."

"Nurses and doctors are OK and so are the interpreters, but the receptionists are not always nice."

"One of the things is that cleaning (trash) is an issue. The floors are dirty at Creighton."

"I was sent to University (UNMC). I was waiting for the results, and they told me they lost the blood. They took it again, and again I waited. It was late and I couldn't wait any longer, so I had to go to emergency. The nurse told me I had to register again or she wouldn't be responsible. For this I had a huge bill. I didn't want to go to emergency. I was pressured to go and register in emergency. Then the doctor came, and I was checked again. I was only going there for my blood test, and I ended up with a huge bill."

"When I had a C-section, I didn't have any pain medicine (morphine). They didn't find it. I had to suffer the pain."

As the comments indicate, the Hispanic women have not had good experiences with health care in the Omaha; however, the majority of both men and women in our survey rated both doctors and nurses as adequate or better. We assumed that their negative experience may have been related to communication problems. The facilitator asked the discussants about language problems. Only one person responded: "I went to St. Joe Hospital. I had to check on a personal illness. This doctor was Asian. He didn't give me an Rx or anything to me. He recommended me to another doctor that was his relative. He wanted me to follow an Asian therapy." When asked if there was a language barrier, this respondent said "No, there was an interpreter there."

When the men were asked if they needed an interpreter, one person said he acted as an interpreter for his mother, otherwise she would need one. Another man said that when his wife was in the delivery room at St. Joe's, they provided her with an interpreter. These men may not view communication or lack of an interpreter as a problem because they have limited contact with the healthcare system; only one Hispanic man was not married, and only 5 of the 12 women were single, divorced, or separated. One man admitted that his wife took care of the family's healthcare needs.

When the women were asked about language problems, several said yes, there was a problem, but only one mentioned having problems with interpreters: "I went to a hospital and asked for an interpreter. Everyone was busy. Someone spoke a little, and so he volunteered."

Although only one woman mentioned a problem with an interpreter, several women commented on the difficulty of completing the paperwork. The women said:

"I always get help to complete the forms."

"Sometimes we understand, but it is difficult to write it in English."

"My experience with the doctor was that I was told, 'We are not Chicano, and so you have to learn English.' "

The men also thought completing paperwork created challenges. One said he used an "interpreter." The others said:

"The forms are in Spanish."

"With the changes in insurance and the doctors' requirements, some language is hard to understand in either Spanish or English."

"Sometimes the translations are wrong."

"They use a computer, and they use the Spanish from Spain, which is very different than what we use here."

Written and verbal language, with or without the use of an interpreter, is a problem for the Hispanic population; however, only two people in the survey said they were unable to complete the paperwork when they visited a healthcare facility.

When the discussion moved to communication with doctors, the responses were mixed. The men said:

"Sometimes the terminology they use is too scientific."

"Regularly I go to the One World Center where they are bilingual."

"All the time I have been to the doctor with my family, no problems."

"I always get answers to what I ask for."

"Sometimes they listen too much and they go by what you are saying and they do not go beyond what we are saying. If we say we need an antibiotic, they do not focus any further."

The women, when asked if they had problems communicating with doctors, answered no, not always, and OK for some. The other comments included:

"Sometimes you get the medicine but do not get full explanations every time. I want to know the secondary effects. If they give me something I don't know about, I announce that I don't know. Sometimes you cannot do that because they write out the prescription and then leave—the doctor is gone and you cannot ask questions. If you ask the nurse, she will say 'I don't know.' "

"Another thing I have noticed—the appointment is at 11:00, and you get in 1¾ hours later—then the doctor only spends a couple of minutes with you. It is unfair to wait 1¾ hours; but if we are a little late, we have to reschedule."

"The service has been improved even though there are more people to attend to."

Most of the women and men said the doctors had shown cultural sensitivity to their Hispanic culture; however, two men disagreed. One man said, "I think they do not understand what we expect . . . Mom and Dad used to have a close relationship with the doctor. We expect the doctor to remember us. We want to have a rapport with the doctor. Some illnesses are repeated. The doctors take up to 15 minutes and that is it . . . They do not have two hours to spend with me, and that is why the nurses do a background check. The time we spend with the doctor is limited. For example, I have a doctor that is treating me for ten years now; I have been following her from office to office . . . She works at UNMC (Dr. Rodriguez). This doctor pays attention to what I have to say. She asks questions about the family even when people are waiting." The other man said, "Some doctors think they speak Spanish and they think they know our culture. I have seen ladies in the operating room with no one from their culture. Sometimes someone only speaks Spanish—being alone with no one in your culture is frightening. Some people that speak Spanish cannot always interpret exactly what we mean in our culture."

The two men were not addressing cultural sensitivity but quality of care and communication. However, the fact that only two people felt healthcare providers were not culturally sensitive may be related to the fact that many of these respondents get their health care at the Chicano Indian center, where language is not a problem.

The Hispanic men indicated in the survey and during the focus group discussion that they had experienced no pressure from healthcare providers to assimilate. However, the Hispanic women said yes during the discussion. Their comments were:

"Sometimes you have to stay with your own cultural beliefs. If you come into the office in a binder (for chronic back pain), they practically tear it off."

"I agree with the doctors, because the doctors need to be informed about the home remedies before they see us. The doctors are right in being upset if we do not tell them what the remedy is for."

"The only thing we are lacking is more information about diets and diabetes."

"I would suggest going to a nutritionist, but it is expensive."

"I applied for Medicaid, and it was given to only one of my sons and not my daughter—both were United States citizens. The one that got sick was the one not approved."

The women do not think their Hispanic culture is a problem, but they do perceive that many in the health care profession do. The women also shifted the discussion to alternative medicine, so the facilitator probed. The following is the list provided by both groups (however, the men provided more remedies than women): lemon mixed with honey for a sore throat; herbal teas, especially chamomile tea; plants in the backyard; grandma's remedies; cinnamon, aloe vera ointment for hemorrhoids; savila for kidney stones; and cactus.

The men said the choice of using a folk remedy or going to the doctor depended on what was wrong with them:

"If I have the flu, I go to the doctor."

"For some things I will take aspirin or Tylenol."

The women noted that American chamomile tea is toxic and should not be given to babies.

The Hispanic focus groups ended with the women being asked about the leading cause of death in their community and the men being asked about participating in future healthcare research. The women said the leading causes of death were diabetes, heart attacks, strokes, and cancer. These causes were given during the completion of the survey, so they are probably repeating what they heard earlier. One woman said that Nebraska ranked first for asthma. She asked the facilitator, "Is this true?"

Only two men responded to the question concerning participation in future healthcare research. One man said it depended on what was required and his schedule. A second man said he needed to know how the results would be used and what impact it would have on the community.

In summary, although the Hispanic respondents indicated on the survey that they were satisfied with health care in the Omaha community, the focus group discussion indicated that there is need for improvement. This population, similar to African Americans, is concerned with the consistency of health care and the cost. Language is still a problem even with an interpreter, because the interpreter may not be familiar with the specific culture or dialect. And although the majority of the respondents said in the survey that they were willing to participate in a healthcare study, only two males commented on their participation, and this was not an affirmation. We can only assume that the discrepancy between the survey results and the focus group may be related to the fact that during the focus group session participants were sharing their past experience with healthcare providers and the survey is representative of their most recent experience. We learned that many of the participants visit a healthcare facility that serves primarily the Hispanic population, and even with bilingual staff there are still language problems. The Hispanic population, like the Native American population, is more satisfied when the healthcare provider is affiliated with an organization whose primary goal is serving their population. In addition, the Hawthorne effect may have been operating because the survey results indicate satisfaction with health care in Omaha, but the focus group indicates many communication problems.

Sudanese

The Sudanese focus group was also divided into men and women and conducted on two separate days. There were 10 men and 7 women. Thirteen of the participants were married, one was separated, one was widowed, and two were single. Only four of the Sudanese had no children under 19. Five of them had less than a 9th-grade education, three some high school, five were high school graduates, three had some college, and one had a bachelor's degree. Most of the women had less than a high school education. Only two individuals identified their religion as Muslim; the rest said Protestant or Catholic. None of the Sudanese said English was their first language, and all of the women needed an interpreter.

Due to the fact that all of the women required an interpreter, an excessive amount of time was spent completing the survey, which limited the time for the focus group. As a result, there were many questions that were asked of the men that were not asked of the women. The men were asked, but not the women, where they got their health care. They said Creighton Medical Center and Immanuel Hospital, but added, "Here in Omaha's Sudanese community we have a problem with unborn children. Some are born with heart disease. We don't know what is wrong with unborn children. They suffer with heart ailments; TB for the elders, they cough a lot. Another problem—we have a communication problem with the doctors."

The men were asked if they knew what the leading cause of mortality was for their people. One person said, ". . . lack of communication . . . no hospital, so many die of diseases and some people can die because they get no treatment."

When asked about the difference between their country, the Sudan, and this country, the United States, they said,

"The majority here has needed to see a doctor, but we do not know what the cause of disease is."

"Lack of cleanliness brings about the virus . . ."

"We have mental problems."

"Lung cancer."

". . . malaria."

The men seemed to imply that people are sicker here than in the Sudan. The facilitator did not probe regarding the "virus," so we do not know if they meant HIV/AIDS or influenza. Perhaps the perception that people are sicker here is due to better access to health care.

When the facilitator asked the men why there were communication problems, they said,

> ". . . Sudanese women—they don't go to school and cannot understand English."

> "Sudanese women cannot be examined by male doctors. They fear with the private body."

Most of the men agreed that English was their second language and not their first, and as a result there were communication problems, especially for women. However, the women did not agree with men about male doctors. The women said,

> "We want a woman doctor because it is very easy to talk to a woman doctor. I am very shy to talk to a man . . ."

> "We have man doctor in Sudan. The woman doctor in Sudan is not good."

> "I go to either. I don't feel bad. Here in this country we have to have a translator if we have a problem. Lots of women are shy when we talk to a man. It is not easy to explain private things to a man doctor in the United States. It is difficult to talk about pooping all the time and diarrhea to the doctor. We could tell a man doctor with a woman translator; however, that is the key—we must have a woman translator."

The facilitator probed the communication problem. All the women agreed that there were problems with translations. They said the interpreters must know the many dialects in order to be effective. The women also said they spoke English among themselves when there was a problem understanding the different dialects or languages. One woman spoke of a situation in which a woman mistakenly had an oophorectomy and now cannot have any children (and yes, the term was translated *oophorectomy* by the Sudanese interpreter).

The men also discussed communication problems that their families were having:

> "I am suffering from headaches . . . the doctor prescribes sleeping pills. I have a hard time taking the medication and going to work. The same thing happened with my wife. We stopped the medicine, and we were no longer sleepy."

> "My son cannot breathe. I thought it was a stuffy nose. He went to doctor many times and was given an aspirator device. I changed doctors. The doctors just prescribed more medicine. I gave the medicine to the child; took him back. The doctor said to explain again. Doctor says he thinks an oper-

ation is needed. The doctor did surgery, but it took almost eight months to fix the problem. The doctor thought the problem was his lungs instead."

"I am concerned with the Sudanese women or African women in general. Most Sudanese cannot speak English. When you try an interpreter for women, they cannot interpret for them. She (the Sudanese woman) will not tell all her problems except to the husband."

As is indicated from these comments, the men are articulating the medical problems of their families. Most of the men spoke English but were still having communication problems with healthcare providers. For example, one man said, "My wife has been sick eight months. She has mental illness. The doctor at Immanuel gave her medicine and says she has schizophrenia. She is still on medication. Now she still has the same problem. I took her to Charles Drew (Health Center). I have no health insurance. The doctor said she will be on the medication forever. I don't know if I explained things clearly to the doctor. It is a big question whether I am communicating clearly to the doctor." This man may not understand that most mental illnesses are incurable, but treatable with medication. Perhaps he was concerned with the cost of the medication. However, another man's comments concerning mental illness was, "Mental illness is a big problem. Oftentimes what they hear is that we have a mental illness because we are sad about the conditions back home." The political turmoil in the Sudan may be related to the high prevalence of mental disorders among the Omaha Sudanese population. Most of the Sudanese are refugees; many were sponsored by religious organizations. However, they still have relatives in Sudan or the refugee camps.

Another man mentioned working conditions in Omaha that may have an effect on the health. "We have joint pain because of the meat companies. We have aches and pains." Many Sudanese work in the meat industry because these are low-skill jobs that they can perform with little knowledge of English. They undoubtedly are doing tedious work that most Nebraskans do not want to do.

Language is the main problem for this population. They are asked to sign forms they cannot read; the doctor prescribes medicine, the purpose of which they do not know; when they take laboratory tests, they can not get the results because the receptionist only speaks English; however, they do get the bill, the cost of which they understand.

Their need for an interpreter has affected the treatment they receive or do not receive. The interpreter may not be available when she or he is needed, causing patients to wait hours for treatment or causing treatment to be postponed. One discussant said UNMC had only one Sudanese interpreter. This interpreter is mostly likely utilized by most of the healthcare centers in Omaha.

The issue of mental health came up again with the interpreter. One articulate respondent said, "Our community has a different way of saying depressed. . . . Depressed means 'mad' in our language. When asked, a Sudanese person will say 'no' when asked if he is depressed. Mental health issues should be concerned with ethnic concerns." This man became the spokesperson for the Sudanese population.

"HIV is a problem because of lack of education, and it is increasing. Our people do not know where this comes from. The disease is invisible. To prevent it, the Sudanese people need to understand it. If we see it, it makes sense. We cannot see the symptoms. We need more information on preventing STDs. We need to be made aware that it is dangerous."

"Alcohol is a problem. The people need education to learn what alcohol will do to them. Interpreters are another problem. It is damaging to say the wrong word. Taking one pill three times a day can be translated into three pills in one hour. That person almost died. We need health care to pay attention to the Sudanese community and its medical issues."

This respondent was also addressing the issue of cultural competency of the healthcare providers. The Sudanese are the most recent immigrants to the Omaha community—the medical community as well as the wider community are still assessing the Sudanese' healthcare needs. When asked if the healthcare community ignores their culture, the answer was yes. The comments included:

"We don't have enough information about health care . . ."

"Diseases—diabetes and high blood pressure are common. We are not eating many healthy foods."

"We need to educate our community to protect themselves from diabetes"

"We need a counselor on how to prevent HIV. . . .to show us how to protect ourselves"

"When a woman gets pregnant, they often have a C-section, even if they had five children before."

"When we visit a doctor, we might have to wait one or two hours to see a doctor . . ." [During the discussion the wait was said to be associated with the unavailability of an interpreter and that "there is just one female interpreter. Sudanese people need to be taught how to deal with issues in society."]

As indicated earlier, the males were better educated and more proficient in English than the women, thus many of the questions that were asked of the males were not asked of the women. However, some of the comments made by the women when completing the survey instrument shed some light on the problems that they have encountered.

The women acknowledged that a midwife is used for childbirth and that many women do not want a male doctor to examine their "private parts." They also indicated that herbal remedies were used back home that are not available here. They said they were familiar with HIV but if they had it, they would not discuss it. They said they were not treated well because they did not understand or speak English and that doctors made them feel bad; the women also agreed with the men that they were concerned about being diagnosed as depressed, and that when people die they don't know why—they don't know the cause of death.

The women were not asked about assimilation. However, based on the comments, we can assume that they would agree with the men, who said they felt pressure to behave like Americans. One final question from a male participant was whether there would be more seminars like this one. The facilitator said yes, that CUMC recognized that it was not adequately meeting the needs of the Sudanese community. I think it would be more accurate to say that the Omaha medical community has not adequately met the needs of this Sudanese community.

Vietnamese

The Vietnamese group consisted of four women and six men. Seven of the 10 were married, 2 were single, and 1 was divorced. Five of the Vietnamese had no children under the age of 19. Five had some high school, one had some college, two had associate's degrees, and one had a bachelor's degree. All said English was not their first language.

Most of the Vietnamese were recruited by a Vietnamese Catholic priest. His name was given to the author by a Vietnamese student who had been in two of her classes. The student was the contact person for the Vietnamese community. As a result, seven said they were Catholic, two indicated they were Buddhists, and one said "other." The student was Catholic and attended the Catholic Church where the focus group was conducted.

Six of the Vietnamese said they had been treated at CUMC, and four said their last visit to a healthcare provider had been the emergency room at CUMC. Seven rated the visit to the doctor as good; three said excellent. The rating of the nurses was divided among adequate, good, and excellent. Nine of the 10 said they would be willing to see the same healthcare provider at their next visit.

Eight of the 10 said they had forms to complete; 7 said they were able to do so without help. Only 1 of the 3 who needed an interpreter said she did an adequate job. Thus, the questionnaire indicated that the Vietnamese population was satisfied with their healthcare experiences. However, at the beginning of the focus group, the Vietnamese interpreter requested that the following information be put on record:

"The groups thank Creighton for the focus group session; however, they wanted the following concerns expressed:

1. It is important for healthcare providers to learn more about the Vietnamese culture. They have at-home medication remedies. Spooning and coining can cause hematomas. It is viewed by the Americans as abusive. Healthcare groups need to understand and respect this when this cultural group tries to cure ailments before seeking traditional American health care.

2. Make sure that the law enforcement representatives respect this and not take away the children or put them (the parents) in jail.

3. The Vietnamese people have been here since 1975. They wonder: "Why is there still not the proper respect for their traditions?"

This statement indicates that the Vietnamese community is still upset over Child Protective Services removing a Vietnamese child from the family because a public school teacher observed round, red marks on his body, which was the result of the family administering a home remedy called *coining*. The incident occurred in 2002 and was well publicized in the press and local television news. The Vietnamese parents were accused of child abuse and had to hire an attorney to regain custody of the child. To the Vietnamese, this was an indication of the cultural incompetence of the public school system. Coining and spooning are traditional remedies that have been practiced for centuries by the Vietnamese. Perhaps this is why more than 50% of the Vietnamese in our survey said that healthcare providers were not familiar enough with Vietnamese culture to treat someone from their ethnic or racial group, and four said that some illnesses are better treated by a healthcare provider of the same race or ethnic group.

The Vietnamese were willing to participate in our survey and focus group in order to inform the larger community about the culture and health concerns of the Vietnamese in Omaha. The first question asked by the facilitator was where the respondents got their health care and the quality of that care. Our discussants said, " clinics," and that the care was good. However, they added that the personnel at these clinics perceive them as a minority in the community. They believed that if an individual has health insurance, they get better service. They claim that it helps to go to the same clinic all the time so that the healthcare providers know you and give you better care. Sometimes they wait as long as an hour and a half for care, but if they are late the healthcare providers make "a big issue of it."

The second set of questions had to do with language and interpreters. Our discussants said that sometimes a friend or family member will act as an interpreter; if you know you will need an interpreter, you should let them (the health provider) know. However, interpreters are usually not available late in the evening, and the use of an interpreter is no guarantee that the doctor will understand you or you him (or her). In other words, the patient does not know if the interpreter is translating his or her needs correctly. Later in the discussion, the question was raised regarding the use of children as interpreters. Several discussants said they had used children as interpreters, but they claim that children were used more often by older persons as interpreters. One person said, "The children are born here and some can interpret. Sometimes, however, the medical language is something that the children have not been exposed to." The discussants indicated that they would like an interpreter appointed to help the Vietnamese community, especially the elderly and in emergency cases.

It is worth mentioning that the Vietnamese interpreter for this group was a radiologist employed by Creighton University Medical Center. She is sometimes asked to interpret for patients at the university, but she is not a trained interpreter. Several of the discussants were proficient in English; most of these comments were expressed by them and not the interpreter. Later in a translation session with the interpreter, which was arranged by the author to translate questionnaires written in Vietnamese, the interpreter expressed her dissatisfaction with the way the coining incident had been handled. The author of this chapter indicated that the university planned to utilize results from these kinds of studies to improve doctor/patient communication and foster cultural competency among healthcare providers.

The discussants were asked if a Vietnamese doctor would improve the quality of health care. Comments included:

"Some Vietnamese don't want to go to a Vietnamese doctor. They don't want to express their illnesses to a Vietnamese doctor."

"I prefer to go to a Vietnamese doctor. I have a family doctor and a specialist, who are Vietnamese that I go to."

Someone else said that she hoped the group would focus on recruiting at least one healthcare interpreter. This prompted the facilitator to probe further regarding communication problems. Someone who had been used as an interpreter in the past said that "sometimes the patient does not tell the doctor everything. Sometimes Vietnamese want to be treated right away and not have to answer too many questions. Some patients do not want to tell the whole truth to the doctor."

The facilitator continued to probe for communication problems. She asked if there was "a problem telling everything that would help a doctor understand what your illness is." She also asked if the healthcare provider was "sensitive to things unique to your culture." The discussants said they tell everything to the doctor through the interpreter so that they can get proper care, but that if the interpreter is not able to communicate, then the patient will not receive proper care. They said they were concerned about the waiting time, but that the doctors were sensitive, pleasant, nice, and respectful. "The problem of all the people that came today (to the focus group) is that we need a specialized (trained) interpreter with our mother language (Vietnamese) so that our illnesses can be accurately described. It must be someone with medical terminology knowledge."

Many of the Vietnamese did not speak English; they wrote their answers to the questionnaire in Vietnamese. Their assimilation into American culture is minimal, at best; their cultural belief and practices are still basically Vietnamese. A 1999 study found that the Vietnamese living in Philadelphia used coining, cupping, acupuncture, tiger balm, healing ceremonies, various herbal remedies, and root medicine to treat colds, flu, and headaches; the use of traditional medicine was attributed to lack of health insurance, inadequate transportation, and language barriers.[20] When our discussants were asked about alternative medical practices, they said,

> "Normally we do the home remedy 2-3 days until the illness subsides. Otherwise, we go to a health care provider."

> "Right now I have a cold, and I use a home remedy first. If I go to a doctor, I have transportation problems and interpreter problems. So I get well on my own first."

When probed about problems associated with home remedies, the following statements were made:

> "The wife used home remedy and had a bruise. The doctor wanted to know about it."

> "The school nurse sometimes see marks."

> "The law is sometimes involved."

These statements indicate some of the problems that have occurred regarding the use of Vietnamese folk remedies. Many law enforcement officials and healthcare practitioners would interpret the bruise and marks as wife or child battering or child abuse and/or neglect, and *not* the side-effects of a folk remedy. Additional comments by our discussants included,

> "How would the doctor really understand when the doctor asks what medicines you have taken? Sometimes the doctors are afraid that the herbs would counteract the medicines."

"They feel that the doctor will feel differently about their home remedy treatments."

"I had a muscle spasm. When you are sick, your body is different. I use spooning (a coin, spoon, or bone to rub against the skin that is medicated by ointment) to help with the circulation and to warm up the body. If the doctors understand why we use the home remedies, the two could work well together." [The discussant is referring again to the 2002 incident previously described in this chapter. Obviously that incident would not have occurred if the school officials had been familiar with Vietnamese traditional medicine.]

The assimilation issue was probed via the facilitator asking the discussants if they felt pressure to act like Americans. One discussant said, "I have studied both Chinese and American medicines. Some things are not good for the kidney or liver. But it is good to see the doctor first." Another discussant said, "The doctors use the analysis charts for Caucasians, and then compares those with your child. But they are . . . Caucasian measurements." This individual is referring to the growth chart commonly used in well baby clinics by most pediatricians.

Probably the most significant comment concerning assimilation was, "we like to be treated with modern medicines. The only thing is . . . language barrier . . . holds some back with using home remedies." Translation: improvement in communication skills between healthcare providers and the Vietnamese community may result in less home remedies and more modern medicine.

The final questions asked by the facilitator for the Vietnamese population was if they knew the causes of illness and death for their community and would they be willing to participate in healthcare research. Their answers for causes of morbidity and mortality included hepatitis, accidents, tuberculosis, and heart problems. In addition one person said, "Since we have come over here, we consume the same foods, so the illnesses are the same as Americans." Another response was, "We eat a lot of rice and vegetable, so our women have less rate of breast cancer." The Vietnamese focus group said they would be willing to participate in healthcare research and thanked the research team for their interest in Vietnamese community.

SUMMARY

The major problem faced by all participants was communication. The Vietnamese have similar communication problems as Native Americans, Hispanics, and the Sudanese; English is not their first language. Dissatisfaction with health care is usually related to communication: patients do not understand the provider and the provider does not understand the patient, and the accuracy of the medical interpretation may be an issue.

Communication was also a problem for the research team. In all groups, the Hawthorne effect affected the answers: the survey findings reflected what the respondents thought the researcher wanted to hear—that they were satisfied with their healthcare experience. The focus group represented the reality of their experience: they were not satisfied. The lack of consistency in the findings indicated that we did not communicate well the purpose of our study.

Communication was also a problem for the African American respondents, where English *was* their first language. This group was better educated but equally critical of the healthcare system and reluctant to participate in healthcare research. They also, like the Vietnamese, Native Americans, Sudanese, and Hispanics, rated the Omaha healthcare system as adequate or better in the survey, but they expressed their dissatisfaction during the focus group. However, the African American participants were better able to maneuver the healthcare system. They were able to find culturally competent health care through trial and error and research (asking other people /patients).

To improve relations with ethnic/racial minority groups, healthcare providers should reach out to the community: provide workshops on a given population's health, sponsor health fairs, and train more minority healthcare personnel.

However, the cost of health care encourages many people to self-medicate. Self-medication for some of the discussants involves traditional medicine, the efficacy of which has not been tested. Many of the participants revealed their reluctance to discuss home remedies with their healthcare providers. We have no way of knowing if the cost or illness is aggravated or mitigated by self-medication or traditional medicine. The lack of adequate health insurance is not just a local problem, but a national one. More than 46 million Americans have no health insurance. The study participants may not be the only ones foregoing a visit to the emergency room or hospital in order to avoid a huge medical bill.

The most significant finding from this research is that respondents are more satisfied when the healthcare provider is ethnic-based. Respondents who attended clinics primarily for Native Americans or Hispanics found their providers to be more culturally competent. If we want to reduce the health disparities that exist in our community, we may need to produce more culturally competent healthcare providers, regardless of their race or ethnicity.

REFERENCES

1. James C, Thomas M, Lillie-Blanton M, Garfield R. *Key Facts: Race, Ethnicity, & Medical Care.* The Henry J. Kaiser Family Foundation; January 2007.

2. Buchwald D, Mendoza-Jenkins V, Croy C, McGough H, Bezdek M, Spicer P. Attitudes of urban American Indians and Alaska Natives regarding participation in research. *Gen. Intern Med.* 2006;21(6):648–651.

3. Call KT, McAlpine DD, Johnson PJ, Beebe TJ, McRae JA, Song Y. Barriers to care among American Indians in public health care programs. *Med. Care.* 2006;44(6):595–600.

4. Jones DS. The health care experiments at Many Farms: the Navajo, tuberculosis, and the limits of modern medicine, 1952–1962. *Bull Hist Med.* 2002;76(4):749–790.

5. Moreno-John G, Gachie A, Fleming CM, et al. Ethnic minority older adults participating in clinical research: developing trust. *J Aging Health.* 2004;16(5 Suppl):93S–123S.

6. Robertson NL. Clinical trial participation. Viewpoints from racial/ethnic groups. *Cancer.* 1994;74(9 Suppl):2687–2691.

7. Rotenberg KJ, Cerda C. Racially based trust expectancies of Native American and Caucasian children. *J Soc Psychol.* 1994;134(5):621–631.

8. Harmon A. Gatherers hit a snag: The tribes don't trust them. *New York Times.* December 10, 2006:1.

9. Baker R. Minority distrust of medicine: A historical perspective. *Mount Sinai J Med.* 1999;66(4):212–222.

10. Blendon RJ, Scheck AC, Donelan K, et al. How white and African Americans view their health and social problems: Different experiences, different expectations. *JAMA.* 1995;273(4):341–346.

11. Corbie-Smith G, Thomas SB, St. George DM. Distrust, race, and research. *Arch Inter Med.* 2002;162(21):2458–2463.

12. Earl CE, Penney PJ. The significance of trust in the research consent process with African Americans. *West J Nurs Res.* 2001;23(7):753–762.

13. Gamble V.N. A legacy of distrust: African Americans and health care. *Am J Prev Med.* 1993;9(suppl. 12):35–38.

14. Armstrong K, Ravenell K, McMurphy S, Putt M. Racial/ethnic differences in physician distrust in the United States. *Am J. Public Health.* 2007;97(7):1283–1289.

15. Voils CI, Oddone EZ, Weinfurt KP, Friedman JY, Schulman KA, Bosworth HB. Who trusts healthcare institutions? Results from a community-based sample. *Ethn Dis.* 2005;15(1):97–103.

16. Cook CT, Kosoko-Lasaki O, O'Brien R. Satisfaction with and perceived cultural competency of healthcare providers: The minority experience. *J Nat Med Assoc.* 2005;97(8):1078–1087.

17. Mayo E. *The Human Problems of an Industrial Civilization.* New York: Macmillan; 1933.

18. O'Brien R, Kosoko-Lasaki O, Cook CT, et al. Self-assessment of cultural attitudes and competence of clinical investigators to enhance recruitment and participation of minority popuplation in research. *J Nat Med Assoc.* 2006;98(5):674–680.

19. Kosoko-Lasaki O, Cook CT, O'Brien R, et al. Promoting cultural competency in researchers to enhance the recruitment and participation of minority populations in research: Development and refinement of survey instruments. *Eval Prog Plan.* 2006;29:227–235.

20. Pham TM, Rosenthal MP, Diamond JJ. Hypertension, cardiovascular disease, and health care dilemmas in the Philadelphia Vietnamese community. *Fam Med.* 1999;31(9):647–651.

Chapter 15

Health Disparities: The Nebraska Perspective

Reverend Raponzil L. Drake, DMin
Anthony Zhang, MA
Diane Lowe, BA

H *ealthy People 2010* has two overarching goals: (1) increasing the quality and years of healthy life and (2) reducing health disparities. The second goal of *Healthy People 2010*, to eliminate health disparities, includes differences that occur based on gender, race or ethnicity, education or income, disability, geographic location, or sexual orientation. Compelling evidence indicates that race and ethnicity correlate with persistent, and often increasing, health disparities among U.S. populations in all of these categories, and it demands the attention of our nation. Despite steady improvements in the overall health of the United States, racial and ethnic minorities continue to experience a lower quality of health services, are less likely to receive routine medical procedures, and have higher rates of morbidity and mortality than nonminorities. Various health sources, including the *Nebraska Healthy People 2010 Report*, the Nebraska Office of Minority Health *2003 Health Status Report, 2006 Strategic Plan*, and *Health Facts for Racial/ethnic Minorities*[1-3] web resource, all indicate that the same is true in Nebraska.

Who Are the "Cornhuskers"?

Nebraska is a culturally diverse state enriched by German, Irish, English, Swedish, and Czech populations and increasing populations of American

Indians, Hispanics or Latinos, Africans, and African and Asian Americans. Each of these groups represents varying colors, cultures, and languages.

While Nebraska has not had the population growth of other states, growing at a rate of roughly 3% annually,[4] there are very significant recent demographic changes. Population growth of racial and ethnic minorities in Nebraska are similar to national growth for these populations, with greater than 30% growth of Hispanic and Asian populations from 2000–2006. (See **Table 15–1.**)

In the mid-1990s, the U.S. Census Bureau projected that Nebraska's minority populations would reach a high of 15% of the total population by the year 2025.[5] In 2005—*20 years ahead of the projection*—the racial/ethnic minority population of Nebraska was estimated to be 14.6%. From 2000–2005, Nebraska's racial/ethnic minority population grew 20% from 214,152 to 256,969.[6] It is now estimated that the number of Hispanic Americans in Nebraska will reach approximately 145,000 by 2025, a 16% increase over the 2005 data. The number of Asian Americans will reach about 40,000 by 2025, a 41% increase over the 2005 data. The African American population is projected to grow by 44% (109,000 people) from 2005–2025, and 50% growth of the Native American community is predicted (25,000 people by 2025).[6] By contrast, the white population is projected to grow 10%.

The Federation for American Immigration Reform (FAIR) estimated in July 2005 that the number of foreign-born residents in Nebraska was about

Table 15–1 *Nebraska Population by Race and Ethnicity*

Race	Estimates (2000)	% Population (2000)	Estimates (2006)	% Population (2006)	Change (2000–2006)	% Change (2000–2006)
Nebraska total	1,713,426		1,768,331		54,905	3.2
White	1,587,380	92.6	1,622,682	91.8	35,302	2.2
African American	70,186	4.1	77,636	4.4	7,450	10.6
Native American	15,534	0.9	17,103	1.0	1,569	10.1
Asian*	23,771	1.4	30,478	1.7	6,707	28.2
Hispanic	95,194	5.6	130,304	7.4	35,110	36.9
White non-Hispanic	1,498,111	87.4	1,500,725	84.9	2,614	0.2
Minority Population	215,315	12.6	267,606	15.1	52,291	24.3

*Including Native Hawaiian or Other Pacific Islander.
Source: U.S. Census Bureau. Population estimates, 2000–2006.

92,187. This represented 5.2% of Nebraska's overall population, and an increase of 226.9% above the 1990 population of foreign-born residents in the state (28,198 residents).

There are large concentrations of racial/ethnic minorities in the urban areas of Omaha and Lincoln. Lancaster County in Nebraska (Lincoln), ranks 14th nationally in per capita refugee resettlement: 84% of foreign-born Nebraskans entered the state since 1990.[7] There are Sudanese and Somali families all across Nebraska.

But there is also increasing diversity across the state in large and small towns, where many minorities and immigrants are employed in meat packing and agriculture. Of the 93 counties in Nebraska, 29 had minority populations greater than 5%; by 2005 the number had risen to 34 with 2 more with 4.8% population.[8]

This cultural diversity also brings great linguistic diversity. It is estimated that more than 60 languages are spoken in the school systems of Omaha and Lincoln! There are reflections of this linguistic diversity across the state **(Table 15–2)**.

Health Disparities in Nebraska

Accompanying this increase in diversity are striking disparities in health for Nebraska's racial/ethnic populations, disparities that are often associated with poverty, level of education, employment, and physical environment. Access to care, maternal and child health and well-being (particularly infant mortality), life expectancy at birth, and potential years of life lost are among the key health disparities in Nebraska, as elsewhere.

Maternal and Child Health

Disparities of maternal and child health are often considered benchmarks of unmet health needs.[9] In Nebraska during 2000–2004, infant mortality for African Americans was 2.9 times higher than for whites (16.9 per 1,000 live births), and for Native Americans it was 2.4 times higher than for whites (5.9 per 1,000 live births).[10] A newborn is considered low birth weight if he or she weighs less than 5.8 pounds (or 2,300 grams) at birth. These babies experience higher rates of illness and death than other infants. Many of the risk factors found to be related to low birth weight are preventable. During 2000–2004, African Americans had the highest incidence of low-birth-weight babies in Nebraska: 125.1 per 1,000 live births. For whites, the rate was 65.8 per 1,000. Mexican American mothers are almost three times as likely as non-Hispanic white mothers to begin prenatal care in the third trimester or to receive no prenatal care at all. Latino children are less likely to be fully immunized than non-Hispanic white children.[10]

Table 15–2 *Languages Spoken in Nebraska*

Afrikaans	Mandarin/Chinese
Albanian/Shiquip	Marathi
Amharic/Ethiopian	Mongolian
Arabic/Egyptian/Lebanese/Syrian	Native American
Armenian/Haieren	Nepalese/Nepali
Bengali/Bangla	Nuer
Cambodian/Khmer	Other
Chinese/Cantonese	Pashto/Pashtu
Dutch	Polish
English	Portugese
Farsi/Persian/Dari	Romanian/Moldavian
Filipino/Tagalog	Russian
French	Samoan
German	Serbo-Croatian/Bosnian
Hindi/Indian/Urdu	Slovak
Hmong	Spanish
Indonesian	Tajik
Japanese	Thai/Tai/Thaiklang
Kanjobal	Tonga/Tongan
Korean	Turkish
Kurdish/Zimany/Kurdy	Ukrainian
Lao/Laotian	Vietnamese
Malay/Bahasa/Malaysia	

Source: Nebraska Department of Education.

Life Expectancy at Birth and Years of Potential Life Lost

During 2000–2002, the life expectancy at birth of Native Americans was 67.9 years, more than 10 years less than that of white persons (78.3). The life expectancy at birth of African Americans was 71.6, 6.7 years less than that of whites. During 2000–2004, African Americans lost more than twice as many years of potential life (12,131.4 per 100,000) as whites (5,786.5 per 100,000).[11]

Access to Care and Poverty

During 2001–2006, 45.2% of Hispanic or Latino American adults in Nebraska reported having no health insurance, compared with 10.9% of white adults; 36.8% of American Indian or Native American adults and 22.6% of African Americans in Nebraska reported no health insurance.[11] During 2003–2006, 20.3% of Native American adults (compared with 9% of white adults) in Nebraska reported that they were unable to see a doctor at some time in the previous 12 months because of costs of care; 18.3% of Latino or Hispanic American adults and 15.6% of African American adults reported that they were unable to see a doctor because of the cost of care.[11] In 2004–2005, the proportion of African Americans living in poverty in Nebraska was 34%, 3.8 times the rate of whites (9%). The percentage of Latino or Hispanic Americans living in poverty was 26%. In Nebraska, at least 145,000 people under the age of 65 are uninsured. The majority of the uninsured have incomes below 200% of the federal poverty level, although more than 63% are employed. In Nebraska, 27% of the total Latino population is uninsured.

Other Health Disparities

During 2000–2004, Native Americans had the highest rates for diabetes-related deaths (260.9 per 100,000), three times the rate for all other Nebraskans combined. African Americans and Hispanic Americans had rates of 162.8 per 100,000 and 109.3 per 100,000, respectively. During these same years, Native Americans had the highest mortality rate due to heart disease (276 per 100,000) of any racial/ethnic group in Nebraska. African Americans had the highest rate of cancer (all sites) of any racial/ethnic group in Nebraska, 255.2 per 100,000 compared with an overall rate of 182 per 100,000.[11]

African Americans and Native Americans have the highest incidence of HIV/AIDS; African Americans have a relative risk of 11.2%; Native Americans, 5.4%; and Latino Americans, 4.7%. In 2005, the incidence of sexually transmitted disease was 14.1 times higher for African Americans than for white Americans in Nebraska. During 2001–2006, 47.9% of Native American adults reported smoking cigarettes compared with 20.5% of whites. The Latino population in the United States has a disproportionately high prevalence of asthma, chronic obstructive pulmonary disease, HIV/AIDS, obesity, suicide, teenage pregnancy, and tuberculosis.

Unequal Treatment: Confronting Racial and Ethnic Disparities in Health Care, a research report of the Institute of Medicine (IOM), contrasts the medical and health care received by whites and the care received by racial/ethnic minorities. Study researchers controlled for factors that affect quality of medical and health care, such as insurance (uninsured and underinsured), type of insurance, (private vs. Medicaid and Medicare), socioeconomic status, current health status, and so forth. The IOM reported that the quality of health care for racial/ethnic minorities is frequently poorer than for persons who are white.[12]

What Is Nebraska's Commitment Today? What Are We Doing?

Public health stakeholders in Nebraska—including the governor, legislators, academia, the state department of health, local public health departments, and professional associations—have identified health disparities and cultural competency as high priorities. But having an impact will require public investment. Every health program and section of Nebraska Department of Health and Human Services (NDHHS) might include in their respective budgets, and set aside some amount of each grant received, funds to support cultural competency and health disparities reduction. In addition to *disease* surveillance, surveillance of language needs, quality of care, cultural barriers, and best health practices should be adopted as routine functions of *health* surveillance.

The NDHHS identified and ranked cultural competence a key factor in the quality of healthcare delivery, 1 of the 10 essential functions of public health and one of the top three priorities for the future of public health[13] in its application for the Turning Point Grant received from the Robert Wood Johnson Foundation.

Prior to receiving the Turning Point Grant, it was determined that the staffs of 16 local public health departments serving 22 of Nebraska's 93 counties lacked skills and training in core competencies in public health.[14] Chief among these inadequacies was lack of cultural competence skills. As early as 1997, the need to build effective strategies to meet the needs of racial/ethnic minorities, and to create a system of culturally competent, linguistically appropriate strategies, training, and programs for health promotion, disease prevention, and medical care was documented, and public health leaders and stakeholders identified cultural competence as a top priority for public health in Nebraska.

But the need for cultural competency in the elimination of health is not only a public health concern. It is also of concern in health care and health services. During 2006, the Office of Minority Health, with other community health organizations, established the Medical Translation and Interpretation (MTI) Leadership Group, which developed a provider survey to assess the language needs of patients.

Participants included physicians, pharmacists, and other healthcare providers in Lincoln-Lancaster County, Nebraska. Of 550 surveys distributed, 173 responses were received. Only 61 respondents offered written health information and forms; 100 did not offer translated materials. A total of 130 respondents indicated that 1% to 10% of their patient population has limited English proficiency (LEP). Only 11 respondents had no LEP patients. When asked what method was most used to provided interpretation and translation services, 118 said they are more likely to use friends and family; of this number, 49 felt that practice was adequate. When asked about the costs associated with interpretation and translation services, 49 respondents reported spending a combined minimum of $219,000. In identifying the greatest barriers in communicating with LEP patients, 28 said lack of time, 44 said lack of interpreter services, 43 responded that cost was the greatest barrier, and 24 responded that they are not responsible for being able to communicate with LEP patients. When asked if licensed medical providers are legally required to provide interpretation and translation services, 81 responded yes, 21 responded no, and 66 were uncertain.[15]

Nebraska's Office of Minority Health and Health Disparities

In an effort to eliminate health disparities, Nebraska created an Office of Minority Health (OMH) in 1992. Several years earlier, a Minority AIDS Task Force in Lincoln worked to raise awareness about this and other minority health issues. In 1991 a Nebraska Minority Health Coalition was created, made up of representatives from community-based organizations and advocacy groups. This coalition approached the Director of Health for the state of

Nebraska about the need for a minority health office. In 1992, the first *Minority Health Status Report*, published by the Nebraska State Department of Health's Bureau of Health Policy and Planning, described significant disparities affecting Nebraska's racial/ethnic minority populations. These important developments led to the establishment of the OMH.

In 1997, the OMH, following a major reorganization of state government, was expanded to a staff of four: an administrator, administrative assistant, a program specialist for Native American populations, and a program analyst. The Native American Public Health Act was also passed, and now in its 10th year, awards $100,000 annually to each of Nebraska's four federally recognized tribes—Ponca, Omaha, Winnebago, and Santee-Sioux—and to Native American populations in the Chadron area.

A significant asset to minority health in Nebraska is the Chief Medical Officer, Dr. Joann Schaefer, and her commitment to the elimination of health disparities. Her support for culturally competent, linguistically appropriate communication and care is strong and public. Schaefer reminds Nebraskans, especially public health professionals, that racial/ethnic minority populations have diverse beliefs and values about health, disparate incidences of disease, and sometimes different responses to therapies. As more leaders are courageously outspoken about the disparities in quality of care and barriers arising from language and cultural differences that prevent communication between patients and providers, health outcomes will be markedly improved.

State Financing for Nebraska's Public Health

In May 2001, the Nebraska legislature passed the Nebraska Health Care Funding Act, Legislative Bill 692,[16] which provided $47.5 million to fund several public health initiatives, including mental health and substance abuse services. Of this amount, $10 million was awarded to universities for health-related research projects; $14 million for biomedical research, of which $700,000 was earmarked for research to improve racial/ethnic minority health; $1.58 million for minority health initiatives in counties with 5% or more racial/ethnic minority populations; $1.725 million for five community health centers; $1.8 million for local public health departments; $1.4 million for two federally qualified health centers; $5 million for the Children's Health Insurance Program; $658,000 for the purchase of pandemic influenza anti-virals; and $220,000 for the operation of satellite offices of minority health In Congressional Districts 2 and 3 to coordinate state policy pertaining to minority health. Additional funding to staff the office of public health, respite care, and developmental disabilities was also included in this legislation. Tobacco settlement funds and intergovernmental transfer trust funds were and continue to be the source of this funding. This funding demonstrates Nebraska's commitment to public health and minority health.[16]

Despite these laudable efforts, health disparities continue. More can and must be done. Funds awarded based upon 1990 and 2000 U.S. Census totals do not take into account the growth of minority populations, nor do they take into account the rising costs of health care and the uninsured.

Health Education of Racial/Ethnic Minorities

Health education targeted to racial/ethnic minority populations represents the primary intervention strategy of OMH to increase health literacy, improve compliance with recommended health behaviors, and improve health outcomes. Focus areas include adult immunizations, asthma, bioterrorism, cancer awareness/screening, cardiovascular health, chronic disease management, diabetes, domestic violence, eye exams, food safety, health access/insurance, healthy lifestyles, healthy relationships, hearing exams, HIV/AIDS/STDs, maternal and child health, men's health, mental health, nutrition, obesity/weight loss, management, oral health, orthopedics, pandemic flu, physical activity, prescriptions and medications, sex education/pregnancy prevention, sexual assault/harassment, smoking, substance abuse, tuberculosis, and women's health.

Health education is delivered using bilingual guides and community health workers and is offered at ethnic community centers, health clinics, home visitation programs, and mobile health clinics. It is often tied to events such as festivals/cultural events, health career fairs, health conferences/institutes, "lunch and learn" programs, newsletters, and nutrition and health forums.

Partners in public education include human service agencies, community-based organizations, faith-based organizations, colleges and universities, local health departments, behavioral health providers, businesses, child care providers, city government agencies and programs, community and cultural centers and coalitions, community wellness programs, domestic violence agencies, employers of large groups of minority persons, federally qualified health centers, financial institutions, insurance companies, interpreter service providers, libraries and local foundations, media, Native American tribes, nursing homes, probation offices, and juvenile justice officials.

There are several keys to ensure effective health education efforts. Health education efforts to racial/ethnic minorities must be culturally competent and linguistically appropriate; must be visible, inviting, and easy to access; and should provide supportive environments for the individuals to adopt and sustain healthy behaviors. Health educators should understand the cultures, including differences between our healthcare system and that of the countries of origin of those being reached. Representatives of the minority groups should be involved in planning, and education programs should use presenters who are credible, trusted, and accepted by the community. Information should be available in various languages, and programs should provide ongoing education at regularly scheduled times; health education can be combined with healthcare services. Other keys to success include using culturally centered social marketing strategies; depoliticizing health issues; offering realistic, specific alternatives for nutrition and physical activity; and recognizing that housing, food, and transportation are health issues.

The Need for Public Health Leadership

Although the efforts just described are laudable, health disparities persist in Nebraska. The demographic changes and the health disparities associated with them present great challenges for public health leadership in Nebraska. Leaders must establish appropriate policy priorities, including elimination or reduction of health disparities, commitments to research, health education, and public outreach and education. Reducing these persistent disparities will require enhanced public education; improved access to health care; and culturally competent, linguistically appropriate health care. Public health leaders must also address the system deficits of a shortage of medically trained interpreters—a health workforce that does not mirror or reflect the racial/ethnic diversity of the patients and consumers served and that does not adequately engage the public in discussions of the future of a far more diverse America and Nebraska. Programs to enhance recruitment of racial and ethnic minorities to the health workforce as trained and licensed medical interpreters, public health nurses, program managers, physicians, dentists, and administrators are essential.

These challenges also demand promotion of cultural competence of Nebraska's health care, education, and service workforces. Only by adopting more aggressive policies and becoming more culturally competent will healthcare providers and public health leaders be able to close the health disparity gaps and respond to the needs of more than 260,000 minority residents of Nebraska.

Failure to respond to these challenges carries significant economic and societal costs: lost time from work and higher costs and insurance claims because of increasing rates of morbidity of increasing numbers of persons who are under- and uninsured. Health disparities, if left unattended, threaten to burden the public health infrastructure and severely affect state and local economies.

Further, there is a clear question of social and economic justice. Emily Friedman, in *White Coats, Many Colors*, observed, ". . . Although less than 20% of Americans over age 65 are members of minority groups, nearly 40% of those under 25 are."[9] When the first wave of baby boomers face retirement, nursing home or assisted living, and other medical or social service needs, they are likely to be supported by people who do not match their cultural backgrounds or race and ethnicity, many of whom are paid low wages and/or are under- or uninsured and suffer great disparities of healthcare access and health.

But leadership can be very difficult, even painful. To change the health system in ways to serve those most in need, some people and organizations may sustain losses. Marty Linsky, of the John F. Kennedy School of Government, Harvard University, and co-author of *Leadership on the Line: Staying Alive through Leading*,[17] insists that today we must differentiate between the exercise of authority and the exercise of leadership and be willing to go beyond the scope of one's authority in the exercise of leadership.[17] Today's public health leaders must prepare all 93 counties in Nebraska to recognize and acknowledge the changing demographics, that Nebraska, like the nation, is not an *English-only* domain, that racial/ethnic minorities have poorer health outcomes whether in Ord, Ogallala, or Omaha. Courageous leaders must be willing to say to white-run, white-administered boards of health, hospital boards, and nursing home boards, that changes are needed to make Nebraska the best it can be—and to identify what those changes must be. Heifetz and Linsky remind us that needed changes must be implemented at a rate that can be absorbed.[17] Healthcare providers, following Heifetz and Linsky's model of leadership on the line, must recognize the dangers of marginalization, diversion, attack, and seduction.[17] It is tempting to ask that minority stakeholder groups take on all responsibility for any minority health initiatives or to make health disparities and cultural competence lower priorities when faced with seemingly more pressing public health issues.

Supporters and allies may applaud our risk-taking leadership, but we, the public health leadership of Nebraska, must understand the disequilibrium, pressure, and stress placed on our state system of health care in leading adaptive change. We must calibrate the pressures, distribute the losses, and allocate the costs—remembering to allocate some of the loss to ourselves. We do, after all, have a share or stake in the systems we want to change.

Ray Schulte, a change consultant for The Center for Parish Development, proposes another attitude and behavior for leading systemic adaptive change:

resisting acclimatization to the way things presently are.[18] In the exercise of leadership, resistance to change may manifest as people and organizations attempt to "cool us off" or "heat us up." They work like thermostats to regulate behavior. Chris Argyris, after 15 years of studying business leaders, describes this as *single-loop learning*.[19] Leadership is difficult because learning has been reduced to problem solving. Problems are defined as external to ourselves and our organizations. By default, we lose the leverage needed to make and lead adaptive change as we then fall into defensive reasoning. Argyris calls this pattern of inculcated behavior "single loop learning strategies." She then defines her single loop learning this way: ". . . a thermostat that automatically turns on the heat whenever the temp drops below 68 degrees is a good example of single loop learning. A thermostat that could ask, 'Why am I set at 68 degrees?' and then explore whether or not some other temperature might more economically achieve the goal of heating the room would be engaging in double-loop learning."[19]

With respect to the communities within the public health infrastructure in Nebraska—individual voters, county boards of health, hospital administrators, the professional public health workforce, elected and appointed officials, academia, and professional associations—leaders exist who are asking the questions necessary to sustain engagement for the critical decisions needed to advance cultural competency as a first necessity in the elimination of health disparities. Culturally competent, linguistically appropriate health care throughout Nebraska is a vision that must be addressed systemically, must be institutionalized within Nebraska's health systems, and modeled by healthcare professionals who individually interact with patients and clients. As leaders, Nebraska's healthcare professionals and the systems within which they work must become not only culturally competent, but culturally proficient (standard of excellence).

Many healthcare organizations face problems in recruiting and retaining employees. Nebraska's Office of Rural Health tracks medically underserved areas of the state and administers the student loan repayment program for healthcare and medical students, who in exchange for loan repayment, agree to serve in medically underserved areas. Imagine a policy that directed those funds to re-train, and prepare for examination, physicians who are immigrants but whose credentials are not recognized in the United States. Imagine a program for mentoring racial/ethnic minority children and youth, offering stipends for working in labs and public health departments statewide. Racial/ethnic minorities and immigrants represent a great potential resource for the healthcare workforce.

We should also recognize that elderly persons, persons who are deaf or hearing impaired, persons who are from different regions of the United

States, persons of different socioeconomic status, and so forth, may also require a different kind of care if it is to be culturally competent. Bridging the language/cultural gaps among those who have limited and no English proficiency will help in the elimination of health disparities related to problems of access and socioeconomic status.

Who Benefits from Greater Leadership and Elimination of Health Disparities?

Improved access to quality health care greatly diminishes morbidity and mortality, and improved provider–patient relationships increase the likelihood that patients will actively cooperate in efforts to improve their health. Patient-centered approaches to health care lessen the disease burden on patients, increase patient compliance with treatment regimens, and reduce the chance of poor diagnoses due to miscommunication.[20] A culturally competent healthcare workforce is good for all Nebraskans. That workforce will improve the standards of care for all patients, not just those who are of different races or ethnicities, cultures, or languages.

Improving health care for all racial/ethnic minorities will result in a healthier workforce in Nebraska. It will result in fewer days lost from work and will enhance productivity. Improving the health of Nebraska's increasingly diverse workforce will give a competitive edge to Nebraska in the global economy by reducing the cost of labor. Eliminating health disparities is a win for all Nebraskans.

Offering culturally competent, linguistically appropriate care also decreases the risk of malpractice and other liabilities that can result when patients and physicians, or other healthcare providers, face linguistic and cultural barriers.

What Are the Obstacles to Effective Change?

However good our intentions, it is important to identify any obstacles to change and the means to surmount them. Obstacles to enhancing cultural understanding and competence and reducing health disparities include cross-cultural conflicts and misunderstandings, specific beliefs and attitudes of certain cultures, language and literacy barriers, poverty and other socioeconomic issues, limited program resources, health system hurdles, and certain public policies.

Cultural differences may result from ignorance; disrespect; feelings of oppression, hostility, indifference, or insensitivity; or lack of trust. There are also negative feelings, relationships, and dynamics between minority groups and the white, non-Hispanic majority and among the different minority groups.

Beliefs and attitudes that may hinder health education and foster continued health disparities include prejudices, poor cross-cultural communication resulting in misunderstanding, lack of understanding or acceptance of the concept of preventive health behavior, fatalistic attitudes towards illness, unwillingness to seek care until the problems are severe, inadequate health knowledge and literacy, strong beliefs in traditional remedies, the lack of a cultural concept of mental health, and cultural rules about women and what may or may not be discussed.

Language and literacy barriers include lack of health education materials in specific languages, particularly those of small minorities; availability and cost of interpreters and translators; difficulty recruiting outreach workers who speak the languages necessary to communicate to particular groups; providers who do not provide interpreters or do not know how to work with interpreters; use of children to interpret; interpreters' lack of medical certification or adequate training in health concepts and terminology; low literacy levels; and messages that are too complex.

Socioeconomic issues may complicate the delivery of health education—and the willingness of minority populations to hear and implement that education. Families and individuals struggling with poverty and fighting to meet basic needs such as food, housing, and transportation often do not place high priority on health education or health care. Recommendations of healthy diets may seem irrelevant to people who experience food insecurity. Transportation and child care also present barriers to heath education and health care among those living in poverty. Health coverage is often lacking, which severely limits options to access health services. Funding for medications or other treatments may not be adequate.

A major barrier in outreach to immigrant communities is that many immigrants are undocumented, cutting them off from many assistance programs. Fear of deportation keeps them (and even some with documentation) away from programs that would serve them. Past experiences with healthcare providers, even in refugee camps, greatly influences health-seeking behaviors of immigrants and refugees.

Resource limitations that constitute barriers to adequately serving racial/ethnic communities include financial, personnel, and data inadequacies. It is difficult for public agencies and organizations to obtain the level of funding needed to meet their health and educational program needs; it can be especially difficult to obtain funding to sustain programs for the long term, which is needed to be truly effective. High staff turnover frequently disrupts community connections, and limit of staff (people and time) restricts the amount of health education available and timely access to health services. Some funding sources are inflexible about how their funds can be used, some require excessive paperwork, and some include rigid evaluation requirements. Lack of adequate minority population data that are current, local, and specific to different minority groups is another challenge.

The fragmented, complex healthcare system is difficult enough to navigate for those who are advantaged by income, education, and health coverage, and speak fluent English. For immigrants and refugees, and other racial/ethnic minorities, health education is even less accessible through most healthcare services (even if they can access those services) because of the language and culture barriers discussed earlier.

Health education within the healthcare system is largely treatment based and confined to matters directly related to the diagnosis and treatment of specific health problems. Although disease prevention gets considerable publicity, the U.S. healthcare system is more oriented toward medical treatment than toward education and preventive measures. Prevention measures are primarily in the form of medical screenings and exams that can detect problems, which, if treated early, may prevent serious complications or will be more likely to be successful.

Patients who seek preventive health advice from professionals such as nutritionists or physical fitness experts are not likely to have their costs covered by health insurance. Covered health services are likely to be available only when serious health problems occur as a result of poor diet and inactivity. The system offers treatments to quit smoking or control alcohol and drug addictions, but it has less involvement in efforts to prevent substance abuse.

Public policies and the lack of enforcement of policies may present obstacles to reaching racial/ethnic minorities. One example of this is the lack of compliance and enforcement of Title VI of the Civil Rights Act and the culturally and linguistically appropriate services (CLAS) standards, which require health providers to provide interpreters and translators for their limited- and non-English speaking patients. In addition, Title VI violation complaints often do not result in provider compliance.

Public policies may also be barriers to increasing the number of minorities in the health professions. Higher education and employment obstacles for undocumented immigrants reduce the numbers who can pursue health careers. The certification process for health professionals trained in other countries prevents many from pursuing U.S. qualifications. There are health professionals trained outside of the United States who could provide health care to limited- or non-English speaking patients, but they are unable to meet the requirements for certification.

There are restrictions on providing services to undocumented immigrants. In particular, the requirements of a Social Security number for many assistance programs makes it difficult for organizations to reach this population group with health education and assist them with access to the healthcare services they may need.

Who Else Can Help?

There is a broad variety of ways to address these obstacles and expand efforts to reduce health disparities, many of which could be the role of OMH. One means is to involve new partners or expand involvement of existing partners. There are many possibilities: the business sector, especially major employers of minorities such as Nebraska's meat packing industry; local chambers of commerce; the financial sector; local and financial foundations; colleges and universities, local and county governments; faith- and cultural-based community organizations; media; civic or other charitable organizations; child care providers; nursing schools; minority health professionals and community leaders; and law enforcement.

The OMH can better support local efforts by improving relations and communications with partners, facilitating networks and collaboration, improving data collection, providing a link to the legislature and other policymakers, assisting with message dissemination, taking the lead on cultural competency, assisting in efforts to increase the number of racial/ethnic minorities in health professions, leading assessment and strategic planning, assisting with program and project development, coordinating and providing technical assistance with funding, training, and increasing health services for racial/ethnic minorities.

In the fall of 2006, the Nebraska OMH sponsored focus groups across the state to discuss health education for racial/ethnic minority populations. Eighty-seven organizations participated in the focus groups, providing valuable information for planning and prioritizing the public health needs of Nebraska. The focus groups elicited a wide range of suggestions that reflect the extent to which resources and technical assistance are sought by public health stakeholders in Nebraska. Some are mentioned here:

- Place more trust in local partners and find ways to work within partners' rules to help them help their community.
- Convene groups to exchange information on resources and best practices and facilitate partnerships.
- Sponsor meetings to support dialogue—round tables, working teams, and so on on minority health.

- Advocate for and help provide accurate, up-to-date local-level minority population data that are specific to different populations.
- Provide up-to-date information on health disparities, gaps, and number of uninsured and underinsured specific to communities.
- Develop a website to be a clearinghouse for minority health information; include useful links, a calendar of events, a catalog of multilingual resources, health status reports, best practices, collaboration opportunities, locations of health services, and funding opportunities.
- Develop a unified, single set of health education resource materials.
- Set the tone for leadership.
- Provide analysis of key issues.
- Raise OMH public profile and awareness.
- Give voice to community perspectives.
- Develop leaders and recognize leadership.
- Target younger people with health education and involve parents through groups like 4H.
- Provide statewide health education campaigns and more public health announcements in multiple languages, especially English and Spanish.
- Visit reservations and tribal leaders (reservation and nonreservation) to assess resources, gaps, and so on.
- Host an Indian Health Summit, including tribal leadership and key NDHHS people.
- Establish relationships and conduct education with business owners.
- Provide more education to healthcare personnel about cultural issues.
- Include cultural competence in medical school education curricula.
- Include Native American cultures within school curricula.
- Provide specific language materials.
- Establish common goals for minority health that organizations can incorporate into strategic plans.
- Sponsor a 2020 visioning process.

Clearly, there are myriad opportunities for improving the access of Nebraska's minorities to high-quality, patient-centered, and culturally and linguistically appropriate care that will reduce the health disparities in the state's increasingly diverse populations. There are many opportunities and many interested parties—including the Minority Health Advisory Committee of Nebraska, the Nebraska Minority Public Health Association, the Tribal Health Departments, the Public Health Association of Nebraska, the Mexican American Consulate in Omaha, the Nebraska Association of Translators and Interpreters, Creighton University School of Medicine, University of Nebraska Medical School, the Center for the Elimination of Health Disparities—from which cultural and community centers, healthcare providers, and organizations can learn more about health disparities and cultural competency in health care.

SUMMARY

In a speech delivered to a gathering of Latino professionals, the chief administrator of Nebraska's Department of Health and Human Services, Jacquelyn Miller, quoted *The Human Right to Health: The People's Movement for Human Rights Education*[21]: "The United Nations has declared that 'health is a human right.' " Miller continued,

> . . . every woman, man, youth and child has the human right to the highest attainable standard of physical and mental health, without discrimination of any kind . . . enjoyment of the human right to health is vital to all aspects of a person's life and well-being, and is crucial to the realization of many other fundamental human rights and freedoms . . . The United Nations further declared that Human Rights related to health include: the human right to the highest attainable standard of physical and mental health, including reproductive and sexual health; the human right to equal access to adequate health care and health-related services, regardless of gender, race, or other status; the human right to the equitable distribution of food; the human right to access to safe drinking water and sanitation; the human right to an adequate standard of living and adequate housing; the human right to a safe and healthy environment; the human right to a safe and healthy workplace and to adequate protection for pregnant women in work proven to be harmful to them; the human right to freedom from discrimination and discriminatory social practices; the human right to education and access to information related to health, including reproductive health and family planning; and the human right of a child to an environment appropriate for physical and mental development.

She boldly stated, *"I contend that if health is a human right, then a health disparity is a human rights issue and the struggle to achieve health equity for all is an issue of social justice."*[22]

In America today, one in four people is a racial/ethnic minority; by 2070, it will be one in two.[9]

Be an advocate—speak up, speak out!

REFERENCES

1. The *Nebraska Healthy People 2010 report 2006 Strategic Plan.*
2. Nebraska Office of Minority Health *2003 Health Status Report.*
3. *Health Facts for Racial/ethnic Minorities.*
4. U.S. Census Bureau. 2006. *Annual Estimates of the Population of the United States, Regions, and States and for Puerto Rico: April 1, 2000.* http://www.census.gov/popest/geographic. Accessed May 2007.
5. U. S. Census Bureau. 1996. http://www.census.gov. Accessed May 2007.
6. U.S. Census Bureau. 2006. *Population Estimates, Census 2000.*
7. U.S. Census Bureau. 2006. *American Community Survey.*
8. Nebraska Office of Minority Health, Department of Health and Human Service. Worksheet: Minority health initiative counties. 2005.
9. Friedman E. *White Coats, Many Colors: Population Diversity and Its Implications for Health Care.* Chicago: American Hospital Association; 2005.
10. Nebraska Department of Health and Human Services. *Vital Statistics 2000–2004.*
11. Nebraska Behavioral Risk Factor Surveys and Minority Oversample Behavioral Risk Factor Surveys. 2006, combined.
12. Institute of Medicine. *Unequal Treatment: Confronting Racial and Ethnic Disparities in Health Care.* Washington, DC: National Academies Press; 2002.
13. Palm D. Designing and Building New Local Public Health Agencies in Nebraska. *J Public Health Manag Pract.* 2005;11(2):139–148.
14. Mainer JS, Kramer S. *Mausner and Bahn Epidemiology: An Introductory Text.* Philadelphia: W.B. Saunders; 1985.
15. Medical Translation and Interpretation Leadership Group. 2007. Available at: http://www.members.cox.net/mtigroup/2007_mti_website_017.htm. Accessed January 2, 2008.
16. Legislative Bill 692 originally, now Legislative Bill 321, as of the close of the One Hundredth Session of the Nebraska Unicameral Legislature.
17. Heifetz RA, Linsky M. *Leadership on the Line: Staying Alive through the Dangers of Leading,* Boston: Harvard Business School Press; 2002:14, 20.
18. Schulte R. *A Strategic Church Transformation Process.* Chicago: The Center for Parish Development; 1997 (as shared in oral exercises in workshops settings).
19. Argyris C. Teaching smart people how to learn. *Harvard Bus Rev.* 1991;69(3):99–109.
20. U.S. Department of Health and Human Services. 2005 National Healthcare Quality Report.
21. The People's Movement for Human Rights Education Organization. The Human Right to Health. http://www.pdhre.org/rights/health.html. Accessed June 2007.
22. Miller JD. Achieving Better Health Outcomes for Nebraska.

Chapter 16

Cultural Proficiency and Health Disparity: The St. Louis, Missouri, Perspective

Michael T. Railey, MD

S t. Louis, Missouri, was once the eighth largest city in the United States, with 857,000 residents. The city now ranks as the nation's 50th largest, behind, for example, Fresno, California; Mesa, Arizona; and Colorado Springs, Colorado—none of which had 100,000 residents in 1950.[1] Today St. Louis is known for its healthcare disparities. Fifty years after being among the nation's top 10 cities, significant indicators—including life expectancy, infant mortality, maternal mortality, HIV/AIDS, other sexually transmitted diseases, and disability days—demonstrate some of the worst medical outcomes in the state and often in the nation.[2] What happened?

As one might expect, the answers to the question of what happened are multiple. The population declined from 850,000 in 1950 to approximately 340,000 in 2007. All population changes have not been bad, though. The St. Louis metropolitan area has evolved to encompass unprecedented diversity. The city and county are no longer simply black and white. Asian Americans, Hispanics, Chinese Americans, and Bosnians populate the communities. At the time of this writing, the Bosnian population in St. Louis is the largest in the world outside of Bosnia itself.

This burgeoning diversity has created a great need for cultural competency among healthcare providers. This chapter will discuss how the St. Louis medical community must better understand, interpret, and administer to the different ethnic groups within the city. To improve the health of the population, the medical community must recognize the multicultural identity of the population it serves. There must be collaborative efforts of the county, public health officials, and the populace to improve the delivery of health care to its neediest clients. To enable the reader to understand better the challenges confronting St. Louis, this chapter presents a brief history of the city.

The Emergence and Growth of the City of St. Louis

Founded in 1764, St. Louis has been known as the "Gateway to the West" for two centuries. Early settlers included whites, African slaves, Creoles, freed slaves, and American Indians. The 1799 U.S. Census listed the population as 56 free blacks, 268 slaves, and 601 whites.[3]

The Louisiana Purchase of 1803 positioned St. Louis as an important trade center. By 1879, the St. Louis riverfront was a portal for thousands of blacks fleeing oppression and the limited opportunities of the South in search of a better life. The river city became a hub for transportation and accessibility to Western markets. Referred to as the town of "shoes and booze," business dynasties such as Anheuser-Busch (beer) and the Brown Shoe Company established headquarters in St. Louis. The city had a reputation for getting things done and moving goods and merchandise to the West.

During this time, educational problems for the underserved of St. Louis began. The challenge of educating disadvantaged citizens was not adequately addressed then and is not now. Education of St. Louis blacks was stymied in 1847 when the Missouri Assembly passed a law stating that no person should keep, or teach in, any school for the instruction of Negroes or mulattos in how to read and write. Twenty-eight years later, in 1875, the state legislature reversed its ruling and directed the city's school board to provide a high school for black children.[3] Ten years later, in 1885, the first official matriculates of Sumner High School graduated, more than 20 years after the Emancipation Proclamation. The St. Louis City School Board has struggled since its inception to train and educate its students adequately.

In 2007 there is still controversy about how to improve education and prepare well-qualified high school graduates for college and the job market. Experts agree that an excellent education lays the foundation for a successful life and that education is related to health status. A poor educational system results in poor health of the population; this is the St. Louis experience.

Financial Development and Socioeconomic Disparities

In September 2006, the *St. Louis Post-Dispatch* published an article on the salaries of local chief executive officers (CEOs): 54 CEOs had a median income of $3.13 million.[4] The average worker in St. Louis earns $37,900, meaning CEOs earned 83 times the earnings of the average worker. This represented an 11% increase in CEO pay from 2004. Nationally, the rate of growth in executive pay has exceeded the growth of the ordinary workers' pay. St. Louis is a prime example of the rich getting richer and the poor getting poorer. A common question among native St. Louisans is, "What high school did you go to?" The answer immediately identifies an individual's socioeconomic status and where one can afford to live. If unable to secure a home in an excellent school district, children run a great risk of a substandard education.

The relationship between social class and health status is well documented. Income inequalities are related to health disparities. Significant selected health disparities of St. Louis are depicted in **Table 16–1**. Table 16–1 displays only disparities between the white and African American populations. This is not to imply that other special populations are not significant. St. Louis County is 1.7% Hispanic and 3% Asian. The city of St. Louis is less diverse, with a majority of African American (53%) and lower percentages of Hispanics and Asians than St. Louis County. There are more than 80,000 uninsured in the County of St. Louis. Clearly, the culture and presence of the black population has a tremendous effect on economic and health status measures. Until this population is better served and disparities reduced, progress will be hindered.

From 1999 to the present, there is remarkable consistency of disparities with relatively small variations in outcome measures. The health status of the underserved populations of St. Louis, in particular the black population, has remained abysmal, reflecting the economic and financial circumstances.[2] Comparing St. Louis with state and national measures, St. Louis has the worst health indicators in the state, and in some instances, the nation.

Health Disparity in St. Louis: How Did It Happen?

There has been much speculation about the causes of ethnic and racial health disparities. One was the *defective gene hypothesis*.[5] It was believed that some populations harbored defective genes and their problems were uniquely theirs, minimally affected by environment and circumstance. Blacks were

Table 16–1 *Selected Healthcare Indicators for St. Louis*

Health Issue	St. Louis City, White	St. Louis City, Black	St. Louis County, White	St. Louis County, Black
Inadequate prenatal (per 100 live births)	8.2	23.6	3.7	14.3
Asthma ER (under 15) (per 1,000)	6.9	38.1	6.4	36.6
Teen pregnancy (per 1,000; ages 15–17)	20.5	62.6	9.3	42.2
HIV/AIDS—hospital (per 10,000)	3.1	8.9	.3	4.9
Mental Disorders— Hospitalization (per 10,000)	146.2	230	9 7.3	142.5
Deaths of chronic diseases (per 100,000)				
Heart disease	261.5	282.3	215.8	351.2
Stroke	47.1	64.6	46.3	84.9
Diabetes	25.3	50.2	18.5	51.3

Source: Missouri Department of Health and Senior Services. Missouri Information for Community Assessment (MICA). Minority Health Disparities in St. Louis County and St. Louis City, 2005.

thought to be intrinsically inferior. This explanation is belied by the fact that when African Americans' living conditions improved, their health also improved.

Another explanation was the *ghetto miasma hypothesis*. It was proposed that there was something in the air; a "ghetto miasma" that caused health disparities.[6] People living in crowded conditions, sharing the same air were prone to poor health. A third hypothesis was *moralistic*. Poor people got what they deserved because they were lazy, drank, smoked, and had poor hygiene. Poverty and chronic diseases were acts of God, brought upon disobedient people as punishment.

Today we know that health disparities are related to social factors, including income, education, occupation, family status, and coping with daily stressors.[7] The high stress of low-income living and a lack of access to adequate preventive health care is an important contributing factor. One can easily understand that chronic worry and inability to make ends meet grind away at the human body, contributing to hypertension, obesity, and heart disease as a result of depressed, sedentary living. Neighborhoods affordable by those of lower socioeconomic status are generally devoid of access to private gym memberships and jogging paths. Having no insurance or being underinsured limits access to adequate and timely health care. This is further compounded by patients' lack of knowledge and verbal and body language skills that would enable them to communicate effectively with the front office personnel and healthcare providers. The process of making appointments can be daunting. Many become frustrated and give up, complaining that they were unable to get an appointment.

These problems are deeply rooted. Solutions must be carefully crafted and implemented by culturally effective and acceptable means.

The Genesis of Disparities

Healthcare disparities in St. Louis can be attributed to many causes. As noted earlier, African Americans are the largest ethnic group in St. Louis city, the largest minority in the county, and subject to the greatest health disparities. The genesis of poor health outcomes among African Americans includes many lifestyle factors. The eating habits of the early African Americans in St. Louis, as with any group of people, were based on ancestral traditions, teachings, and habits. During slavery they subsisted on "scraps" from the master's table, second-line (imperfect) crops, and pork. Organ meats (such as brains or liver), fried foods, highly salted vegetables (greens) and unusual animal parts generally discarded by the master were prepared in ingenious fashions to add flavor. Cattle and beef were usually consumed by whites. Pig snoots, pig feet, brains, chitterlings, and tripe became the cuisine of the African American culture.

A very interesting article from the 2001 *Journal Archaeology*, entitled "Ham Hocks on Your Cornflakes," examined the role of food in the African American identity.[8] Excavations in Annapolis, Maryland, and 13 other sites in the Chesapeake region were explored. Findings were consistent; food remains showed a definite pattern. Pork was much more commonly consumed than beef, and shallow-water fish not purchased from markets where whites typically shopped predominated. Apparently by the late 19th century as whites turned to beef, blacks did not. "For many people, eating particular foods serves not only as a fulfilling experience, but also a liberating one—an added way of making some kind of declaration. Consumption then is at the same time a form of self-identification and of communication." Blacks living under the oppression of slavery, with very few options, gathered at the end of the day for a communal meal with friends and family. They most likely found spiritual strength and regeneration through eating and camaraderie. This experience over generations became a part of the culture.

Unfortunately, this choice of foods exacts a devastating price. High salt intake, high fat, cholesterol, and triglycerides accelerate atherosclerosis and contribute to the genesis of hypertension, diabetes, coronary artery disease, and stroke. For those descendants, white or black, who are not able to free themselves from this trap of culinary suicide, the outcome is predictable. A foundational cornerstone of healthcare disparities is set firmly in place.

The Question of Racism

America was founded in theory and constitutionally on the powerful premise that all men are created equal. Unfortunately, the ugly specter of racism, no matter how generated or manifested, is detrimental to the peaceful coexistence of diverse cultures. Race relations have been a problem since the founding of the United States. The history of St. Louis reflects the influence of racism and cultural bias and must be considered a contributor to the health disparities that exist today.

Examination of a few major historical events over the past 150 years on a timeline is useful (**Table 16–2**). From the landmark U.S. Supreme Court Dred Scott decision in 1857 to multiple efforts to desegregate St. Louis public schools, African Americans in St. Louis have remained at the lower end of the socioeconomic scale. This is also reflected in self-esteem. Although the Emancipation Proclamation declared that slaves were free in 1863, it was more than 20 years before St. Louis established the first black high school. St. Louis was slow to provide educational opportunities to its poorer populations and slower still for African Americans.

Between 1915 and 1919, there were 18 major interracial disturbances in America. The race riot of 1917 in East St. Louis claimed more African American lives than any other riot in American history.[9] The riot was significant in determining why East St. Louis now has the largest proportion of blacks (98%) of any city in the United States. East St. Louis and the neighboring city of Alton, Illinois, have long been blighted.

Racism in St. Louis has gone from "overt to covert" as revealed in a 1991 television documentary with journalist Diane Sawyer.[10] Numerous episodes of

Table 16–2 *Timeline*

Dred Scott	Emancipation Proclamation	Black High School	Riot	World War II	Desegregation	Race Documentary
1857	1863	1885	1917	1941	1952	1991

business and social transactions were observed and secretly taped. Men of different races, purposefully equipped with similar "presenting" stories, sought to acquire apartments, automobiles, and other goods and services. It was consistently observed on camera that responses to African Americans were decidedly different than responses to whites. In one instance, a white man was offered an apartment for rental while a black was told it had just been rented. Denials and rationalizations were used by those involved when confronted. This type of covert discrimination is frequently hard to prove and even harder to eradicate. In light of these racist practices, it is reasonable to hypothesize that racism is a significant contributor to disparate health outcomes; these may result from different referral patterns, treatment decisions, and even diagnoses.

Education and Its Role in Healthcare Disparity in St. Louis

The St. Louis Public School Board is responsible for educating more than 33,000 students of the city of St. Louis. For a system more than 169 years old and the largest in the state, it has demonstrated very little progress toward excellence in education for all. During a period of four years between 2003 and 2007, the district has been through four superintendents.[11] The schools have been doing poorly, both physically and academically for years, with a proposed mandated state takeover in 2007. The cause for lack of progress is difficult to define. One may consider a number of reasons ranging from poor leadership to politics to financial problems and mismanagement. Obviously, children have suffered the most in this process as the schools consistently fail to educate students adequately. Health literacy, which plays such a significant role in securing access and then converting that access to improved outcomes, is, in part, affected by educational attainment, educational quality, and socioeconomic status. When education falters, poor health outcomes will not be far behind.

Cultural Proficiency in Clinical Medicine

Armed with a better understanding of the many factors involved in caring holistically for patients, the culturally proficient processes of being a provider (physician, physicians assistant, nurse practitioner, etc.) can be examined. When a patient accesses the healthcare system seeking assistance, the medical person in charge is required to conduct a history and physical examination in a manner that maximizes data gathering and minimizes time loss. It is within the context of this original encounter that cultural competency, or incompetency, becomes evident, and it is vitally important to setting the relational foundation necessary to achieve a successful outcome.[12,13] In the manner of greeting the patient, the interaction begins on a positive or negative basis. Although pleasantry and good manners are important, they are inadequate to conduct a *culturally competent interview*, defined as one in which the patient is made to feel comfortable and an atmosphere is created with which the patient is comfortable and confident in describing his or her health problem and discussing his or her perspective and understanding of it.

Cultural competence requires patience, knowledge, attitude, and skill to assure patients that their interpretation of circumstances and their belief system will be accepted and respected.[11] There is no place for ethnocentrism. A therapeutic encounter, or environment, is shaped by body language, spatial positioning, and word selection. There should not be an air of skepticism or a lack of acceptance by the provider.

These concepts are best illustrated by the encounter between a proficient clinician and a minority patient. Alyssa is a 19-year-old African American woman presenting for evaluation of a vaginal discharge. This is her first visit to this office, and she is apprehensive not only about seeing a new doctor but about having a stranger examine her in a "personal manner." Having to discuss intimate matters with a stranger may also be very uncomfortable. Greeting Alyssa with a smile and an open, extended hand, the clinician makes certain she is positioned so that they face each other at fairly equal head (upper torso) levels and that their bodies are turned appropriately toward one another. No notes are initially made. The physician begins with nonthreatening conversation about any difficulties in transportation and getting to the exam room. Alyssa's living situation is explored. The clinician takes careful mental note of the fact that she lives with her grandmother. After determining Alyssa's perspective of her problem and why she has come to see a doctor, the clinician asks what she thinks causes the problem and what her greatest fears are about it.

Sensing apparent real interest and concern in the tone and type of questions asked, Alyssa is encouraged to "take a chance" and is honest about her fears of pregnancy and sexually transmitted disease, possibly acquired from a person she knows she should not have been intimate with. She is even more concerned with her growing frustration with wanting to have someone to love her for herself and with her repeated "poor selections" of men at such an early age. The clinician's mental note of Alyssa living with her grandmother yields additional important knowledge; it is determined that she lost her mother to cancer at a young age and her father is incarcerated. In the short span of 5 to 7 minutes, the groundwork has been laid for a trusting, truthful relationship between provider and patient—and a good clinical outcome.

The St. Louis Perspective: How Can We Make It Better?

The challenge facing health care and, in particular, educational institutions is how to educate health professionals and provide them with the skills, attitude, and knowledge to provide culturally competent care, as illustrated in the example interview with Alyssa. In caring for underserved and diverse populations, these skills are vital and not common with many practicing physicians. This challenge is exacerbated because caring for underserved populations often means the income generated is minimal and the skills needed are maximal.[12]

St. Louis has two medical schools and must begin to capitalize on these assets. Medical school leadership and faculties must change their attitudes toward cultural competency. An initiative at St. Louis University years ago to increase cultural sensitivity of the teaching faculty was met with little enthusiasm or participation. No record of faculty who attended any of the course work was kept, nor was the instruction mandatory. To my knowledge, no further attempts have been made. I am unaware of any program similar to this at Washington University. Both universities have infrastructures in place, with deans of multicultural affairs who can influence recruitment. In my opinion, teaching professors and the "culture" of St. Louis medical schools should include more instruction in the management and understanding of health disparities and cost-effective care for the underserved. The small percentage of minority physicians on faculties must change, not only in Missouri but across the country.[12] Care of underserved patients—with its difficulties, frustrations, and poor rewards—should become part of the education process to prepare professionals of the future and reduce real-life culture shock and consequent avoidance of these kinds of patients. Students should be taught that the poor and disadvantaged are a part of their professional responsibility.

Further, current practitioners should strive to understand their own weaknesses of cultural proficiency. The availability of physician, nurse, and ancillary medical personnel in St. Louis is adequate. Another effort the health professions institution can and should make is to offer more continuing professional education about cultural competence, in particular with reference to the large minorities of St. Louis.

Another area of potential improvement in the cultural competence of health professionals is selection for admission to health professions schools. Studies have revealed that choices physicians make about employment very much depend on their experiences prior to matriculation in medical school. When schools select students who have previously expressed a desire to serve the underserved, the chances of that happening after completion of residency training are enhanced. It is also known that culturally proficient and competent instructors influence students and residents. They may also exert negative influences. At my med school, I will never forget a top-notch fellow student who was literally grabbed and shaken by a professor exhorting him to not consider family medicine as his specialty choice because this would be a waste of good talent. He acquiesced and selected a cardiology residency and fellowship. The notion that a specialist is a brighter and more worthwhile physician than a primary care doctor is dangerous, elitist, and detrimental to the development of culturally competent physicians.

Capitalizing on the presence of the Area Health Education Center (AHEC), which is located at St. Louis University, could be very beneficial if a campaign could be initiated and maintained to reach local doctors with the need to assess their personal cultural proficiency and follow up on any deficits to improve.

Area medical societies (there is a black or African American medical society and a larger more dominant and traditionally white medical society) should provide presentations demonstrating cultural competence and incompetence and how techniques and skills may be improved. This would contribute to addressing the problem in St. Louis in a professional and, one hopes, nonthreatening manner. The AHEC would also contribute to the retraining of physicians and other health professionals.

St. Louis faces challenges other than those of professionals. The public school system must provide better education about access to health care and provide education to improve health literacy. Whether this will involve a state takeover of the St. Louis school system is yet to be determined.

If local medical societies take ownership of health disparities and influence the schools to provide proper eating, exercise programs, and health education throughout the school years, they could make an important contribution in diminishing health disparities. Further, if the schools can improve English proficiency, which has been shown to improve health literacy and ability to negotiate the healthcare systems of America, their impact will be enhanced.

SUMMARY

The initiatives within the medical and educational arenas will be enhanced or hampered by the commitment of city and county governments. Government must become a stakeholder and provide financial backing and efforts to create a better financial base for all of St. Louis. In my opinion, all health departments should have weekly access to radio stations to provide programming, teaching, health education, emergency preparedness, and dissemination of other important health information to the public. There are more than 1 million residents in St. Louis County and 340,000 in the city. The need for resources is great, and the community has the resources. It needs to use them. St. Louis has maintained at least four major professional sports franchises for years (baseball, soccer, football, and hockey). The presence of these money generators, which all do well, should be one of the sources of funds.

For those currently suffering from health disparities, the use of healthcare coaching using persons of similar ethnicity and racial background to assist them "negotiate" the system would be valuable. Coaches from the community are easily trained and may be of great benefit to patients.

The St. Louis perspective for improving cultural proficiency and diminishing healthcare disparities provides important insights. To effect change will require many collaborating agencies and organizations in a unified effort. **Figure 16–1** illustration depicts how stakeholders in the St. Louis area could work together to resolve this vital problem.

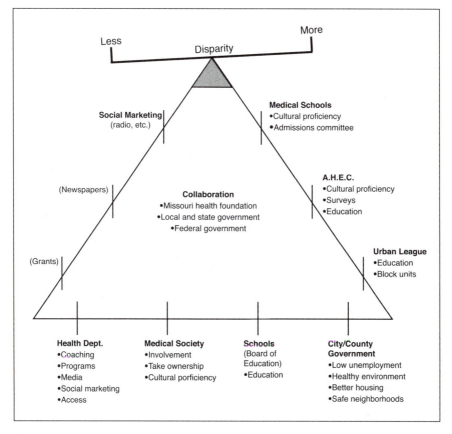

Figure 16–1   *St. Louis Disparities*

REFERENCES

1. Living Wage, Dying City: St. Louis. *The Public Purpose.* December 2000:40.

2. Missouri Department of Health and Senior Services. Missouri Information for Community Assessment (MICA). Minority Health Disparities in St. Louis County and St. Louis City, 2005.

3. Wright JA. *Discovering African American St. Louis: A Guide to Historic Sites.* St. Louis: Missouri Historical Society Press;1994.

4. Executive Pay. *St. Louis Post-Dispatch.* www.stltoday.com. September 10, 2006.

5. Ibrahim S, Kwoh CK. Special feature: Theories on African-American/White differences in the incidence of cardiovascular disease: A historical perspective. *ABC Digest Urban Cardiol.* 2000;7(3):16–23.

6. Epstein H. Ghetto miasma—Enough to make you sick. *New York Times. Sunday Late Edition* October 12, 2003; sec.6:75.

7. Hixon AL, Chapman RW. Healthy People 2010: the role of family physicians in addressing health disparities. *Am Fam Phys.* 2000;62:9.

8. Warner M. Ham hocks on your cornflakes. *Archaeology.* 2001:48–52.

9. Leonard M. Race riot. East St. Louis *Post Dispatch*; 1917.

10. Sawyer D. Two and one half weeks in St. Louis: True colors. *Primetime Live ABC News.* September 26, 1991.

11. St. Louis Public Schools circle the drain. http://ShrewdnessofApes.blogspot.com/ 2007/03. March 23, 2007.

12. Sutton M. It's not just political correctness: It's good medicine. Cultural competence. *Fam Pract Mgmt.* Oct 2000:58.

13. King S, Nanda N, et al. Promoting culturally congruent relevant care. Nov/Dec 2000:9–20.

Chapter 17

Health Disparities in the Pediatric Age Group

Cristina Fernandez, MD
Cathy Hudson, MD
Karl S. Roth, MD

The history of the United States is the history of immigration, chiefly of the poor and the disenfranchised. Thirteen years after the Declaration of Independence, the fledgling United States Congress passed the Naturalization Act of 1790, giving "any alien, being a free white person" the right to citizenship. Any schoolchild is aware that the initial immigration to the North American continent, beginning with the settlement of Plymouth, was given its impetus by the desire to seek religious freedom and a better life. Because the earliest immigrants came from an agrarian European society, "better life" was defined for them by cheap land for farming and plentiful raw materials for necessary craftsmen, such as blacksmiths and carpenters.

However, in the early 19th century, several factors in Europe conspired to drive successive waves of immigrants to American shores, chiefly the East Coast. Among these was the rising cost of land, the growth of the Industrial Revolution with its accompanying urban crowding and, perhaps most significantly, the post-Napoleonic European political foment and persecution and the Irish Potato Famine. It should be noted that none of these driving forces would be likely to encourage the wealthy to become immigrants, but rather the poor. Consequently, in the decades between 1830 and 1880, a total of approximately 7.5 million underprivileged people, chiefly Irish and German, landed in Boston and New York City. Because they were too poor to move inland, they settled as best they could in the tenement sections of the cities, creating vast areas of abject poverty and public health problems.

The prevalent attitude of the well-to-do toward these tenement slums was that the unfamiliar cultures, the crime, and the saloons were threats to the Republic and that the rampant disease sweeping through them was just dessert for such a sinful way of life.[1] Little imagination is required to see the analogy between this and the attitude of modern society toward those unfortunates who contracted HIV in the late 1990s. Among these "sinful" folk was a German refugee, a radical socialist and friend of Karl Marx, Dr. Abraham Jacobi.

Dr. Jacobi arrived in New York City in August 1853 and settled into the German-American community of "Klein Deutschland" (Little Germany). Children below the age of 10 made up one-third of the population,[2] and the infant mortality was appallingly high. Jacobi proposed the concept of a free dispensary in the midst of this public health nightmare; in doing so, he established the functional basis for what we know today as "the clinic" in academic medical centers throughout the United States. It was through the uncompromising efforts of Abraham Jacobi and his German immigrant associates to improve the health and living conditions of the poor that the foundation for the care of American children was laid, and he is widely acknowledged as the Father of American Pediatrics.

What is most relevant about the facts just related to the subject at hand is the historic precedent of highly educated and idealistic fellow refugees from a scientifically advanced society bringing their concepts and training to bear on an intolerable human condition. The impetus to do so was the Utopian socialist view of what must be done to bring value to the life of each human being in society. Moreover, it should be kept in mind that in all of this, race was a minimal consideration, while culture did not enter into the equation at all because the changes were initiated within the teeming German immigrant slums by one of their own. In American society today, there is considerable pluralism involving race, religion, language, and socioeconomic background of new immigrants, not to exclude people already here. Application of the precepts of pediatric care laid down by Jacobi a century and a half ago, in the context of a modern society virtually inconceivable to someone in the 1850s and working in a teeming urban slum, may not be the best way of going about things. In saying this, we acknowledge intrinsic flaws within the medical care delivery system, making it an "unfriendly" place for certain subpopulations, perhaps for a variety of reasons.

On the other hand, a survey of the literature on the subject of healthcare disparities in the United States finds a striking paucity of regard for the intrinsic cultural barriers that may exist toward *seeking* medical care as we offer it. There is a pervasive belief, usually introduced as a subtle premise, to most arguments that the fault must lie with the delivery system and the financing of medical care. Ergo, if only there were sufficient money and enough good doctors, everyone would avail themselves and their children of the medical care that our society offers. We were unable to find any study that approached the question of healthcare disparities in pediatrics from the perspective of what intrinsic reasons within a culture might inhibit a search by parents for medical care for their children.

It is, of course, this utter dependency upon parents to decide when/where/how to access care that most distinguishes the questions of healthcare access in pediatrics from those in other areas of medicine. Children, innocent of questions relating to immigration status, employment status, etc., nonetheless when ill require health care and their cultural/language barriers and socioeconomic status are irrelevant; all such choices have been made for them. However, it is precisely for this reason of dependency that the parents' reasons for choosing *not* to seek medical care become so vitally important to our understanding. As a consequence, we felt it essential to incorporate a discussion of this specific issue into this chapter for the readers' consideration and possible future research.

Background

Provision of medical care for the poor through "charity" is well documented as early as 800 A.D. in Syria and Baghdad under the Caliphate, a social attitude that found its way into Europe through Moorish Spain and the medical centers in Aragon, Catalonia, and Valencia.[3] In an ethical sense, charity can be viewed from at least two different perspectives: there is that of the provider, who gives for personal and/or professional reasons, and that of the recipient, who generally has little choice in the matter because options are so limited and a search for relief from suffering so compelling. Thus, little attention need be paid by the provider to attitudes of the recipients because the relationship is a vertical one with the power at the top. This model of charitable care for the poor was moved forward in history, finding its way to Britain in the 18th century; there were 40 charitable institutions founded between 1719 and 1800.[4] As we have seen (vide supra), the same model was imported to the United States by Abraham Jacobi in caring for the poor of Klein Deutschland in the 19th century. Thus, it is not surprising that there is a well-entrenched assumption that clinics exist today as a means to discharge the social responsibility of caring for the poor and the disenfranchised.

However, what is different about our society today is its relative heterogeneity, in comparison to that of 9th-century Baghdad or 18th-century Britain. The United States is experiencing massive immigration of the poor of other countries; unlike previous immigrations, however, the majority of these individuals are not only identifiable by poverty, but by color, religion, and language as well as culture. This heterogeneity has forced institutional changes; unfortunately, categorizations such as black, Hispanic, African, and so forth, which are often pertinent to medical matters, have also found their way into our social lexicon, where they have no relevance at all. Since the social turbulence of the 1960s, delivery of health care has been accepted as requiring understanding/consent on the part of both the provider and the recipient. Hence, translators have gained an important role in this regard, an example of additional expense that must be met by the society in discharging its responsibilities. However, the interposition of a translator could be seen as tipping the balance of power in the doctor–patient relationship still further in the direction of the former, an unfortunate adverse consequence of attempting to "do the right thing."

Delivery of health care to the disadvantaged, whether through the good graces of a caliph or from a general sense of social obligation, is always likely to be below par compared with that of the well-to-do. This does not, of course, suggest that it must or should remain so, but the necessary implication of fulfillment of a social obligation is that the minimal requirements will be met. Thus, in comparison to what is possible, it will likely always remain less than optimal. In a concise and tightly reasoned essay, Fausto-Sterling has argued that if poverty is the cause for disparity, we must deal with the causes, and if race is a contributor then we must deal, not with race, but with racism.[5] In doing so, we would free ourselves to deal with issues currently being ignored; these include operational and logistical problems within the delivery system, as well as means to introduce adaptability to cultural variations within the heterogeneous groups we wish/need to serve. The consequence of this would be a more flexible and responsive system that, in the final analysis, would be more efficient and directed at the individual rather than the group. The chief barriers to this end are the imbedded attitudes residing within our entire society that are perceived on the highly visible stage of healthcare delivery but are actually played out in more profound levels of the social/political scene.

Literature Review

Beginning in the 1970s there has been a burgeoning literature around the issue of cultural variations and their effect(s) on access to medical care. The inciting event in American history was almost certainly the passage of the Civil Rights Act in 1964, which focused society's attention on the social disparities between black and white Americans.[6,7] Because there had been a steady immigration of Hispanic individuals, contributed to by an influx of people from Puerto Rico over the preceding decade, the Hispanic minority in this country was subsequently included. The unfortunate consequence, however, was that for many years little to no attention was paid to other minority and cultural subgroups, specifically the Native American, African, and Asian peoples. Moreover, the latter categories of people continue to be "lumped" for demographic and Affirmative Action purposes, without regard to the fact that cultural differences between Africans or Asians may be widely disparate. In addition, Laotian or Tibetan immigrants are not considered to be minorities under Affirmative Action, despite the fact that they share little to nothing sociologically or culturally with mainland Chinese. Surely, any rational policy should treat a person from Cambodia, for instance, as a member of a minority group in this country; to do otherwise is to discriminate against someone whose culture and language is vastly different from that of other Asian groups. The point of this is to illustrate that once the door is opened to viewing minority groups in the proper light, the problems of addressing language barriers and cultural diversities in research regarding access to medical care become legion.

In its 1998 report, the Council on Graduate Medical Education (COGME) acknowledged that "new 'minority groups' have been emerging."[8] Thus, individuals from Dominican Republic, Panama, and Central America; blacks from the Caribbean and Africa; and Cambodians and Vietnamese were added to a list that already included Mexican Americans, mainland Puerto Ricans, and American Indians/Alaska Natives. But shall we continue to subcategorize until we reach the point of distinguishing between the black American who grew up and lives in the slums of Detroit (a majority of the residents of the area) from the black American living in Detroit's suburbs who grew up in the slums of Montreal where his parents fled during the Vietnam War? We are already faced with such difficulties in defining "Native American," because some tribes require only descendancy, while others require a minimum of generational ancestry for membership.

Indeed, the literature has become so mired in the fundamental concept that the term *minority* is reserved exclusively for Hispanic, African American, and possibly Native American (when the authors feel charitable) that it is impossible to verify whether or not disparities exist between native-born Caucasian Americans and, for example, a Russian individual from the Caucasus region who speaks with an accent! Such a sad state of affairs can likely be traced to a combination of social research faddishness, likelihood of gaining extramural funding, academic pressures to do so, political opportunism, and personal agendas. In any event, far from clarifying the issues we face in healthcare delivery, such wrongheaded exclusivity, sets us back in any attempts to understand the basic problems and how to deal with them. What is badly needed is a body of literature that examines the global plight of those who are "different" in some apparent respect in getting along in a society that is, like all human institutions, reluctant to acknowledge and accept those differences. Clearly, being caught up in the web of social welfare dependency has ramifications going far beyond those of periodic needs for health care and affecting these unfortunates in virtually every aspect of life from minute to minute.

Armed with these thoughts, an examination of the literature lends itself only to some very general conclusions. One article affirms what intuition would tell us—limited parental proficiency in the English language plays a large role in determination of access to care for children.[9] The authors conclude that English as a Second Language (ESL) class referrals for parents with limited English proficiency have the potential to break down barriers to access to pediatric care. Although there were relatively few parents with limited language proficiency who were not Hispanic in the study, the authors infer the commonsense conclusion that limited ability to communicate in English, irrespective of the language spoken at home, would impair access. However, the difficulty with their conclusion is that attendance at ESL classes requires (1) the will to learn English and (2) the disposable time to be physically present. Success in gaining language proficiency demands that both of these criteria be satisfied; it is not clear that present-day immigrants have either the will or the time, or for that matter, the resources.

How did immigrants of the past gain English language proficiency? In many cases, first-generation immigrants did not, instead establishing themselves as members of ghetto neighborhoods in which people shared cultural and language norms. Without the safety net of social welfare, these people were forced to support each other; their children, given the opportunity to assimilate and faced with the harsh realities of failure to do so, preferred to distance themselves from their cultural backgrounds. Thus, English proficiency became an essential means to this end, as well as a communication avenue between their parents and the world outside the ghetto. Having come to America seeking "a better life," the majority of these individuals brought with them the vision that life would be better for their children because of the opportunities available through hard work: a necessary prerequisite to survival in the new country. Disintegration of the classic neighborhood in American society has had an adverse impact on this social structure. Another crucial difference between present immigrant groups, many of whom arrive here to literally escape death, and those of the past is the cultural tradition of education as a means toward self-improvement. This avenue was vigorously pursued by the children of past immigrants, and American scientific and literary history is rich with their creations and discoveries. Today, immigrants from impoverished countries such as Sudan and Mexico have had no opportunity to gain an understanding of the connection among education, language fluency, and social standing. Hence, they have little incentive to pursue education as did the children of immigrants of the early 20th century, which contributes greatly to both illiteracy and failure to assimilate. Yet, the indisputable conclusion must be that English language is a necessary first step toward eliminating healthcare disparities. While the use of interpreters as an interim measure may be essential for delivery of meaningful care to those in need, widespread use of interpreters merely further encourages the dependency so obviously fostered by the social welfare system in general. A necessary consequence of this is continued illiteracy and greater dependency, which, in some respects, may be interpreted as a positive result for continued existence of the social welfare bureaucracy.

At the opposite end of the spectrum of "science" is the paper by Horner and colleagues, purporting to be a report on changing behavior among healthcare professionals.[10] In this paper, published in a most unlikely place, given the importance of the profit motive to managed care organizations, the authors unabashedly state: "The major underlying premise of the working group was that observed disparities in healthcare utilization are primarily a function of healthcare professionals' lack of cultural competence." Such a baseless assertion serves to prove the point made earlier regarding the implicit assumptions made by individuals associating themselves with this question of healthcare access. To go still further, the authors make the egregious statement that: "Patients' racial and socioeconomic characteristics clearly [sic] have been shown to influence physicians' beliefs about their patients' *intelligence* . . ." without any citation! Had this article been published in a newspaper in the Op-Ed section where it more properly belonged, it would have inflamed social debate for months. Such prose cannot qualify as legitimate research by any definition, although it lends weight a priori to the biases of many that the medical profession is to be blamed for lack of access to medical care. In fact, there is a published study purporting to show what was stated in the cited article.[11] The authors, van Ryn and colleagues, evaluated the recommendations made by physicians to white versus black patients regarding the advisability of coronary artery bypass grafting. The physicians were asked to rate each patient regarding certain characteristics (including perceived intelligence), which informed the recommendation. The data, as presented, are egregiously misrepresentational: of 111 white patients 73 (66%) were perceived as intelligent, while of 88 black patients 50 (60%) were rated intelligent, yet the raw numbers of 50 versus 88 are compared for significance!

In contrast to the foregoing, Flores and colleagues[12] have reported on an examination of the factors determining insurance status of Latino children in the United States. Despite the fact that this group of children comprises the largest population of uninsured minors in the United States, the authors found that Latino ethnicity is not associated with insurance status. On the other hand, parental immigrant status, low family income, and increased child age were associated with lack of insurance. Paradoxically, it was also shown that families in which both parents were employed were less likely to have insured their children. One might surmise that the reason is because of a combined income that results in disqualification for Medicaid and inadequate dissemination of information regarding the State Children's Health Insurance Program (SCHIP) provision. However, the overall message to be taken from this report is, as the authors point out, there are specific indicators of high-risk populations that are applicable to the population as a whole. It would be generally beneficial for us to focus on this aspect of the problem, which takes us back to the powerful argument of Fausto-Sterling[5] that we must deal with the core issues, rather than "nibble" at the edges.

Much of what has been said already is corroborated by a review of the existing literature on the subject of pediatric primary care experiences published in 2003.[13] These authors describe a model for links between race and ethnicity and primary care experience in pediatrics. This framework very fairly addresses the possible family/cultural reasons for failing to seek access while making clear the myriad possibilities for failure of the system to provide care that is sought. The point is made that race and ethnicity are so interwoven with socioeconomic status that measurement of one in isolation from another is a very difficult task. Given that a family has sought care, the authors point out that culturally conditioned variation in expectations or preferences may condition their response to any request to rate their experience. Most studies do not attempt to adequately evaluate these factors, making the significance of their conclusions difficult to interpret. In addition, the authors direct attention to the fact that primary care experience rating may be based on a relationship to a single provider, rather than to ease of access, each one an independent variable. They also point to the potentially dichotomous role that health care plans may play in delivery of primary care; that is, by restricting care provision to a specific roster of providers, the relationship between doctor and patient may be strengthened, or it could place an additional burden on minority and/or language-compromised families because of insufficient provision for these issues.

An additional factor, nowhere addressed in the literature surveyed, is the role played by social dependency in evaluation of health care. It is intuitive, although undocumented, that a person forced to exist at a marginal level, dependent on societal "charity," would feel a pervasive sense of unhappiness. The correlation between community conditions and healthcare disparities is strong.[14] Starting from this assumption, to ask such an individual to evaluate one aspect of his or her social situation is to invite expressions of criticism and dissatisfaction to one extent or another. Then, to grant statistical validity to an aggregate of such expressions and draw the conclusion that this specific aspect is fundamentally flawed is pure folly and completely overlooks the human emotional responses the study is designed to evaluate.

Stevens and Shi[13] affirm many of the concerns we have expressed in this chapter as weaknesses in the published studies. They indicate that there is often poor definition of measures of race and ethnicity and that all individuals with the same skin color do not necessarily belong to the same race or socioeconomic status or share the same cultural traditions. A prime example of this is the difference between the immigrant African black person and the African American individual, where there is not even commonality of language/accent of speech, let alone culture. Measurement and evaluation of primary care experience is often partial, with little to no overlap from one study to another, and there is no control in most studies for culture-based differences in perceptions and expectations.

A final factor, and one not considered in any published study, is the impact of care on the child. Few would argue, for example, that attentive and child-friendly dental care in the pediatric patient engenders a life-long attitude toward maintenance of dental health. Certainly, the same should be true of medical care, yet no attention has been given to the child's experience, which might be vastly different from the perceptions of the parent. The preverbal infant, seen by a pediatrician who may be completely unable to communicate with the parent due to a language barrier but who genuinely loves children, may take a very different message from the experience than the mother does. The same could be said about racial and ethnic barriers that need not impair communication between the concerned physician and the child. In this regard, we as a society are imposing far too many of our biases and misperceptions on our children and furthering, rather than conquering, the very prejudice we all decry!

Pediatric Diversity

No me llames extranjero, mírame bien a los ojos, mucho más allá del odio,
del egoísmo y el miedo, y verás que soy un hombre, no puedo ser extranjero.

Don't call me foreign, look deep at my eyes, far away from the hatred,
the egocentrism and the fearful and you will see I am a human being,
I can't be a foreign person.

—Rafael Amor (Argentina Singer)

The United States in the 21st century is continuing to experience a diversity of cultures, religions, race, languages, and shifting socioeconomic patterns that affect the pediatric population. Whereas, in the prior two centuries immigrant populations entered the United States in relatively small numbers and generally underwent extensive assimilation within one or two generations, the latter 20th and early 21st centuries have witnessed a dramatic change in this pattern. Members of minority groups are further increasing in numbers and diversity, while simultaneously tending to become assimilated much more slowly, if at all. By 2050, about 50% of the adolescent population will be of African American, Chicano/Latino, American Indian, or Asian descent. And, according to the 2000 Census, a full one-third of the adolescent population belongs to one or another minority group.[15] Healthcare professionals and local communities are faced with the task of delivering quality health care to an increasingly diverse population with varied beliefs about the definition of "quality health care" as well as multiple ways in which these beliefs affect the execution of the care delivered.

Education

A link among poverty, low educational attainment, and poorer health outcomes, with increased morbidity and mortality, has been well established. Heart disease, diabetes, obesity, HTN, increased lead levels, and low birth weights are all more prevalent among individuals with low income and low educational attainment. By far, Hispanic adults were more likely to have fair or poor health by self-report surveys. However, while federal initiatives have acknowledged the importance of the relationship of socioeconomic inequalities to health, the report of the National Center for Health Statistics (NCHS) does not support the self-reported data. In 2004, the Hispanic/Latino and Mexican American populations were the healthiest of all groups, as judged by the percentage of all persons in fair or poor health and the percentage of all persons with activity limitations due to one or more chronic health conditions.[15] These groups also had the lowest percentage of births with low-birth-weight infants. Indeed, by the same measures, the least healthy population in the United States today is the Native American adult. The percentage of low-birth-weight infants continued to be highest among the African American population. Whites lead both African American and Hispanics in educational attainment at the high school and college level. The percentile of African Americans and Hispanics earning a bachelor's degree is one-half that of whites. Additionally, higher socioeconomic groups have recently achieved greater improvements in health status than lower socioeconomic groups.[16–18]

Perceived Health Disparities

Despite the national statistics cited, a poorer perception of health and disparity in health status persists across all minority groups. This perception of racial and ethnic disparities in health care existed across both high- and low-income groups. Hispanic adults in particular were most likely to report being in fair or poor health (33%), and this rate was significantly different from that of any other racial/ethnic group. In comparison, 23% of blacks and 20% of Native Americans and whites in the low-income bracket reported fair or poor health status. Minority children believe that they are in poorer health than white children, Hispanic children most often reporting that their health status is fair to poor. Perhaps, given the adult perception, the children's reports should surprise no one; the greatest surprise is the self-perception of the Native American adult of relatively good health, simply demonstrating the lack of validity resulting from self-reported studies discussed earlier in this essay.

Other perceived causes of health and healthcare disparities include access to and ease of utilization of health care facilities, caregivers who are not aware of available services, caregivers who feel uncomfortable with providers, provider's beliefs/attitudes/biases, the availability of competent translators, long wait times for a scheduled appointment, long wait times in the doctor's office, inconvenient locations, and lack of adequate transportation.[19,20]

The reader is reminded of the caveats addressed earlier, regarding the reliability of studies based on self-reported data. A report, based on data relating socioeconomic status to mortality, clearly showed that poverty adversely affects longevity in the United States.[21] However, inasmuch as race did not protect the study subjects from this effect, it must be clear that multiple, and thus far unelucidated, factors play a major role in this relationship.

Healthcare Insurance

Some studies have shown that children with private healthcare coverage are more likely to be in excellent health than uninsured children and children on public insurance.[12,13] In 1996, 40% of the nonelderly minority population were uninsured. As an example, only 32% of the eligible Latino children received Medicaid benefits.[22] The children who were uninsured or underinsured were more likely to consider the emergency room (ER) a source of primary care and less likely to identify a particular physician as a source of care. These children also had fewer contacts with a physician in the previous year. Children less than 6 years of age were more likely to be covered by some form of insurance than children aged 6–17 years. However, many of these unfortunate facts have been mitigated by the creation in 1997 of the State Children's Health Insurance Program (SCHIP), authorized by Congress as a jointly funded program designed to provide health insurance for children of the "working poor." The ceiling income for eligibility is a multiple of the federal poverty guidelines and is altered based on the number of dependent children under the age of 18. By 2001, the proportion of eligible Hispanic children uninsured had dropped from 68% in 1996 to 24.9%.[23]

In contrast with the low number of Latino children eligible for Medicaid benefits cited earlier, the greatest proportion of children insured under the SCHIP program in four states (Alabama, Kansas, New York, and Florida) comprise 26% of all enrollees nationwide and are Hispanic.[24] Moreover, SCHIP has been shown to be a potent factor in the reduction of racial/ethnic disparities in health care.[25] However, major uncontrolled variables in any study comparing the Medicaid and SCHIP pediatric populations from the perspective of access to health care are the motivation for assimilation and ability to self-support between the two socioeconomic groups. The former is likely to enhance the willingness to access the system, while the latter is a crucial determinant of eligibility.

SUMMARY

The improvement of the quality of pediatric health/health care for all children, insured or uninsured, involves a meaningful and effective integration of all aspects of the delivery system. A lack of such integration has been a particular problem in delivery of care to special needs patients with complicated medical and behavioral problems. As an example, due to the high rate of low-birth-weight babies in the minority population (vide supra), it may be correctly assumed that a lack of service integration especially affects this group of patients adversely. The ideal healthcare model integrates the patient, care-givers, physician, community, health insurance, economic stability, and cultural awareness and sensitivity in the implementation of a healthcare network that will have better outcomes for today's and tomorrow's children.

Functional integration of the various elements of a community healthcare delivery system as shown should lend itself to eliminating disparities, whether culturally or socioeconomically based. Moreover, blending the clinic settings should achieve better treatment and therapeutic outcomes. Awareness of the barriers in the community (e.g. cultural avoidance of Western health care), as well as those within our healthcare delivery system (e.g. financing, physician continuity, and language) will contribute to more productive discourse and effective outcomes.[15,17] Integration of the healthcare system is also called for in the federal initiative set forth, called *Healthy People 2010*. This initiative was generated as a "blueprint" for elimination of disparities in health and health care in six key areas in which the identifiable socioeconomic and racial disparities are particularly striking: cardiovascular disease, diabetes, infant mortality, immunizations, cancer screening and management, and HIV/AIDS.[27]

For it to be effective, the entire healthcare community will need to accept and implement this initiative. As with any such sweeping change, healthcare providers will need to work cooperatively with other social agencies to continue to make appropriate changes in optimization of the health care of all children. Important factors to be considered and integrated into an effective approach are the cultural heterogeneity within the general population, as well as within many cultural subgroups. Moreover, account must be taken of an historic mistrust, leading, for example, to a stereotyping of individuals, which is an unfortunate problem hampering relations in both directions during a healthcare encounter. It should be kept uppermost in mind that children are not born with prejudices of any sort—they are taught or learn by example, or both. Finally, the healthcare system must divest itself of the philosophy, so prevalent in past years, that "if we build it they will come," because new clinic buildings can no longer compensate for lack of dignity and concern in the treatment of patients. Positive outcomes for the health futures of all children depend on an integrated effort of the entire community and its healthcare delivery system.

REFERENCES

1. Viner R. Abraham Jacobi and German medical radicalism in antebellum New York. *Bull Hist Med*. 1998;72:434–462.
2. Nadel S. *Little Germany: Ethnicity, Religion, and Class in New York City 1845-80*. Urbana: University of Illinois Press;1990:42.
3. Brodman JW. Charity and welfare: hospitals and the poor in medieval Catalonia. Philadelphia: University of Pennsylvania Press; 1998;229.
4. MacDonald FA. The infirmary of the Glasgow Town's hospital, 1733-1800: A case for voluntarism? *Bull Hist Med*. 1999;73:64–105.
5. Fausto-Sterling A. Refashioning race: DNA and the politics of health care. *Differences: A Journal of Feminist Cultural Studies*. 2004;15:1–37.
6. National Vital Statistics System. Health insurance coverage for maternity care: Legitimate live births. United States—1964-1966. *DHEW*. October 1971;(HSM): 72–1009.
7. National Vital Statistics System. Infant mortality rates: Socioeconomic factors. United States. *DHEW*. March 1972;(HSM):72–1045.
8. Council on Graduate Medical Education: Twelfth Annual Report. Minorities in Medicine. Washington, DC: U.S. Department of Health and Human Services, HRSA; May 1998.

9. Flores G, Abreu M, Tomay-Korman SC. Limited English proficiency, primary language at home, and disparities in children's health care: How language barriers are measured matters. *Public Health Rep.* 2005;120:418–430.

10. Horner RD, Salazar W, Geiger J, et al. Changing healthcare professionals' behaviors to eliminate disparities in healthcare: What do we know? How might we proceed? *Am J Manag Care* 2004;10:12–19.

11. van Ryn M, Burgess D, Malat J, et al. Physicians' perceptions of patients' social and behavioral characteristics and race disparities in treatment recommendations for men with coronary artery disease. *Am J Public Health.* 2006;96:351–357.

12. Flores G, Abreu M, Tomany-Korman SC. Why are Latinos the most uninsured racial/ethnic group of US children? A community-based study of risk factors for and consequences of being an uninsured Latino child. *Pediatrics.* 2006,118:730–740.

13. Stevens GD, Shi L. Racial and ethnic disparities in the primary care experience of children: A review of the literature. *Med Care Res Rev* 2003;60:3–30.

14. Laying the Groundwork for a Movement to Reduce Health Disparities. Report II. Prevention Institute. April 2007. www.preventioninstitute.org.

15. National Center for Health Statistics, 2004. http://www.cdc.gov/nchs/fastats.

16. Dumont-Mathieu TM, Bernstein BA, Dworkin PH, et al. Role of parenting advice: A qualitative study with mothers from 4 minority ethnocultural groups. *Pediatrics.* 2006;118:e839–e848.

17. St. Peter RF, Newacheck PW, Halfon N. Access to care for poor children. Separate and unequal? *JAMA.* 1991;268:2033–2034.

18. Rosa UW. Impact of cultural competence on medical care: where are we today? *Clin Chest Med.* 2006;27:395–399.

19. Lieu TA, Newacheck PW, McManus MA. Race, ethnicity, and access to ambulatory care among US adolescents. *Am J Public Health.* 1993;83(7):960–965.

20. Mokad AH, Marks JS, Stroup DF, et al. Actual causes of death in the United States, 2000. *JAMA.* 2004;291:1238–1245.

21. Winkleby MA, Cubbin C. Influence of individual and neighborhood socioeconomic status on mortality among black, Mexican-American, and white women and men in the United States. *J Epidemiol Community Health.* 2003;57:444–452.

22. U.S. Census Bureau. Census Report. Health Insurance Coverage 1996. http://www.census.gov/hhes/hlthins/cover96.

23. U.S. Census Bureau. Census Report. Health Insurance Coverage 2001. http://www.bls.census.gov/cps/ads/2002.

24. Shone LP, Dick AW, Brach C, et al. The role of race and ethnicity in the State Children's Health Insurance Program (SCHIP) in four states: Are there baseline disparities, and what do they mean for SCHIP? *Pediatrics.* 2003;112:e521–e532.

25. Shone LP, Dick AW, Klein JD, et al. Reduction in racial and ethnic disparities after enrollment in the state children's health insurance program. *Pediatrics.* 2005;115:e697–e705.

26. Cultural Competence Education 2005. American Association of Medical Colleges. http://ww.aamc.org.

27. U.S. Department of Health and Human Services. *Healthy People 2010.* McLean, VA: International Medical Publishers; 2000.

Chapter 18

Addressing Health Care in Communities

Ethel Williams, PhD
Frank T. Peak, MPA

> *"Of all of the forms of inequality, injustice in health
> is the most shocking and the most inhumane."*
> —Dr. Martin Luther King Jr.

Disparity in health among minority populations has been well established in the literature. Persons of color are in poorer health, have a lower life expectancy, and less access to health care than white Americans.[1-5] The U.S. Department of Health and Human Services has indicated six focus areas in which racial and ethnic minorities experience serious disparities in health access and outcomes: infant mortality, cancer screening and management, cardiovascular disease, diabetes, HIV/AIDS, and immunization.[6,7] In addition, the Centers for Disease Control and Prevention (CDC) has noted mental health, hepatitis, syphilis, and tuberculosis as diseases and conditions that disproportionately affect minorities.[7]

In 2007, the CDC reported that, "despite great improvements in the overall health of the nation, health disparities remain widespread among racial and ethnic minority populations."[8] Knowledge of disparities dates back several decades. A *Fact Sheet* published by the National Institutes of Health in 2006 reported information regarding minority health 30 years ago. "Americans enjoyed improved health and lived longer lives in the latter part of the 20th century. However, African Americans, Hispanics, Native Americans, and Asian/Pacific Islanders, who represented 25 percent of the U.S. population, continued to experience striking health disparities."[9] While progress has been made in addressing disparities, new approaches to addressing and eliminating the problem must be sought.

Health disparities among minority populations are attributable to many factors. Disparities exist as a result of differential access to care[3,10,11] disparities in the delivery of care,[3,10,12–14] and socioeconomic inequalities to which minority populations are susceptible. Numerous recommendations for eliminating disparities have been offered and attempted. They range from emphasizing the need for minority groups to participate in healthcare research to examining the occurrence of specific health concerns such as diabetes, cancer, hypertension, and heart disease.[15–19] While the importance of these studies and varied approaches to addressing health disparities should not be minimized, additional measures are warranted if disparities are to be eliminated.

The National Association for the Advancement of Colored People (NAACP), in its 2005 *Call to Action to End Health Disparities*,[20] focused on the following points:

1. Increase individual and community awareness.
2. Ensure access to quality health services.
3. Improve delivery of health services.

Similar recommendations were made by the Graduate School of Management at New York University in a 2003 report to the Robert Wood Johnson Foundation. The report, *Addressing Health Disparities in Community Settings*, concluded that successful programs aimed at reducing health disparities centered on "existing organizations mobilizing and managing a broad range of community resources."[21] The importance of the model of an entire community addressing health disparities is a recurring theme.[22,23] Peter Oakley recognized the critical nature of community involvement nearly two decades ago. In discussing health development across the world, he noted that successful development requires community participation.[24] The NAACP broadened the role of community in recognizing the need for "involvement and commitment" of all community stakeholders in addressing health disparities.[25] Florin and Dixon argue that increased involvement of the public leads to more democratic decision making and better accountability while making services "more responsive to the individuals and communities who use them."[26] According to Siegel and colleagues, mobilizing and managing community resources to address health disparities is crucial. This is especially true for populations that face barriers to health care.[21]

Davis, Cohen, and Mikkelsen acknowledged that reducing health disparities can occur through the combination of community action and policy change.[23] In a report by Emmel and Conn, it was suggested that involving communities in the planning and design of healthcare services will ultimately lead to more appropriate and sustainable services.[27] Thus, to eliminate health disparities, it is important to engage communities in exploring and developing strategies.

The Community Approach

Several approaches to defining the term *community* have been used when discussing health care and healthcare initiatives. It is assumed that community is associated with geographic location; however, according to the Institute for Healthy Communities, when the word *community* is preceded by an adjective, it describes a subgroup of populations and organizations: for example, the African American community, the Hispanic community, the public health community. While almost all community health interventions target a specific subgroup, the overall goal is to address the needs of the entire population. The Institute for Healthy Communities defined the term in a broader manner. They included, "[a]ll persons and organizations within a reasonably circumscribed geographic area in which there is a sense of independence and belonging. When determining the parameters of a specific community, it is important to define the community boundaries from the perspective of those who belong to it, not from the perspective of an outsider. . . . [The] delineation of the community must be inclusive of all who function there (education, business and industry, recreation, government, the media, spiritual organizations, human service providers, public health residents, voluntary organizations, and health care provider organizations). The provider organization is not separate from the community; it is a member of the community. The perspective therefore, is not 'we—they,' but 'us.'"[25]

This same inclusive definition was used by the U.S. Department of Agriculture in determining *empowerment and enterprise zones*. Their programs are based on the assumption that residents within a specific area are important to changing the area. However, broad participation of all segments of a community is necessary. This includes private and nonprofit support, religious institutions and organizations, political and government groups, and health and social service groups.[28] In the United Kingdom, the Nuffield Institute for Health determined that communities are defined by their members: "Communities, defined by the members of communities, are made up of the networks and organizations that bind a group of individuals together."[25]

We use an approach that represents elements of each of the preceding definitions as well as the comprehensive conceptualization provided by Israel and colleagues.[29] Drawing on definitions by Sarason,[30] Klein,[31] and Steuart,[32] they suggest that a community is a locale or domain that is characterized by the following elements: (1) membership—a sense of identity and belonging; (2) common symbol systems—similar language, rituals, and ceremonies; (3) shared values and norms; (4) mutual influence—community members have influence and are influenced by each other; (5) shared needs and commitment to meeting them; and (6) shared emotional connection—

members share common history, experiences, and mutual support. Communality may be geographically bounded, but not necessarily (e.g., an ethnic group).

Elimination of health disparities in minority communities requires recognition of the unique nature of health problems associated with each of the minority subgroups (the African American community, the Hispanic community, the Native American community, and the like), marshalling the commitment and resources of all who function there (education, business and industry, recreation, government, the media, spiritual organizations, human service providers, public health residents, voluntary organizations, and healthcare provider organizations). "In the most effective community-based collaborative, a broad range of community people are also invited and encouraged to participate in the planning and implementation process. Those who have participated in effective collaborative efforts suggest that the significance of consumer involvement cannot be overstated. They argue that consumer involvement is absolutely crucial to the legitimacy of the planning process and long-term success of the new service strategy. They believe that strong consumer involvement pays identifiable dividends."[33]

The Need for Community Empowerment

The concept of *empowerment* has been explained in a number of ways. Emmel and Conn assert that empowered communities "are able to demand justice, such as a demand for particular quality and responsiveness of service."[27] Drier views empowerment as consisting of several strategies, including community organizing, community-based provision of services, and community development.[34] Each of these strategies has unique components that taken together, stress mobilizing and involving people in the community to define and address their own problems at the neighborhood (geographically defined) level, improve their physical environment, and deliver social services that "improve the lives and opportunities" of the residents. They view the effort to address social problems such as health care as the heart of empowerment.[34] Wallerstein and Bernstein focus on the service delivery aspect of this conceptualization and broaden it to define *empowerment*. They believe empowerment "embodies an interactive process of change where institutions and communities become transformed as people who participate in transforming them become transformed."[35] This kind of empowerment is necessary to address and eliminate health disparities in minority communities. Minority populations must understand problems unique to their subgroup (community) and recognize the need to involve, and then engage, resources within the community (education, business and industry, recreation, government, the media, spiritual organizations, human service providers, public health organizations, voluntary organizations, and healthcare provider organizations).

The challenge of empowering communities is multifaceted when considering minority populations. The challenge associated with the process of empowerment itself is a huge hurdle. Minority communities lack many aspects of power necessary to bring about change. In a *Health Education Quarterly* symposium on community empowerment and health, Wallerstein and Bernstein explain the quadruple challenge of empowerment. These challenges include (1) how to ensure professionals and organizations value and honor individual contributions, yet address, on a community and societal level, the underlying conditions that further powerlessness; (2) how . . . organizations effectively work with others for community empowerment; (3) the question of power itself—most organization administrators and service providers are not interested in a 'process of empowerment that entitles some people to oppress others as they increase their own power'; and (4) how to sustain long-term commitment to the empowerment process."[35] These challenges alone provide sufficient problems to community empowerment; however, when coupled with the lack of minority participation in decision-making processes, these factors present a formidable obstacle to empowerment.

A number of significant barriers have been identified that negatively affect participation in decision making and empowerment of minorities.[36] Some of the barriers most frequently identified include (1) mistrust, (2) lack of identifiable benefits, (3) conflict in values and benefits, (4) lack of relevant research, (5) methodologies do not reflect the population culture, and (6) lack of guiding principles.

Nine factors associated with racial minorities have been identified by Randall and linked to a negative effect on healthcare training and delivery systems: (1) lack of economic access to health care, (2) barriers to hospitals and healthcare institutions, (3) barriers to physicians and other providers, (4) discriminatory policies and practices, (5) lack of language and culturally competent care, (6) inadequate inclusion in healthcare research, (7) commercialization of healthcare, (8) disintegration of traditional medicine, and (9) disparities in medical treatment.[37]

Minority populations have historically been reluctant to participate in, or have been purposefully excluded from participation in, decision- and policy-making processes that affect health care. Community empowerment is more than elusive when the basic aspects of participation are not evident. In a series of focus groups conducted by the Family Resource Coalition (FRC), a number of barriers to empowerment were identified. These barriers include

(1) a lack of trust between them and the policy makers or service providers; (2) lack of understanding how their families or neighbors will benefit from the work; (3) feeling intimidated and inferior when confronted by professionals who do not speak their language, or who do not speak it on their level; (4) an inability to see a well-defined role for themselves in the "real" decision-making process; (5) recognition by minorities that healthcare providers and policy makers hold strong positions on "the issues," and feeling that the views they hold are not welcome; (6) being intimidated in the governance process and the use of Robert's Rules; and (7) a belief that participation is a waste of time because, although they may have the opportunity for input, the key decision makers reserve the right to make all final decisions.[38]

To be effective in attempting to eliminate health disparities, policy makers must understand and address these barriers.[8] The CDC recommends providing communities with the knowledge and tools they need to create change. In *Walking the Walk*, California Tomorrow reported that currently, "Service delivery systems have little or no accountability to local residents/community members" and that for the future "[c]ommunity members/local residents should have and exercise the power to shape how services are delivered, their structure and location, and to initiate the creation of new programs/projects. Community members/local residents must realize that they have the power to close programs/projects and to reallocate resources if they are ineffective or harming the well-being of residents."[39]

This is not a new perspective. There are models of best practices that date back to the era of segregation, when minority communities (especially the black community) had few options other than those provided in their community network. A historical observation of the practices deemed successful may provide some insight into possible ways of eliminating current disparities in health and health care.

History

According to the NAACP, "Long before it became a broad-based public concern, efforts were under way to ensure that economic and social barriers would not lead to an increasingly severe health crisis in the minority community."[20] Efforts in addition to those addressing social and economic concerns have long existed. Perhaps the most memorable are programs developed for the black community by the Black Panther Party in the late 1960s and 1970s. The Black Panther Party instituted or envisioned starting these programs as part of a process to help African Americans and other oppressed peoples meet their basic necessities so that they might organize to acquire the resources for self-determination and empowerment. Among these efforts were:

George Jackson Medical Clinic, designed to provide free medical treatment and preventive medical care for the people.

The Sickle Cell Anemia Research Foundation, established to test and create a cure for sickle cell anemia through research and providing information to the black community.

People's Free Dental Program, created to provide free dental check-ups, treatment, and an educational program for dental hygiene.

People's Free Optometry Program, created to provide free eye examinations, treatment, and eyeglasses.

People's Free Ambulance Program, created to provide free, rapid transportation for sick or injured people without time-consuming checks into the patients' financial status or means.

Child Development Center, created to provide 24-hour child care facilities for infants and children between the ages of 2 months and 3 years.[40]

Some of these programs still exist or were models for many of today's human and community service programs. These programs assembled resources existing within the black community as well as the participation and input of the affected population (blacks) in decision making. These examples are not the earliest models. During the 19th century, the black community produced models worthy of emulation. These models grew out of necessity due to a segregated society. Many of these models are preserved for posterity through the University of Michigan's Kellogg African American Health Care Project. Notable examples include:

- Dunbar Memorial Hospital, 1918–1927, resulted from planning by a biracial committee intent on establishing a nonprofit institution that served Detroit's African American population.
- Howard University Medical School, 1868, Washington, DC.
- Meharry Medical College, 1876, Nashville, Tennessee.
- Knoxville College Medical Department, 1895, later Knoxville Medical College, Knoxville, Tennessee.[41]

Many of these endeavors did not survive. "As with most efforts that have been established by and from within the (indigenous) populations who have and continue to suffer from disparities and access to healthcare, they were undermined and eliminated by the broader society through policies and other means that fail to support or validate the need for their existence."[41] This is an additional barrier to overcoming health disparities.

Historical examples have not gone unnoticed. Recent activities in cities and states across the United States have begun to demonstrate the importance of empowering communities. For example, REACH (Racial and Ethnic Approaches to Community Health), a program initiated by the CDC, emphasizes and supports community-driven activities aimed at reducing health disparities. The CDC provides training, technical assistance, and support to REACH communities and helps these communities develop, implement, and sustain effective community interventions. As a result of this initiative, REACH has documented the following objectives:

- Empowering community members to seek better health.
- Bridging gaps between the healthcare system and the community by encouraging residents to seek appropriate care and changing local healthcare practices.
- Changing local social and physical environments to overcome barriers to good health.
- Mobilizing evidence-based public health programs that fit the unique social, political, economic, and cultural circumstances of specific communities.
- Moving beyond interventions that address individual behavior to the systematic study of community and systems change.[8]

Communities across the United States have recognized the importance of these CDC initiatives. REACH Communities (2006) include but are not limited to:

Access Community Health Network (IL)

African American Health Coalition (OR)

Albuquerque Area Indian Health Board (NM)

Association of American Indian Physicians (OK)

Black Women's Health Imperative (LA)

Boston Public Health Commission

Center for Community Health, Education, and Research (MA)

Charlotte Mecklenburg Hospital System (NC)

Chicago Department of Health (IL)

Choctaw Nation of Oklahoma

Chugachmuit Native Organization (AK)

Community Health and Social Services (MI)

Community Health Councils of Los Angeles

Eastern Band of Cherokee Indians (NC)

Florida International University

Fulton County Department of Health and Wellness (GA)

Genesee County Health Department (MI)

Greater Lawrence Family Health Center (MA)

Hidalgo Medical Services (NM)

Institute for Urban Family Health (NY)

Latino Education Project (TX)

Los Angeles Biomedical Research Institute at Harbor–UCLA Medical Center

Lowell Community Health Center (MA)

Matthew Walker Comprehensive Health (TN)

Medical University of South Carolina

Migrant Health Promotion (TX)

Missouri Coalition for Primary Care

National Indian Council on Aging (NM)

New Hampshire Minority Health Coalition

Oklahoma State Department of Health

San Francisco Department of Health

Seattle–King County Department of Health (WA)

Special Services for Groups (CA)

Trustees of Columbia University (NY)

United South and Eastern Tribes Inc. (TN)

University of Alabama at Birmingham

University of California, San Francisco

University of Illinois at Chicago

University of Nevada, Reno[8]

Community Solutions to Health Disparities

The initiatives previously discussed provide a foundation for addressing some of the barriers to eliminating minority health disparities. What emerges from community empowerment attempts is knowledge and experience that barriers can be eliminated only through a process that provides safe environments and a level of trust that makes the people feel appreciated; that convinces them that their input is of value, is valued, and will be utilized; that they will not be ridiculed or punished for their participation; and that they will not be oppressed and penalized by the system for exercising their responsibilities in pursuit of social equity.

Strategies for reducing health disparities must be community specific. Environmental factors must also be addressed if minority communities are to eliminate disparities. Suggested means for communities and community networks to effect change have successfully included the following:

1. *Overcome mistrust by creating community partnerships.* Specific efforts must be made to partner with minority organizations to allay fears, dispel myths, and educate the community on the importance of research. According to the U.S. Department of Health and Human Services, "community health is profoundly affected by the collective behaviors, attitudes and beliefs of everyone who lives in the community. Partnerships, particularly when they reach out to non-traditional partners, can be among the most effective tools for improving health in communities."[42]

2. *Community assessment and education.* What was very clear from each of the focus groups assembled by the Family Research Coalition was their limited amount of knowledge about healthcare research. It is important to assess the level of understanding for each community. Assessment strategies include focus groups, discussions with minority organizations, and community surveys. Educating communities on the importance of research and individual participation can come only after some level of trust has been established.[38]

3. *Physician education.* A number of studies show the tremendous need for doctors and all healthcare providers to be culturally competent. They should also have access to linguistically competent translators and translations.[2,10,36] Focus group experiences also point to the need for healthcare providers to understand the lack of trust of the healthcare system and the unique characteristics of each minority group. Individuals are more willing to interact (be involved in research) if the mores of their group are understood and respected. Focus groups with doctors also pointed out the need for more diversity training.[15] Training in medical school and beyond are crucial steps for better relationships.

The National Center for Cultural Competence suggests that doctors and other healthcare professionals:

- Have a defined set of values and principles and demonstrate behaviors, attitudes, policies, and structures that enable them to work effectively cross-culturally.
- Have the capacity to (1) value diversity, (2) conduct self-assessment, (3) manage the dynamics of difference, (4) acquire and institutionalize

cultural knowledge, and (5) adapt to diversity and the cultural contexts of the communities they serve.

• Incorporate the preceding in all aspects of policy making, administration, practice, and service delivery, and systematically involve consumers, key stakeholders, and communities.[36]

In focus groups consisting of minority representatives and the community healthcare and other social service organizations that serve them, the Eastern Nebraska Community Network determined that in order for minority communities to be empowered to address health disparities, the following conditions are crucial:

Language and Cultural Sensitivity

The need for language and cultural sensitivity training for staff in organizations providing service to the community is paramount. In an often paternalistic system, input of community members is often discarded or discounted.

Personnel Hiring and Training

Hiring and training of personnel who represented the consumer population must be a priority.

Communication and Relationship Building

Positive communication and relationship building between members of the community and service providers is mandatory. Without this positive start from the beginning of the relationship, the community feels alienated and isolated.

Sustainability

If support and process reinforcement does not come from agency administrators and executives, if buy in and vested interest does not come from the community, change is not likely to occur or be maintained in provider agencies.[43]

If health disparities among minority populations are to be eliminated, community empowerment is essential. Eliminating the barriers previously described is a part of the solution, but just the beginning. The CDC has underscored a number of principles for the community health programs, specifically the REACH programs, that they deem vital to understanding, and thus eliminating, minority health disparities. These 10 principles embody the need for a community approach to addressing health disparities.

They recognize the necessity of removing barriers that impede attaining healthy minority communities.

1. *Trust.* Building a culture of collaboration with communities that is based in trust.

2. *Empowerment.* Giving individuals and communities the knowledge and tools they need to create change by seeking and demanding better health and building on local resources.

3. *Culture and history.* Designing health initiatives that acknowledge and are based in the unique historical and cultural context of racial and ethnic minority communities in the United States.

4. *Focus.* Assessing and focusing on the underlying causes of poor community health and implementing solutions that are designed to remain embedded in the community's infrastructure.

5. *Community investment and expertise.* Recognizing and investing in local community expertise and working to motivate communities to mobilize and organize existing resources.

6. *Trusted organizations.* Embracing and enlisting organizations within the community that are valued by community members, including groups whose primary mission is not related to health.

7. *Community leaders.* Helping community leaders and key organizations be catalysts for change in their communities.

8. *Ownership.* Developing a collective outlook that promotes shared interest in a healthy future through widespread community engagement and leadership.

9. *Sustainability.* Making changes to organizations, community environments, and policies that will help ensure that health improvements are long-lasting and that community activities and programs are self-sustaining.

10. *Hope.* Fostering optimism, pride, and a promising vision for a healthier future.[8]

In the report to The California Endowment (TCE), PolicyLink—a communication, research, and capacity-building organization—acknowledged that health disparities in minority communities "require multilayered and focused efforts over a long period of time."[22] They suggested a partnership among community leaders, nonprofit organizations, healthcare providers within the minority community, the public, and for-profit leaders and organizations. According to Eisen, "community empowerment is both the process and outcome of organized community leaders gaining control over their lives."[44]

SUMMARY

The community approach to addressing minority health disparities is empowering minority communities to identify and find solutions to problems unique to them. It must be a joint effort among the community, the institutions, and organizations that are a part of the community served. The more institutions and organizations in the minority communities identify themselves with the community, the greater the commitment will be. Communities must be empowered to meet the challenges today and in the future. "The future belongs to those who prepare for it today" (Malcolm X).

REFERENCES

1. Agency for Healthcare Research and Quality. Key themes and highlights from the National healthcare disparities report. 2006. http://www.ahrq.gov/qual/nhdr06/highlights/nhdr06high.htm. Accessed March 12, 2007.
2. Watson SD. Race, ethnicity, and quality of care: Inequalities and incentives. *Am J Law Med.* 2001;27:203–224.
3. Lillie-Blanton M, Brodie, M Rowland D, Altman D, McIntosh M. Race, ethnicity, and the health care system: Public perceptions and experiences. *Med Care Res Rev.* 2000;57:218–236.
4. Cornelius I. Ethnic minorities and access to medical care: Where do they stand? *J Assoc Acad Minority Phys.* 1993;5:16–25.
5. Donovan, JL. (1984). Ethnicity and health: A research review. *Soc Sci Med.* 1984;19:663–670.
6. Disparities in health care: AHRQ focus on research. http://www.ahrq.gov/news/focus/disparhc.htm. Accessed February 19, 2007.
7. Center for Disease Control and Prevention. *Eliminating racial and ethnic disparities.* 2007. http://www.cdc.gov/nccdphp/publications/aag/reach.htm. Accessed February 9, 2007.
8. Center for Disease Control and Prevention. *Racial and Ethnic Approaches to Community Health (REACH) U.S. Finding Solutions to Health Disparities.* 2007. http://www.cdc.gov/nccdphp/publications/aag/reach.htm. Accessed February 9, 2007.
9. National Institutes of Health. *Health Disparities Fact Sheet.* October 2006:1.
10. Hewins-Maroney B, Schumaker A, Williams E. Health seeking behaviors of African Americans: Implications for health administration. *J Health Human Serv Admin.* 2005;28:68–95.
11. Weinick R, Zuvekas S, Cohen J. Racial and ethnic differences in access to and use of health care services. *Med Care Res Rev.* 2000;57:36–55.
12. Jackson J. Urban Black Americans. In: A. Harwood, ed. *Ethnicity and Medical Care.* Cambridge, MA: Harvard University Press; 1981.
13. Mayberry RM, Mili F, Olifi E. Racial and ethnic differences in access to medical care. *Med Care Res Rev..* 2000;57:108–146.
14. Shi L, Starfield, B. The effect of primary care physician supply and income equality on mortality among blacks and whites in U.S. metropolitan areas. *Am J Public Health.* 2001;91:1246–1250.

15. Cook C, Kosoko-Lasaki O, O'Brien, RL. Satisfaction with and perceived cultural competency of healthcare providers: The minority experience. *J Nat Med Assoc.* 2005;97:1078–1087.

16. Glenn-Vega A. Achieving a more minority-friendly practice. *Fam Pract Manag.* 2002. http://www.aafp.org/fpm. Accessed February 19, 2007.

17. Jackson V. Cultural competency. *Behav Health Manag.* March/April 2002:20–26.

18. Francis C. Medical ethics and social responsibility in clinical medicine. *J Urban Health.* 2001;78:29–45.

19. Hanley JH. Beyond the tip of the iceberg: Five stages toward cultural competence: Reaching today's youth. *Community Circle of Caring J.* 1999;3:9–12.

20. National Association for the Advancement of Colored People. *Call to action on health.* 2005:18–50. http://www.naacp.org/departments/health/health_index.html. Accessed February 9, 2005.

21. Siegel B, Berliner H, Adams A, Wasongarz D. *Addressing health disparities in community settings.* New York: New York University Press; 2003:63.

22. Bell JD, Bell J, Colmenar R, et al. *Reducing Health Disparities through a Focus on Communities: A Report to the California Endowment.* Oakland, CA: PolicyLink; 2002.

23. Davis R, Cohen L, Mikkelsen L. *Strengthening Communities: A Prevention Framework for Reducing Health Disparities.* Oakland, CA: Prevention Institute; 2003.

24. Oakley P. *Community Involvement in Health Development: An Examination of the Critical Issues.* Geneva, Switzerland: World Health Organization; 1989.

25. The Institute for Healthy Communities. *Community Health Policy.* Hospital and Health System Association of Pennsylvania; 1999:2.

26. Florin F, Dixon, J. Public involvement in health care. 2004:1. http://www.bmj.com. Accessed March 31, 2007.

27. Emmel N, Conn C. *Towards community involvement: Strategies for health and social care providers.* Leeds, U.K.: Nuffield Institute for Health, University of Leeds; 2004. www.nuffield.leeds.ac.uk/downloads/comm_involve_guide1.pdf. Retrieved February 19, 2007.

28. USDA, Rural Development. *Key Principles: A Discussion of the Program's Guiding Principles.* http://www.ezec.gov. Accessed February 27, 2007.

29. Israel B, Checkoway B. Schulz A, Zimmerman M. Health education and community empowerment: Conceptualizing and measuring perceptions of individual, organizational, and community control. *Health Educ Qrtly,* 1994;21:149–170

30. Sarason S. *The Psychological Sense of Community: Prospects for a Community Psychology.* San Francisco, CA: Jossey-Bass; 1984.

31. Klein, D. *Community Dynamic and Mental Health.* New York: John Wiley and Sons; 1968.

32. Steuart, G. Social and cultural perspectives: Community intervention and mental health. Paper presented at the Fourteenth Annual John W. Umstead Series of Distinguished Lectures, Raleigh, NC; 1978.

33. Egan G. *Change Agent Skills in Helping and Human Service Settings.* Monterey, CA: Books/Cole; 1985.

34. Drier P. Community empowerment strategies: The limits and potential of community organizing in urban neighborhoods. *Cityscape,* 1996;2:2. http://www.huduser.org/Periodicals/CITYSCPE/VOL2NUM2/dreier.pdf.

35. Wallerstein N, Bernstein E. Introduction to community empowerment, participatory education, and health. *Health Educ Qrtly.* 1994;21:141–148.

36. National Center for Cultural Competence. *Conceptual Frameworks/Models, Guiding Values and Principles.* http://gucchd.georgetown.edu/nccc/framework.html#lc. Accessed March 9, 2007.

37. Randall V. *Why Race Matters. Race, Healthcare and the Law.* Dayton, OH: University of Dayton Press. http://academic.udayton.edu/health/03access/data.htm. Retrieved March 9, 2007.

38. Family Resource Coalition; 1999.

39. Chang H, Nguyen L, Murdock B, et al. *Walking the Walk: Principles for Building Community Capacity for Equity and Diversity.* California Tomorrow; Spring 2000.

40. Williams K, Johnson VW. Eliminating African American health disparity via history-based policy. *Harvard Health Pol Rev.* 2002;3:1–3. http://www.hcs.harvard.edu/~epihc/currentissue/fall2002/williams-johnson.php. Accessed February 9, 2007.

41. *Kellogg African American Health Care Project.* Ann Arbor: University of Michigan Press. http://www.med.umich.edu/haahc. Accessed March 9, 2007.

42. U.S. Department of Health and Human Services. *Healthy People 2010: Understanding and Improving Health.* Washington, DC: U.S. Government Printing Office; 2000:2.

43. Peak F, Peak C, Wax H. *Consumer Involvement: A Focus Group Report.* Eastern Nebraska Community Network; 2000:unpublished.

44. Eisen A. Survey of neighborhood-based, comprehensive community empowerment initiatives. *Health Educ Qrtly.* 1994;21:236.

Chapter 19

The Relevance of Economics for Public Policies in Multidisciplinary Health Disparities Research

Albert A. Okunade, PhD, MS, MBA
Chutima Suraratdecha, PhD, MBA

The world has achieved considerable gains in health status measured by average life expectancy at birth. Rising real incomes and medical insurance have fueled the growth of innovative medical technologies that prolong life span and raise quality of life.[1] Smallpox, poliomyelitis, and measles have been eradicated or are on the verge of complete elimination. While health outcomes (e.g., life expectancy, infant mortality) have improved over the years, gaps in health indicators continue to widen within countries (based on areas of residence or segregation, gender, ethnicity, age, income, education, etc.) and across nations (related to per capita income or national wealth) with the indigent and vulnerable subpopulations the particularly adversely affected.

The critical need to understand and devise effective instruments for ameliorating U.S. health inequalities and their systemic social and economic damages is implicit in the fairly recent "Call for Papers" announcement on a theme issue of the *Journal of the American Medical Association* to be devoted to healthcare access. More specifically, the uninsured and underinsured population segments in the United States in 2003 were estimated at 61 million persons aged 19 to 64 years old.[2] This statistic has grave implications, especially for the poor, as shown in a study finding that new cases of tuberculosis and drug-induced death rates are among the largest health disparities for four of the five investigated racial and ethnic groups.[3]

The role of economics as a *discipline* (defined as the science of making an efficient resource allocation decision in the presence of resource scarcity and competing uses) is fundamentally primal in healthcare disparities research and related public policies. This is important because gender, ethnic, geographic, and other disparities in economic resources (e.g., earnings, assets or wealth, and networking or social capital) and healthcare inequalities (e.g., in access, delivery, and outcomes) are highly correlated.

Health care must be prioritized efficiently and equitably. Therefore, an increasingly vocal sect among the practitioners of scientific economics also insists on achieving equity goals in addition to those targeting cost containment and efficient resource management. Greater investments in education and health build human capital accumulation. In effect, resource allocation policy decisions in health care, similar to those in the education or schooling sector, are areas highly influenced by equity concerns in some public policy debates. This is because an individual's health status or educational investment or attainment yields personal benefits (e.g., better health, greater incomes) and also confers other positive (i.e., external) benefits on the larger society (e.g., children vaccinated against polio also tend to improve the health status of other children; a healthier workforce is more productive and pays higher income taxes to finance the provision of public goods that include the interstate highways and indigent health care). Persistent health disparities domestically and internationally lead to greater economic concerns driven by interest in equitable distribution and concern for justice. Understanding the evidence about disparities is likely to aid in the design of more effective policies and to improve healthcare delivery (how much and how to distribute health care) to reduce inequalities.

Core economic factors have gained increased interest as determinants of health disparities among subpopulations. Clear associations between health outcomes and economic determinants—such as income, employment, occupation, (third-party) insurance coverage, and so forth—are commonly reported in the literature. That is, differences in mortality, disease incidence, prevalence, and burden (i.e., health disparities) occur across socioeconomic classes in a country. At the macroeconomic (or aggregate) level, these factors include employment, government revenue, import, and income distribution. At the microeconomic level (individual, family, or household), important economic factors are income, wealth, and educational attainment, for example.

Among these, data for the appropriate measure of the income variable are theoretically and empirically problematic. Consequently, researchers seek to use a variable related to income (e.g., the percentage of earners at or below the federal poverty level or the share of total income of the richest groups as surrogate measures of income).

This chapter focuses on health disparities from an economic perspective and differentiates the economic factors from other social factors (e.g., ethnicity, location, gender, age, and social classes). The first two sections utilizing economic theory provide fundamental background information on the general conceptual measures of economic status (see Figure 19–1 later in the chapter) and income distribution, the Lorenz curve and concentration curve (see Figure19–2 later in the chapter). Section 3 examines evidence on disparities. Section 4 concludes that health disparities are becoming more important, especially in the policy arena, principally because of the broader impact of disparities on access to care, economic burden, and health outcomes. This chapter complements the other disciplinary approaches to the study and evaluation of health disparities.

Economic Dimension of Health Disparities

The discipline of *economics*, a social science, consists of health, public finance, industrial organization, housing, regional and urban, risk and uncertainty, econometrics, energy, agricultural and resource, health education and welfare, and urban planning. The two major fields are macroeconomics and microeconomics. *Macroeconomics* studies broad economic activities, performance, and trends. In other words, it is "the study of whole economic systems aggregating over the functioning of individual economic units. It is primarily concerned with variables which follow systematic and predictable paths of behavior and can be analyzed independently of the decisions of the many agents who determine their level. More specifically, it is a study of national economies and the determination of national income."[4] Macroeconomic topics include employment, unemployment, inflation, trade deficit, and economic growth, among others. *Microeconomics* is the study of the economic behavior of small economic groups such as firms, families, and individuals. Microeconomics is "the study of economics at the level of individual consumers, groups of consumers, or firms . . . The general concern of microeconomics is the efficient allocation of scarce resources between alternative uses but more specifically it involves the determination of price through the optimizing behavior of economic agents, with consumers maximizing utility and firms maximizing profit."[4]

Identifying the core economic factors that underlie health disparities entails the grouping of countries or populations into different economic categories according to their economic resources (i.e., how economic assets and incomes are distributed). Depending on the level of research unit being investigated, macro- or microeconomics, this is often referred to *economic inequality* or *disparities measurement*.

Economic Status and Its Measurement

An assessment of economic status can be conducted using current earnings or consumption expenditures, permanent income, or wealth as proxies. In general, *consumption expenditure* is measured by the total amount of goods and services that a person receives, in-cash or in-kind, over some defined period of time such as 30 days (1 month) or the 12-month period before the measurement period. *Current income* represents a flow of resources over a period of time, whereas *wealth* captures the stock of assets at a given point in time. According to the U.S. Bureau of the Census, cash or money income includes earnings, interest, dividends, rents, Social Security retirement benefits, pension or retirement income, survivors' benefits, disability benefits, veterans' benefits, workers' compensation, alimony, and some cash welfare benefits. Noncash income includes food, housing, medical care, and social services such as subsidized day care. Theoretically, there are strong arguments for using total expenditure instead of income in household surveys.[5-8] However, collecting income and consumption expenditure data is time-consuming and difficult, and the measure can be volatile.

Wealth refers to economic value of assets or accumulated savings. Wealth measures that are fairly easy to collect include ownership of homes, vehicles, or valuable things that represent a source of economic security for households to meet emergencies and economic shocks; that is, wealth serves as permanent income. *Permanent income* is determined by the consumer's physical and human (education, health) assets, which influence consumer's ability to earn income and make an estimate of anticipated lifetime income. Received economic theory stipulates that household expenditure decisions rely on estimated permanent, and not transitory, incomes. Assets have been documented and measured in various socioeconomic surveys because of ease of measurement and collection, and it captures stable or long-term income of households and individuals. The major sources for income and wealth proxies are national population surveys or socioeconomic surveys, such as the Income, Poverty and Health Insurance Survey in the United States conducted by the U.S. Census Bureau, and the World Bank's Living

Standards Measurement Study (LSMS) household surveys conducted in developing countries.

An extensive body of research in disparities economics has shown a significant relationship between economic status variously measured (income, occupation) and health outcomes.[9–12] According to the Commission on Macroeconomics and Health,[13] the very poor are more often affected by diseases and also bear substantial financial burden for common or catastrophic illnesses. Economic factors are important among the determinants of health disparities in association with other noneconomic factors, such as ethnicity.[14–16] Further, wealth is shown to be more strongly associated with health disparities across ethnicities than income.[17,18] Income deprivation and social cohesion factors are critical determinants of mental health disparities.[19]

Income Distribution

There are alternative conceptual measures of the inequalities or disparities concept. It can refer to inequalities in earned incomes or inequities in income distribution. Our interest here is discussing differences or variations in health status or outcome across different economic groups. Measuring health disparities entails the use of indicators or indexes (e.g., number of physician visits per year) to capture health status.

We examine the identification of economic groups compared and the economic methods used in conducting the comparisons. Quintiles, quartiles, or deciles are commonly defined for continuous variables, such as income. Health outcomes are then compared among the quintiles, quartiles, or deciles. This type of classification is discrete and does not reflect distributional changes over time. Other complicated measures to deal with discrete issues include the Lorenz curve, Gini coefficient, and concentration curve (index).

Lorenz Curve and Gini Coefficient

The *Lorenz curve* is a graphical presentation showing the degree of inequality of a frequency distribution in which the cumulative percentage of health indicators (e.g., mortality rate) is plotted on the vertical or Y-axis against the cumulative percentage of the population ordered/ranked by income or wealth on the horizontal or X-axis. A straight line drawn from the origin to the right top corner (Figure 19–1) indicates perfect equality (i.e., no inequality). The greater the distance of a curve from the diagonal line, the greater the inequality. If the health indicators selected are beneficial to the population, the Lorenz curve will lie below the equality line. In case of deaths, which are prejudicial, the Lorenz curve will lie above the diagonal.

The Gini coefficient *(G)* is a ratio of the area between the Lorenz curve and the uniform distribution line *(A)* to the area under the uniform distribution line *(B)* (**Figure 19–1**). There are alternative calculations of the Gini coefficient. The formula presented here is from Brown[20]:

$$G = 1 - \sum_{i=0}^{k-1}(Y_{i+1} + Y_i)(X_{i+1} - X_i)\sum_{i=0}^{k-1}(Y_{i+1} + Y_i)(X_{i+1} - X_i)$$

where G = Gini coefficient
Y = Cumulated proportion of health outcome
X = Cumulated proportion of population

The values of G range from 0 (perfect equality) to 1 (perfect inequality), and a smaller coefficient suggests greater equality in income or wealth.

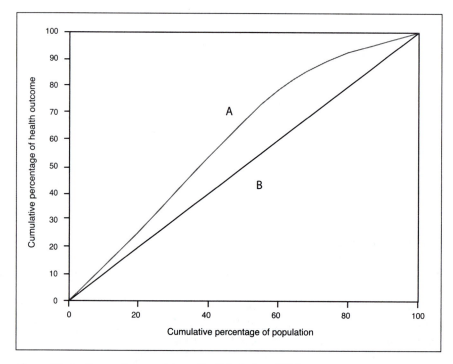

Figure 19–1   *Lorenz Curve and Areas for Calculation of Gini*

Concentration Curve and Concentration Index

Unlike the Lorenz curve, the *concentration curve* ranks populations by their economic status, not health. The concentration curve plots the cumulative percentage of the population ranked by economic status from the most disadvantaged (relatively the poorest) to the least disadvantaged (the richest) against the cumulative percentage of health outcomes **(Figure 19–2)**. If poor health is concentrated among the lower economic classes, the concentration curve lies under the diagonal. The concentration index is calculated the same way as the Gini coefficient, with the exception that its values range from −1 to +1. When the curve lies above (below) the diagonal or the equity line, the coefficient is negative (positive).

The *concentration index* measure tends to provide a more accurate indicator of socioeconomic inequalities in health than the Lorenz curve,[21,22] especially when heath and income are positively related.[23] As a result, applications of the concentration curve and the concentration index are more common and internationally available.

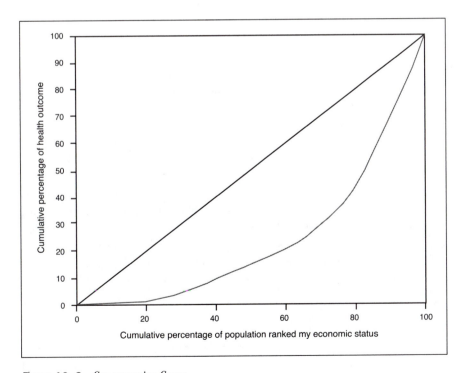

Figure 19–2　*Concentration Curve*

Some Evidence on Economic Studies of Health Disparities

Using data from the National Health and Nutrition Examination Surveys and the Hispanic Health and Nutrition Examination Surveys, the concentration index was used to measure changes in socioeconomic inequality and prevalence of being overweight in U.S. adolescents.[24] The authors report that socioeconomic disparity varied across ethnic and gender groups, and the changing pattern of these disparities over time suggests that obesity prevention and management efforts should target each of the socioeconomic classes. Jiménez and colleagues[25] constructed the concentration curve to depict income-related inequalities in health and use of health care in Canada. They found that variations in income-related health inequalities are likely attributable to differences in resources between rich and poor individuals within a province and that the difference in inequalities between provinces is the source of income-related inequities in healthcare use. Concentration indexes calculated from nationwide survey data in Finland, Norway, and Sweden suggest that lower socioeconomic status is associated with reporting more illnesses.[26] Another study measured economic-related inequalities of neonatal, infant, and child mortality in Matlab, Bangladesh, using a concentration index; it concluded that nontargeted health intervention programs do not reduce the poor–rich gap.[27] Hosseinpoor and colleagues[28] used the concentration index to measure socioeconomic-related inequalities of infant mortality in Iran. They confirm that socioeconomic inequality of infant mortality is determined by health systems and nonhealth sector factors, such as education and infrastructure.

An analysis of economic inequality based on using the multilevel, multinomial logistic regression model to investigate income equality (Gini coefficient of per capita consumption expenditure) and burden of under- and overnutrition in 77,220 never-married women, aged 15–49 years, from 26 Indian states suggests that the burden of suboptimal nutrition is likely to occur in high-income, inequality states.[29] In a population-based study using data of more than 3,000 Canadians and more than 5,000 U.S. adults, also based on a logistic regression model, researchers found that significant disparities related to race, immigrant status, and income exist in both countries but are greater in the United States.[30]

Some Policy Reflections

Health inequalities remain a central concern of health policy[31] because of the widening inequality of healthcare access, provision, financing, and outcome. Because of the economic and social implications of health inequalities, public health policy makers, practitioners, and employers are increasingly interested in crafting policies to close the widening gaps. These efforts cut across local communities and countries around the globe. Some studies contend that health policies and programs themselves contribute to disparities in health and wealth, especially in low-income settings.[32] They recommend instituting community-based initiatives, especially those based on micro-financing and removal of user fees for health services, as more potent policy instruments for reducing the health ills (disparities relative to others) of the poor.

Finally, the U.S. healthcare system, with its largely employment-based health insurance coverage design, is both fragmented and expensive, leading to wider health inequities between the well-off and the poor who are unemployed or hold hourly jobs without health coverage. The latter group comprises those covered under Medicaid (a federal–state partnership indigent care insurance), Medicare (if disabled and nonelderly), or uninsured. On the contrary, Australia's public–private health system, compared with the United States and other OECD (Organization for Economic Cooperation and Development) countries, has been lauded for ensuring high and fairly equal access to physicians, hospitals, and dental care.[33,34]

SUMMARY

In conclusion, human health status is a stock concept. The health stock depreciates due to intensity and duration of use, simple passage of time, and lack of optimal upkeep of the cell body or soma. A person's health status can be enhanced through sustained engagements in healthier lifestyle habits (e.g., improved quality of nutritional intake, maintaining healthy energy balance and as such normal body mass index [BMI]) and obtaining quality health care (e.g., regular physician visits). These two broad strategies for improving personal health status require investments of economic resources. In effect, income disparities between the rich and the indigent population subgroups represent resource disparities that underlie disparities in healthcare access, process, and outcome. The number of years spent in formal schooling is also positively and highly correlated with health status; therefore, health disparities are further associated with disparities in the educational attainments of the rich and the poor.

The strong link of health disparities and resource holdings of the high- versus low-income groups leads to the practical policy suggestion that appropriate incentives be offered to the poor to invest in marketable skills and quality schooling in order to earn real incomes that rise consistently with the higher labor productivity phase of the worker's life cycle. A consistent rise in the educated worker's earned incomes, rather than income transfers from the public coffers that remain flat, opens up the likelihood of obtaining employer-based or private-purchase health insurance if employed full-time. Moreover, educating the poor to engage in healthy lifestyle habits (e.g., smoking cessation, regular physical exercise) would tend to shift the decision-making horizons of the poor from the short to long run. This way, the poor would be more likely to invest in better health human capital, seek more and better quality education or schooling, and undertake less risky lifestyle behaviors to raise longevity and quality of life. If so, resource-based health disparities are likely to narrow in the future as the educational attainment, incomes, and health status improve for the poor relative to the well-off population segment. Meanwhile, from a recently proposed policy perspective, the U.S. government could begin to address income-based health disparities by designing a two-tier national healthcare system based on educational attainments and earned incomes.[35]

REFERENCES

1. Okunade AA, Murthy V. Technology as a major driver of health care costs: A cointegration analysis of the Newhouse conjecture. *J Health Econ.* 2002;21:147–159.
2. Drummond R, Fontanarosa PB. Call for papers: Theme issue on access to health care. *JAMA.* 2006;295:2182–2183.
3. Keppel KG. Ten largest racial and ethnic disparities in the United States based on Healthy People 2010 objectives. *Amer J Epidemiol.* 2007;166:97–1034.
4. Bannock G, Baxter RE, Davis E. *Dictionary of Economics.* New York; Penguin: 2003.
5. Houthakker SH. The econometrics of family budgets. *J Royal Stat Soc.* Series A (General). 1952;115:1–28.
6. Prais S, Houthakker H. *The Analysis of Family Budgets.* London: Cambridge University Press; 1955.
7. Houthakker SH. An international comparison of household expenditure patterns, commemorating the centenary of Engel's Law. *Econometrica.* 1957;25:532–551.
8. Tobin J. A statistical demand function for food in the U.S.A. *J Roy Stat Soc.* Series A (General). 1950; Series A:113–141.
9. Adler NE, Newman K. Socioeconomic disparities in health: pathways and policies. *Health Affairs.* 2002;21:60–76.
10. House JS, Williams DR. Understanding and reducing socioeconomic and racial/ethnic disparities in health. In: Smedley BD, Syme SL, eds. *Promoting Health: Intervention Strategies from Social and Behavioral Research.* Washington, DC: National Academies Press; 2000.
11. Lantz PM, House JS, Lepkowski JM, Williams DR, Mero RP, Chen J. Socioeconomic factors, health behaviors and mortality. *JAMA.* 1998;279:1703–1708.
12. McDonough P, Duncan GJ, Williams DR, et al. Income dynamics and adult mortality in the U.S., 1972–1989. *Am J Public Health.* 1997;87:1476–1483.

13. CMH (Commission on Macroeconomics and Health). *Macroeconomics and Health: Investing in Health for Economic Development. Report of the Commission on Macroeconomics and Health.* Geneva: World Health Organization; 2001.

14. Bond-Huie SA, Krueger PM, Rogers RG, Hummer RA. Wealth, race, and mortality. *Soc Sci Quart.* 2003;84(3):667–684.

15. Hayward MD, Crimmins EM, Miles TP, Yang Y. The significance of socioeconomic status in explaining the race gap in chronic health conditions." *Am Soc Rev.* 2000;65:910–930.

16. Kington RS, Smith JP. Socioeconomic Status and Racial and Ethnic Differences in Functional Status Associated with Chronic Diseases." *Am J Public Health.* 1997;87:805–810.

17. Robert SA, House JS. SES differentials in health by age and alternative indicators of SES. *J Aging Health.* 1996;8:359–388.

18. Scholz JK, Levine K. U.S. black-white wealth inequality: a survey. In: Neckerman K, ed. *Social Inequality.* New York: Russell Sage Foundation; 2004.

19. Fone D, Dunstan F, Lloyd K, Williams G, Watkins J, Pamer J. Does social cohesion modify the association between area income deprivation and mental health? A multilevel analysis. *Int J Epidemiol.* 2007;36:338–345.

20. Brown M. Using Gini-style indices to evaluate the spatial patterns of health practitioners: Theoretical considerations and an application based on Alberta data. *Soc Sci Med.* 1994;38:1243–1256.

21. Wagstaff A, Paci P, Van Doorsler E. On the measurement of inequalities in health. *Soc Sci Med.* 1991;33:545–547.

22. Wagstaff A, Van Doorslaer E. Measuring inequalities in health in the presence of multiple-category morbidity indicators. *Health Econ.* 2007;16:281–289.

23. Bommier A, Stecklov G. Defining health inequality: Why Rawls succeeds where social welfare theory fails. *J Health Econ.* 1994;21:497–513.

24. Zhang Q, Wang Y. Using concentration index to study changes in socio-economic inequality of overweight among US adolescents between 1971 and 2002. *Int J Epidemiol.* 2007;36:916–925.

25. Jiménez RD, Smith PC, Van Doorslaer E. Equity in health and health care in a decentralized context: Evidence from Canada. *Health Econ.* 2007; forthcoming.

26. Lahelma E, Manderbacka K, Rahkonen O, Karisto A. Comparisons of inequalities in health: evidence from national surveys in Finland, Norway and Sweden *Soc Sci Med.* 1994;38:517–524.

27. Razzaque A, Streatfield PK, Gwatkin DR. Does health intervention improve socioeconomic inequalities of neonatal, infant and child mortality? Evidence from Matlab, Bangladesh. *Int J Equity Health.* 2007;6:4.

28. Hosseinpoor AR, Van Doorslaer E, Speybroeck N, et al. Decomposing socioeconomic inequality in infant mortality in Iran. *Int J Epidemiol.* 2006;35:1211–1219.

29. Subramanian SV, Kawachi I, Smith GV. Income inequality and the double burden of under- and over nutrition in India. *J Epidemiol Com Health.* 2007;61:802–809.

30. Lasser KE, Himmelstein DU, Woolhandler S. Access to care, health status, and heal health disparities in the United States and Canada: Results of a cross-national based survey. *Am J Public Health.* 2006;96:1300–1307.

31. Rainham D. Do differences in health make a difference? A review for health policymakers. *Health Pol.* 2007;84:123–132.

32. Molyneux C, Hutchison B, Chuma J, Gilson L. The role of community-based organizations in household ability to pay for health care in Kilifi District, Kenya. *Health Pol & Plan.* 2007;22:381–392.

33. Van Doorslaer E, Clarke P, Savage E, Hall J. Horizontal inequities in Australia's mixed public/private health care system. *Health Pol.* 2008;86(1):97–108.

34. Kumar R, Jaiswal V, Tripathi S, et al. Inequality in health care delivery in India: The problem of rural medical practitioners. *Health Care Analysis.* 2007; 15:223–233.

35. Okunade, Albert A. "Canadian-ize" the US health care system for the poor. *Health Affairs eLetters.* 2006. Available at: http://content.healthaffairs.org/cgi/eletters/25/4/1133.

Chapter 20

Conclusion: Global and Domestic Health Disparities– Possible Solutions

Cynthia T. Cook, PhD
Richard L. O'Brien, MD, FACP
Sade Kosoko-Lasaki, MD, MSPH, MBA

The United States is not a homogeneous society, but a multicultural, multiethnic, and economically diverse nation. Although the majority population is non-Hispanic white, this population has been declining since 1970 because of low fertility rates and a decline in European immigrants. In 1970, 83% of the U.S. population was non-Hispanic white, today it is 67%. Hispanics are now approximately 14% of the population, blacks 13%, Asians 5%, and Native Americans 1% (an increase of 50% since 1970).[1]

Hispanics are the largest and fastest growing minority and are also the largest foreign-born group in the United States. In 2002, 52% of the foreign-born came from Latin America, 27% from Asia, 15% from Europe, and only 3% from Africa.[2] The challenge for healthcare professionals today is to provide culturally competent care to a multicultural, multiethnic, and economically and educationally diverse population. Unfortunately, immigrants coming from the most economically disadvantaged regions, like their economically disadvantaged American counterparts, may require the most health care but are least likely to have access to or be able to afford it. Consequently, health disparities and the need for culturally competent care will continue to exist as long as we remain a multicultural, multiethnic, and economically diverse country.

Wars, famine, poverty, political instability, human rights violations, and economic and educational opportunities are the catalysts that keep immigrants, documented and undocumented, coming to the United States. The global flow of migration is from low-income to high-income countries in search of economic, social, and political opportunities. People tend not to migrate for health care, although residing in a high-income country may provide access to needed health care.

The health disparities that are prevalent in the United States are related to social factors: access to health care, lack of health insurance, education, occupation, income, race and/or ethnicity, residential segregation, and racism. It is well documented that people who are employed usually have health insurance and, therefore, access to adequate health care. We also know that education, income, occupation, and race or ethnicity affect life expectancy, morbidity, and mortality rates and that minorities and recent immigrants are more likely to live in poverty as a result of little or no education, low or no job skills, and/or lack of English proficiency, which predisposes them to health disparities. Health disparities may be more a social issue than a medical one. To decrease health disparities, we need to provide adequate education, income, and health care for the ever increasingly diverse population of the United States.

Universal health care may be one answer, but not "the" answer to health disparities. The 46 million people who do not have health insurance are the working poor, the self-employed, and the young who think they are invulnerable to disease, illness, and death. Some of the poor and most of the elderly are eligible for Medicaid and/or Medicare. However, even among the medically insured there are disparities. The Whitehall study was the classic example of social class and/or occupation having a stronger impact on morbidity and mortality than access to adequate health care; the British study found the higher the occupational status the lower the death rate from coronary heart disease.[3,4] The stressors of daily life appear to have a negative impact on the poor and a positive impact on the well off. Nevertheless, immigrants keep coming to the United States and suffering health disparities, especially if they are poor and remain poor.

There will be health disparities, both domestic and global, as long as there are economic disparities. In 2005, it was estimated that more than one-half of the world's population lived on less than $2 a day.[5] The average per capita gross national income per purchasing power parity (GNI PPP) for the developing world was $4,760 (excluding China); the more developed world's GNI PPP was $29,680.[6] Obviously the developed world, including the United States, has more resources to improve and maintain the health of its populations.

The health of a country's population can be measured by life expectancy, infant mortality, and maternal mortality. The higher the per capita income of a country, the higher the life expectancy and the lower the infant and maternal mortality. Even though within some high-income countries (the United States in particular), there are some groups (African Americans and Native Americans in particular), whose health status is similar to low- or middle-income countries (i.e. low life expectancy, high infant mortality, and high maternal mortality) compared with the dominant white population. A disproportionately large number of African Americans live at or below the poverty level and may be more prone to the stressors of daily life, which includes poverty, as well as racism.

Nevertheless, most high-income, developed countries have a relatively high health status—life expectancy, 77 years; infant mortality rate, 6 per 1,000 newborns; and maternal mortality ratio, 20 per 100,000 live births—whereas the developing world or low-income countries are characterized by low life expectancy (64 years), high infant mortality rates (61 per 1000 live births), and high maternal mortality ratio (440 per 100, 000 live births). However, the greatest disparities between the developed and developing world are illustrated by sub-Saharan Africa, where the life expectancy is 49 years, the infant mortality rate is 92, and the maternal mortality ratio is 920;[6,7] all of which have been affected by the HIV/AIDS pandemic.

The leading cause of mortality in the United States, the richest country in the world, is heart disease. The leading cause of death in sub-Saharan Africa, the poorest region in the world, is HIV/AIDS. Death from chronic illness such as heart disease, cancer, and diabetes is more characteristic of high-income countries, whereas in low-income and developing countries, infectious diseases are common causes of mortality: HIV/AIDS, respiratory infections, diarrhea diseases, malaria, tuberculosis, and malnutrition.[5,8,9] In fact, the majority of children's deaths under age 5 in Africa and Asia are due to infectious diseases, whereas infections cause only 5% of deaths under age 5 in the United States and other high-income countries.[10] Health disparities within the United States are miniscule in comparison to global disparities. The developing world does not have the luxury of evaluating whether their healthcare providers are culturally competent, although international healthcare providers find it necessary to be familiar with the local culture so as not to offend, and to practice health care in a culturally acceptable manner.

Why the disparity between rich and poor countries with respect to the causes of mortality? First, most high-income countries began economic, demographic, and epidemiological (mortality) transitions in the 19th century. Prior to the 19th century, Europe and North America were in stage 1 of the demographic transition (high birth rate, high death rate, little or no population growth) and stage 1 of the epidemiological transition (the high death rate was from pandemics, famine, and war). Stage 2 of the demographic transition is the Industrial Revolution, which coincides with urbanization. People have a more nutritious and stable diet, and public health measures in the form of safe food, water, and sewage systems are implemented. The result is a reduction in the death rate, higher birth rates, and population growth. This is juxtaposed with stage 2 of the epidemiological transition, characterized by receding pandemics, less frequent wars and famine, and people less frequently dying from infectious diseases. The third stage of both these transitions characterizes the developed world today; there is a low death rate and birth rate; very little population growth; and disease prevalence shifts from infectious, communicable diseases to chronic, noncommunicable ones.

Most of the developing world is stuck in stage 2 of the demographic transition (high birth rates but low death rates) and stage 2 of the epidemiological transition (less frequent pandemics from infectious diseases). However, sub-Saharan Africa is in stage 2 of the demographic transition and stage 1 of the epidemiological transition: economic development is low and the population is still dying from infectious diseases as well as from famine and wars.

SUMMARY

Economic development and stable governments are the answers to global health disparities. Reducing health disparities domestically and globally is a moral imperative demanded by justice and a clear commitment to human rights and dignity. Article 25, Section 1 of the Universal Declaration of Human Rights states, "Everyone has the right to a standard of living adequate for the health and well-being of himself and of his family, including food, clothing, housing and medical care and necessary social services . . ."[11] Nations have an obligation to provide these rights for their residents, the international community must provide economic and political support for those regions of the world that are economically and politically disadvantaged, and the United States must find a way to reduce the poverty that exist within its borders. Only then will health disparities be reduced. But the moral imperative rests not only on governments, but on individual health professionals and the organizations and institutions within which professionals provide their services. Only by understanding and appreciating other cultures, by communicating effectively and sensitively with patients and clients of other cultures, can health professionals satisfy the demands of justice and their own professionalism. Cultural proficiency is essential for professionals to provide care to the world's most vulnerable populations—whether they reside in the United States or the developing world.

REFERENCES

1. Martin P, Midgley E. Immigration: shaping and reshaping America. *Population Bulletin*. 2006;61(4):3–28.
2. U.S. Census Bureau. Recent foreign born by world region of birth: 2002. www.census.gov/population. Accessed December 22, 2007.
3. Marmot MG, Shipley MJ, Rose G. Inequalities in death—Specific explanations of general patterns. *Lancet*. 1984;1(8384):1003–1006.
4. Marmot MG, Smith GD, Stansfeld S, et al. Health inequalities among British civil servants: the Whitehall II study. *Lancet*. 1991;337(8754):1387–1393.
5. Kent MM, Haub C. Global demographic divide. *Population Bulletin*. 2005;60 (4):1–24.
6. Population Reference Bureau. *2007 World Population Data Sheet*. Washington, DC.
7. WHO/UNICEF/UNFPA. *Maternal Mortality in 2000*. Geneva: World Health Organization; 2004.
8. *Statistical Abstract of the United States 2008*. Table 113. Deaths and death rates by leading causes of death and age: 2004. www.census.gov. Accessed December 22, 2007.
9. Causes of death. http://ucatlas.ucsc.edu/health/cause. Accessed December 22, 2007.
10. Kent MM, Yin S. Controlling Infectious Diseases. *Population Bulletin*. 2006;61 (2):1–20.
11. General Assembly of the United Nations. *Universal Declaration of Human Rights*. Adopted December 10, 1948. Available at: http://www.un.org/Overview/rights.html. Accessed December 28, 2007.

About the Authors

Sade Kosoko-Lasaki, MD, MSPH, MBA

Dr. Kosoko-Lasaki, a Nigerian-American, is the associate vice president for Health Sciences, and professor in the School of Medicine, Department of Surgery (Ophthalmology) and Department of Preventive Medicine and Public Health at Creighton University, Omaha, Nebraska.

Dr. Kosoko-Lasaki leads the Health Sciences' Multicultural and Community Affairs Office, with programs like the Health Careers Opportunity Program and the Medical School's Center of Excellence. She also oversees initiatives to recruit disadvantaged students to the health sciences and mentors these students. She has lectured nationally and internationally on cultural proficiency and health disparity issues, focusing on the promotion of "pipeline programs" that prepare and support disadvantaged students from grade 4 through health professional school so they can become successful healthcare providers.

As an ophthalmologist with a public health degree, Dr. Kosoko-Lasaki is passionate about educating people in developing countries about Vitamin A deficiency, the leading cause of preventable blindness in children and a major public health problem throughout the world. She has served as a consultant to UNICEF, USAID, and Helen Keller International in Burkina Faso, Niger, Mauritania, Chad, and the Philippines. Since 1986, Dr Kosoko-Lasaki has researched the prevalence of glaucoma in blacks in St. Lucia, West Indies. With a focus on detecting and treating glaucoma—the most common cause of blindness in African Americans and Hispanics—she has initiated health fairs, screenings, and prevalence surveys throughout the Washington, DC metropolitan area, Nebraska, Iowa, Kansas, St. Lucia, West Indies, and the Dominican Republic. In addition, she created a program for blindness prevention entitled, "Preventing Glaucoma Blindness in Nebraska: A Creighton University Initiative," targeting individuals at risk for glaucoma blindness in Nebraska and its surrounding areas.

Dr. Kosoko-Lasaki is married to Dr. Gbolahan Lasaki, a petroleum engineer. She has three children: Adedayo, Adeola, and Abiola.

Cynthia T. Cook, PhD

Dr. Cynthia T. Cook is an African American medical sociologist and former assistant professor at Creighton University, where she taught sociology of health and illness, global health issues, American cultural minorities, and medical anthropology.

Dr. Cook received her PhD from Texas Woman's University in 2000. Her dissertation topic was "The Role of Health Care in Reducing Maternal Mortality in the Developing World." She has published articles on maternal health in sub-Saharan Africa, the effects of skilled health attendants in reducing maternal deaths in the developing world, and the effects of the political economy on the health status of Africa, as well as co-authored articles on cultural competency and health disparities.

Dr. Cook has done independent research on healthcare facilities in Ethiopia, traditional healers in South Africa, and polygamy in Ivory Coast, and she was the evaluation specialist for the Creighton University Cultural Competency study. She has been published in the *Journal of the National Medical Association*, *International Journal of Medicine and Law*, *Journal of Evaluation and Program and Planning*, *The Journal of Black Studies*, *The International Third World Studies Journal and Review*, and the *Journal of Asian and African Studies*.

Dr. Cook is presently an assistant professor in the Department of Sociology and Criminal Justice at Florida A&M University in Tallahassee, Florida.

Richard L. O'Brien, MD, FACP

Dr. O'Brien is a university professor and a member of the Center for Health Policy and Ethics, Creighton University. He is a third-generation American descended from Irish famine immigrants, who settled in the Midwest where they were railroad laborers and farmers. He received his medical degree from Creighton, trained in internal medicine on the First (Columbia) Division at Bellevue Hospital in New York, and was a postdoctoral fellow in enzyme chemistry at the University of Wisconsin.

During the Vietnam War, he was assistant chief of the Department of Molecular Biology at Walter Reed Army Institute of Research where, with colleagues, he determined the mechanism of malarial parasite resistance to quinine and chloroquine. He was on the faculty of the University of Southern California (USC) School of Medicine, where he taught medical students and graduate students in experimental pathology and biochemistry, and conducted laboratory research in cellular and molecular biology and cellular immunology. He was instrumental in the development of the USC Comprehensive Cancer Center and the Kenneth Norris Jr. Cancer Hospital and Research Institute. He was deputy director of the Cancer Center from 1974 to 1981 and director of the Center and the Norris from 1981 to 1982. From 1982 to 1992, he was dean of the Creighton University School of Medicine, and from 1984 to 1999 he was the vice president of health sciences at Creighton. In 1985 he established the Center for Health Policy and Ethics; he has been a member of the Center since 1999. Dr. O'Brien is currently engaged in studying ethics of health policy development, ethics of human subject research, and reduction of health disparities.

About the Contributors

Janet E. Bonet, BA

Janet E. Bonet studied interpretation and translation in Mexico at the University of the Americas from 1975 to 1982, returning home to Omaha, Nebraska, in 1983 to a burgeoning community of Hispanic, Asian, and African immigrants. She has been instrumental locally and nationally in increasing public awareness of interpreting as a profession. In 1986, her interpreting career began; in 1990 she established her business, Protrans; and in 1999, she co-founded the Nebraska Association for Translators and Interpreters, serving six years as President. In 2001, Ms. Bonet became the first Nebraska Supreme Court Certified Court Interpreter and was elected to the National Association for Judiciary Interpreters and Translators Board of Directors in 2004; she has since served on committees for advancement of the culturally and linguistically appropriate services (CLAS) standards and participated in the National Council on Interpreting in Health Care's advisory groups on the national Code of Ethics and Standards of Practice for medical interpreters. Her medical interpreting experience includes 15 years serving agencies and courts in behavioral health, workers' compensation, domestic violence, personal injury, and juvenile sex offender cases. She has translated training and promotional materials, surveys, and legal documents on public health and is a frequent presenter at trainings focused on how to work with interpreters, the significance of Executive Order 13166, the CLAS and NCIHC standards, and the importance of medical interpreter training for language access programs in healthcare facilities and agencies.

Genny Carrillo-Zuniga, MD, ScD

Dr. Genny Carrillo-Zuniga is assistant professor at the Texas A&M Health Science Center, School of Rural Public Health. She is a physician with a master's of science and a doctoral degree in environmental health sciences from Tulane University, School of Public Health and Tropical Medicine. Her current research interests include exposure assessment and health outcomes. Dr. Carrillo-Zuniga's research projects include pesticide exposure in children living in proximity to agricultural fields and lead exposure in children, among other topics. She has participated in the design of a bilingual curriculum in environmental health for Latino communities on the Texas–Mexico border.

Reverend Raponzil L. Drake, DMin

Rev. (Dr.) Raponzil L. Drake is the administrator of the Nebraska Department of Health and Human Services Office of Minority Health, where she is responsible for managing the central and satellite offices, coordinating efforts to address health disparities in racial ethnic minorities, newly arrived immigrants, refugees, and Native American people. She also monitors federal programs and private foundations for funding opportunities; and evaluates state health programs to develop recommendations, policies, and strategies for improving the health outcomes for these populations.

Dr. Drake, a member of the United Methodist clergy for 30 years, is also the pastor of the Fairmont Community United Methodist Church, in Fairmont, Nebraska, where she is responsible for total oversight of the care and nurturing, as well as administrative management, of a small-membership congregation in rural, small-town Nebraska. Dr. Drake earned a BS in accounting at Christian Brothers University, and a master's of divinity and doctorate of ministry at Memphis Theological Seminary. During the summer of 2007, Dr. Drake was privileged to be selected for participation in Harvard University's John F. Kennedy School of Government. She is now an alumnus of the Kennedy School's Senior Executives in State and Local Government program.

Annette Dula, PhD

Dr. Annette Dula believes that bioethics must explicitly address issues of race, class, and culture. One of a small number of African American bioethicists in the United States whose area of interest focuses on racial aspects of bioethics, Dr. Dula is a visiting scholar at the Center for Bioethics and Law at the University of Pittsburgh and an adjunct faculty member at the University of Colorado's Center for Values and Social Policy. A graduate of Hampton University and Harvard University, Dr. Dula was a fellow at the University of Chicago Center for Clinical Medical Ethics and has taught everyday medical ethics to interns and residents in neighborhood clinics. She has been a keynote or invited speaker at the major bioethics societies in the country. She has been invited to speak at universities and medical schools throughout the nation and has served on the bioethics committee of President Clinton's Health Task Force in Washington, DC. She has been published in the *Journal of Healthcare for the Poor and Underserved*, *Hastings Center Report*, the *Journal of Clinical Medical Ethics*, and the *Cambridge Quarterly of Healthcare Ethics*. Her co-edited book, *It Just Ain't Fair! The Ethics of Health Care for African Americans*, was published by Praeger in 1994. Her most recent publication appeared in *African American Bioethics: Culture, Race and Identity*, edited by L. Prograis and E. Pellegrino, in 2007.

Cristina Fernandez, MD

Dr. Cristina Fernandez is associate program director for the joint Pediatric Residency Program at Creighton University/University of Nebraska Medical Center. She works with the underserved population, cooperating with the TB Clinic, and she is building an obesity treatment program called "Healthy Families," a community-based program to decrease obesity. She mentors several residents in asthma and obesity. As assistant professor in the Creighton University School of Medicine, she lectures to medical students, residents, and the community on health disparities topics and is currently involved in a pediatric health disparities project with residents. Childhood obesity is her passion, and she has presented her work at national meetings. She developed a unique clinical–community model in obesity treatment. This model will help children of underserved areas.

Isidore Flores, PhD

Dr. Isidore Flores is a research scientist at the School of Rural Public Health, Texas A&M University System Health Science Center, South Texas Center, McAllen. He earned his PhD in ecological/community psychology from Michigan State University in 1985 and joined the staff of the School of Rural Public Health in 2002. Previously, Dr. Flores worked for the Michigan Department of Public Health, the Midwest Migrant Health Information Office (now called Migrant Health Promotion), the Michigan Public Health Institute, and the Julian Samora Research Institute at Michigan State University.

He has a broad background in research, including experience on projects in Latin America, and over 30 years of work with migratory farm workers—10 of those years in community participatory projects. As director of the Midwest Migrant Health Information Office, he gained experience with the Camp Health Aid Program, which was one of the earliest of the many programs in South Texas involving community health workers (*promotores*). The focus of his current work at the South Texas Center is migration of populations back and forth across the Mexico/U.S. border and its implications for public health. Dr. Flores is known as an insightful advisor to researchers and graduate students in the areas of research design and implementation and program evaluation.

Valda Ford, RN, MPH, MS

Valda Ford is the president and CEO of The Center for Human Diversity Inc.; the host and executive producer of *Valda's Place*—a long-standing cable television talk show; a member of the Council of Public Representatives for the Director of the National Institutes of Health and the National Speakers' Association; and the director of Refugee Initiatives for Unite for Sight.

Ford has created a series of DVDs on cultural competency, intercultural communication, and her work with refugees from Liberia. She makes more than 50 presentations a year to groups as diverse as CEOs, employee diversity groups, and health science students and to international forums dedicated to policy formulation that improves the health of the most vulnerable groups on the planet.

Ford has a master's of public health in health policy analysis and administration from the University of North Carolina at Chapel Hill, a master's of nursing administration from Creighton University, and a bachelor of science degree from Winston–Salem State University. Her career includes nearly a decade of service in Saudi Arabia and the U.S. Virgin Islands. She has made presentations on leadership, public health, and cultural competency in at least 25 states in the United States, as well as in China, the Netherlands, Poland, Ghana, Saudi Arabia, Denmark, Sierra Leone, Sri Lanka, Afghanistan, and Australia.

Vanessa Gamble, MD, PhD

Dr. Gamble, is a university professor of medical humanities at the George Washington University and the first African American woman to hold this prestigious, endowed faculty position. She is also a member of the university's Columbian College of Arts and Sciences faculty in the Department of History. Prior to her appointment to George Washington, Dr. Gamble was director of the Tuskegee University National Center for Bioethics in Research and Health Care. She has also held positions as associate professor of history of medicine and family medicine and was a founding director of the Center for the Study of Race and Ethnicity in Medicine at the University of Wisconsin School of Medicine and as vice president for community and minority programs at the Association of American Medical Colleges. A physician, scholar, and activist, she is an internationally recognized expert on the history of American medicine, racial and ethnic disparities in health and health care, cultural competence, and bioethics.

She is the author of several widely acclaimed publications on the history of race and racism in American medicine, including the award-winning *Making a Place for Ourselves: The Black Hospital Movement: 1920–1945*. Public service has been a hallmark of Dr. Gamble's career. She chaired the committee that took the lead role in the successful campaign to obtain an apology in 1997 from President Clinton for the infamous U.S. Public Health Syphilis Study at Tuskegee. Dr. Gamble is a member of the Institute of Medicine, National Academy of Sciences.

A native of West Philadelphia, Dr. Gamble received her BA from Hampshire College and her MD and PhD in the history and sociology of science from the University of Pennsylvania.

Gordon Gong, MD

Dr. Gordon Gong is senior director for study design and biostatistics at F. Marie Hall Institute for Rural and Community Health, Texas Tech University Health Science Center, Lubbock, Texas. His responsibilities include providing methodological and statistical guidance for study design and data analysis and conducting and preparing research projects in the areas of childhood obesity; community health; human genetics; health disparities among immigrants; and ethical, legal, and social implications in genetic studies with immigrants as research subjects.

Dr. Gong is a cardiologist by training and has wide interests in biomedical sciences including hypertension, osteoporosis, glaucoma, human genetics, molecular biology, signal transduction, and biostatistics, with 40 publications (including book chapters).

In his research and community outreach, he established working relationships with Sudanese immigrant communities in Omaha, Nebraska. During this process, he learned the importance of community outreach and cultural proficiency in research. He and his colleagues have recently published research articles concerning the roles of genetic and environmental factors on body weight index and bone mineral density among Sudanese immigrants in comparison with Caucasians and native-born African Americans.

Margaret A. Graham, PhD

Dr. Margaret A. Graham is assistant professor of anthropology at The University of Texas-Pan American. She received her PhD in anthropology at Michigan State University and held a National Institute on Aging Postdoctoral Fellowship in Sociocultural Gerontology at The University of California–San Francisco. Her research focuses on the anthropology of health and nutrition. She has conducted research in the Peruvian Andes, northern Mexico, the U.S.–Mexico border region, and northern California. Her work has been published in *Social Science and Medicine*, *Ecology of Food and Nutrition*, *Journal of Tropical Pediatrics*, *Field Methods*, and *Health Education and Behavior*.

Gleb Haynatzki, DSc, PhD

Dr. Gleb Haynatzki is an associate professor of biostatistics and lead biostatistician in the School of Medicine at Creighton University, Omaha, Nebraska. He has a PhD from the Department of Statistics and Applied Probability, University of California–Santa Barbara. His main areas of research are statistical modeling of carcinogenesis and osteoporosis and cancer epidemiology. He has worked on numerous biomedical research projects, mostly funded by the National Institutes of Health.

Vera Haynatzka, PhD

Dr. Vera Haynatzka is an assistant professor of biostatistics in the Department of Preventive Medicine and Public Health in the School of Medicine at Creighton University, Omaha, Nebraska. She has a PhD from the Department of Statistics and Applied Probability, University of California–Santa Barbara. Her main areas of research are statistical modeling of carcinogenesis, health disparities in mother-and-child health, and credit risk modeling.

Cathy Hudson, MD

Dr. Cathy Hudson, is an assistant professor of pediatrics at Creighton University School of Medicine, Omaha, Nebraska.

Dr. Hudson received her undergraduate and medical school degree from Creighton University and her pediatric residency from Children's Mercy Hospital in Kansas City, Missouri. Since residency, she has practiced with Creighton University—Children's Physicians as a full-time faculty member. She also teaches medical students and residents in her clinical practice and in the hospital setting.

Dr. Hudson has an interest in the health disparities of the inner-city youth and in the area of child physical and sexual abuse.

Adeola O. Jaiyeola, MD, DOHS, MHSc

Dr. Adeola O. Jaiyeola is director of the Northern Plains Tribal Epidemiology Center, Aberdeen Area Tribal Chairmen's Health Board, in Rapid City, South Dakota. She has a broad range of experience in community and public health. Her expertise includes (1) community health monitoring and assessment; (2) population health/primary care; (3) program planning, implementation and evaluation; (4) public health program supervision and management; (5) surveillance of communicable diseases; (6) communicable disease outbreak investigation and control; and (7) data collection, analysis, and reporting. Between 1988 and 1997, Dr. Jaiyeola worked for the Ontario Ministry of Health in Canada as an epidemiologist intern, an environmental health consultant, and a public health consultant, and she was the regional community medicine specialist for the medical services branch of Health Canada, overseeing public health and clinical practice programs for aboriginal communities in northern Ontario.

She then moved to Fort Worth, Texas, where she served as research epidemiologist and director of the Health Intelligence Center at the Tarrant County Public Health, Fort Worth, Texas, between 1997 and 2006. She led a team of epidemiologists and biostatistician to pioneer the Health Intelligence Center within the Epidemiology Division and was responsible for surveillance activities and community health assessments. During that time, she was the chief editor of two quarterly newsletters and several reports and publications and was the lead in several community health projects including Tarrant County Behavioral Risk Factor Surveillance System (BRFSS) and Tarrant County Monitoring and Assessment Project (MAP).

Since 2006, Dr. Jaiyeola has been serving as director of the Northern Plains Epidemiology Center in Rapid City, South Dakota. She is responsible for carrying out the goals of the Epi Center to assist 18 Northern Plains tribes in a four-state region (South Dakota, North Dakota, Iowa, and Nebraska) in providing research, epidemiology, and public health practice to improve their health. She provides leadership, supervision, and management to a staff of 10 and manages a budget of more than $750,000. She is PI[SN1] for several collaborative research projects between universities and native communities. She has represented her organization and presented projects in several local and national conferences and workshops including the APHA, CSTE, IHS Research Conference, Tribal IRB[SN2] Conference and South Dakota Department of Health Public Health Conference.

Judith Lee Kissell, PhD

Dr. Judith Kissell is director of the Health Administration and Policy Program and resident associate professor, Department of Philosophy, Creighton University, Omaha, Nebraska.

Dr. Kissell is committed to the ethics education of both healthcare students and professionals in the areas of clinical and research ethics. She is particularly interested in introducing healthcare professionals and students to the care of patients who are marginalized by society and who do not have adequate access to health care. She has also written and lectured on problems of research among marginalized populations and particularly immigrant populations.

Dr. Kissell has lectured and authored numerous articles in journals and books in the United States, Europe, and Australia. She is co-editor of *The Healthcare Professional as Friend and Healer, Jesuit Health Sciences and the Promotion of Justice: An Invitation to a Discussion.*

She is currently the director of Creighton University's Health Administration and Policy Program. She is particularly concerned that future administrators of for-profit and nonprofit agencies and institutions be cognizant of ethical issues and of the problems of access to health care in the United States and abroad. Dr. Kissell serves on the Nebraska Board of Dentistry, is an ethics consultant for the Nebraska Board of Medicine and Surgery, and is the Nebraska Public Member for the American Dental Association Examination organization.

Diane Lowe, BA

Diane Lowe is a health program manager for the Nebraska Department of Health and Human Services, Office of Minority Health and Health Disparities. She is responsible for health promotion and education activities targeting racial ethnic minorities, refugees, and newly-arrived immigrants in Congressional District 1. In addition, she is responsible for implementation of the State Partnership Grant to Improve Minority Health. Ms. Lowe holds a bachelor of arts in business, and is finishing her master of arts in management at Doane College in Lincoln, Nebraska.

Nelda Mier, PhD

Dr. Nelda Mier is an assistant professor at the Texas A&M Health Science Center School of Rural Public Health and is based at the South Texas Center in McAllen, Texas. She has a PhD in health education with a minor in health communication and has extensive experience in minority health behavioral research. She is a Mexican American, bilingual researcher who specializes in designing and conducting quantitative and qualitative research using the socioecological approach to address the prevention and management of chronic disease affecting the Mexican American population at the Texas–Mexico border. Dr. Mier has published peer-review articles in many journals, including *Preventing Chronic Disease, American Journal of Health Behavior*, and *Journal of the American Dietetic Association*.

Her research projects include piloting a culturally sensitive physical activity intervention for Mexican Americans, a study on socioenvironmental factors of physical activity among Mexican American adults with diabetes, and a binational project on diabetes and psychosocial factors in a border population, among others.

Ann V. Millard, PhD

Dr. Ann V. Millard is a faculty member in the Department of Social and Behavioral Health at the School of Rural Public Health, Health Science Center, Texas A&M University System. She works at the South Texas Center in McAllen, near the Texas border with Mexico. Dr. Millard's current projects deal with early prevention of diabetes and health of Hispanic migrant farm workers. As an anthropologist, she carried out fieldwork with farmers in rural Mexico, migrant farm workers in Michigan, and *colonia* residents in South Texas.

With a PhD in anthropology from the University of Texas at Austin, Dr. Millard joined the faculty in the Department of Anthropology and the College of Human Medicine at Michigan State University (1980–2002). She edited *Medical Anthropology Quarterly* and was a senior research scholar at the Julian Samora Research Institute. She co-authored *Apple Pie and Enchiladas: Latino Newcomers in the Rural Midwest* and *Hunger and Shame: Child Malnutrition and Poverty on Mt. Kilimanjaro*. In addition, she has written 92 refereed articles, chapters, other publications, and reports on cultural anthropology, population dynamics, and health issues in the United States and abroad. She has carried out ethnographic research and advised on anthropological projects on health and household economics in a number of countries in Latin America, Africa, and Asia. She is a board member of Nuestra Clinica del Valle in South Texas and the American Association of University Women-McAllen Branch. She is currently working on a book on anthropological perspectives on maternal and child health.

Phyllis A. Nsiah-Kumi, MD, MPH

Dr. Phyllis A. Nsiah-Kumi is an assistant professor and investigator–clinician in internal medicine–pediatrics at the University of Nebraska Medical Center in Omaha, Nebraska. She received her doctor of medicine degree from the Case Western Reserve University School of Medicine and trained as an internist and pediatrician at Case Western Reserve University–MetroHealth Medical Center in Cleveland, Ohio. She completed her general internal medicine research fellowship and master's of public health degree at the Northwestern University Feinberg School of Medicine in Chicago, Illinois. She has long had an interest in health disparities, ensuring care for vulnerable populations, and understanding barriers to effective cross-cultural patient–provider communication.

During her fellowship at Northwestern, she worked with a team to develop and test multimedia diabetes education tools for patients with low health literacy. Her work there also included a study of disparities in diabetes incidence in older, middle-age adults and a study of diabetic parents' perceptions of the risk of their children developing the disease. She has also investigated the impact of an educational intervention on resident physicians' use of interpreters in clinical encounters.

Her current research interests include addressing disparities in health communication in clinical and community settings and how African American families with a diabetic family member communicate about diabetes risk and prevention, both with their healthcare providers and within their families.

Albert A. Okunade, PhD, MS, MBA

Dr. Albert A. Okunade is First Tennessee Professor of Economics (endowed), Palmer Professor in Research Excellence (annual), and an affiliate faculty at the Center for Community Health and the Center for Health Care Economics, University of Memphis. He served a faculty sabbatical in residence researching at the Harvard School of Public Health in 2000. Dr. Okunade earned his PhD in economics in 1986 at the University of Arkansas, after earning his BS, MS, and MBA degrees at Wright State University in Dayton, Ohio. He received the University of Memphis Distinguished Research Award in 2002, the Superior Performance in University Research Award (multiple years), and the College of Business and Economics Best Paper Awards for peer-refereed journal publication (multiple years). Moreover, he received the University Honors Program Fellowship Award in 2001 and has ranked as finalist (multiple years) for the University's Distinguished Teaching Award. In the winter of 2006, the *Review of Black Political Economy* ranked his peer-refereed research output in the "top three" among all black economists, U.S.- and foreign-born.

Professor Okunade, the author of more than 100 research papers in leading peer-refereed journals, book, and several book chapters, has presented research papers globally (Canada, Senegal, Italy, Portugal, Spain, United Kingdom, and Finland). He is on the Scientific Advisory Committee of the International Health Economics Association and is a founding Board member of the American Society of Health Economists. He is also secretary/treasurer of African Finance and Economics Association, an Allied Social Sciences Association organization. Professor Okunade is ad hoc referee for leading (peer-review) healthcare and medical journals (*The Lancet*, *MC Health Services Research*, *Clinical Breast Cancer*, *Journal of Health Economics*, *Health Economics*, and *Health Policy*). His research in health care, public finance, and policy has garnered hundreds of citations from his peers, industry, and the wider public.

Rubens J. Pamies, MD, FACP

Dr. Rubens J. Pamies is vice chancellor for academic affairs and dean for graduate studies and professor of internal medicine at the University of Nebraska Medical Center, Omaha, Nebraska. Dr. Pamies received his baccalaureate degree from St. John's University, his medical degree from the State University of New York at Buffalo in 1986, and completed a residency in primary care internal medicine at the Cornell–North Shore University Hospital. In 1989, Dr. Pamies joined the University of South Florida College of Medicine as staff physician and assistant professor. His interest in minority medical education led him to develop the College of Medicine's first Office of Minority Affairs, where he served as director for two years.

Dr. Pamies previously served as chief of service at the Nashville General Hospital, The Edward S. Harkness Professor of Medicine, chairman of internal medicine at Meharry Medical College, and professor of medicine at Vanderbilt University Medical Center (2000–2003). He also served as Case Western Reserve University School of Medicine Associate dean for academic programs and associate dean of student affairs (1996–2000).

Dr. Pamies has a strong commitment to issues in minority education and health. He has been the principal investigator or co-investigator on the following grants: National Institues of Health (NIH)–sponsored Center for Reducing Asthma Disparities, Agency for Healthcare and Research Quality–sponsored Center for Improving Patient Safety, the Racialand Ethnic Approaches to Community Health 2010 Project (Meharry component), the NIH Planning Grant for Clinical Research in Minority Institutions, and the GTE [SN3]Foundation's The Middle School and High School Teacher's Science Academy, receiving approximately $1,480,000 in funding. He serves on countless local and national committees. In September 2005, Dr. Pamies co-authored a book entitled *Multicultural Medicine and Health Disparities*.

Patti Patterson, MD, MPH

Dr. Patti Patterson is professor of pediatrics at the Texas Tech University Health Sciences Center. Dr. Patterson has 20 years of experience in public health, including serving as the commissioner of health, executive deputy commissioner of health and maternal and child health director for the state of Texas. She also developed the F. Marie Hall Institute for Rural and Community Health for Texas Tech University Health Sciences Center.

Dr. Patterson grew up in rural West Texas and holds a medical degree from the University of Texas Medical Branch in Galveston. She was a family medicine resident at Texas Tech Regional Academic Health Center in Amarillo. She is board certified in pediatrics, completing both pediatric residency and chief resident at the University of Texas Medical Branch. She also has a master's degree in public health from the University of Texas Health Science Center at Houston and a bachelor's degree from Lubbock Christian University.

With a continuing concern for international health, Dr. Patterson has participated in 32 medical mission trips to South America, Eastern Europe, and

Africa. Among these she helped set up basic health services, including community health worker programs; provided care for deaf children; and helped establish a regional public health hospital.

Frank T. Peak, MPA

Frank T. Peak is community outreach services administrator for the Creighton University Medical Center Partnership in Health. He has a master's degree in public administration from the University of Nebraska at Omaha. He has a long history in community/political activism and social justice leadership. He is the co-founder and president/CEO of Nebraska Ethnics Together Working on Reaching Kids Inc. (a nonprofit prevention leadership organization addressing substance abuse and other high-risk behavioral issues for youth and communities of color in particular and all youth in general). He has also served as the executive of the Metro Omaha Family Preservation Grant. He has provided research, community needs assessments, and other information-gathering activities and facilitated forums for various organizations and institutions in the field of health and human services. He has presented on cultural competency at local, regional, and national conferences.

Mr. Peak serves as a member of the Statewide Minority Health Advisory Committee of the Nebraska Health and Human Services System Office of Minority Health; is a member of the Douglas County Board of Health; serves by appointment from the Governor of the State of Nebraska to the Executive Committee of the Nebraska Partners in Prevention State Incentive Grant Project; and is a current member of the American Society for Public Administration, Community Campus Partnerships in Health, and the Nebraska Minority Public Health Association (past president). He received the American Society of Public Administrators Lifetime Achievement Award in Social Justice, the Martin Luther King Jr. Humanitarian Award from the state of Nebraska, the Recognition of Excellence Award from the Nebraska Minority Public Health Association, and the Whitney M. Young Jr. Biennial Community Service Award from the Urban League of Nebraska Inc. Mr. Peak is married, and he and his wife are biological, adoptive, foster, and neighborhood parents.

Michael T. Railey, MD

Dr. Michael T. Railey is a native of St. Louis, Missouri, where he initially graduated from the St. Louis College of Pharmacy in 1972. Never intending to stop at pharmacy as a vocation, Dr. Railey went on to graduate from the University of Missouri at Columbia School of Medicine (1976) and the University of Florida Family Medicine Residency program in 1979. After a year of volunteering with the National Health Corps, working a clinic in inner city St. Louis, he has worked in community practices, private, and group practices as his interest in community service grew. Dr. Railey is known for his frequent talks on topics such as stress, managing obesity, hypertension, spirituality, and medicine.

In 1992, he began teaching in the field of training medical students and resident physicians with the family medicine program at Deaconess Hospital, St. Louis. This eventually led to a clinical appointment with St. Louis University School of Medicine for the next seven years, where he served as the director of the Third Year training program for family medicine within the Department of Community and Family Medicine. He received local and national awards for his work teaching medical students. During that time, he has been published in the area of obesity management and wrote a book chapter on obesity in a family medicine text.

After two years as the program director for the Transitional Medicine Residency Training Program at Forest Park Hospital, Dr. Railey recently accepted the position as the director of operations and research with the St. Louis County Health Department.

Karl S. Roth, MD

Dr. Karl S. Roth is chair, Department of Pediatrics, and professor of pediatrics at Creighton University, Omaha, Nebraska.

The Department of Pediatrics is charged with provision of medical care to all children, irrespective of race, creed, religion, or ability to pay. Located in a federally designated, underserved area of Omaha, the Creighton University Medical Center presents a significant challenge in order to fulfill this mission. Understanding the various aspects of barriers to care, as well as cultural reluctance to seek available care, is critical to working successfully with patient populations. Dr. Roth has administrative oversight responsibility for all aspects of pediatric care at the Medical Center.

Dr. Roth also has clinical responsibilities in the area of biochemical genetics, a field that requires special care—not only expensive but relatively unfamiliar to many in the healthcare and state government funding agencies. In this area of medicine, perhaps as much or more than many, healthcare disparities are highlighted for this reason: where the family is privately insured, provision of care is a relatively easy matter, but when public funding is involved, care of an affected child can often turn into a nightmare.

Dr. Roth has published extensively in his field and is a member of multiple national/international pediatric and scientific organizations. He is actively involved in local and regional pediatric issues as a member of the Executive Committee of the Nebraska American Academy of Pediatrics (AAP) Chapter and Voices for Children in Nebraska, a political action group advocating for children.

Esmeralda R. Sánchez, MPH

Esmeralda R. Sánchez is a project coordinator at the Texas A&M Health Science Center, School of Rural Public Health, South Texas Center in McAllen, Texas. She has a BA in psychology and a master's of public health, with a concentration in health policy and management. She is of Mexican American descent and was born and raised in South Texas. Ms. Sánchez has been involved in several research projects addressing the health needs of Hispanics in South Texas and has worked extensively with *promotores* (community health workers). Her research experience includes projects addressing the early prevention of diabetes, nutrition, and physical activity; disease surveillance and building first aid networks in the colonia population of Hidalgo County; and childhood immunizations.

Reverend John P. Schlegel, SJ

The Rev. John P. Schlegel became Creighton University's 23rd president in August 2000. Since coming to Creighton University in 2000, Fr. Schlegel has brought a renewed energy to campus, leading the university through a period of historic growth built on the pillars of academic excellence, life-enhancing research, community, spiritual formation, and the promotion of justice.

Prior to his arrival at Creighton, Fr. Schlegel served nine years as president of the University of San Francisco, another Jesuit institution. Before that, he was Creighton University's assistant academic vice president (1978–1982), academic dean of Rockhurst College (1982–1984), dean of arts and sciences at Marquette University (1984–1988), and executive and academic vice president at John Carroll University (1988–1991).

As president of Creighton, Fr. Schlegel has initiated changes that have enhanced the already nationally recognized academic quality of the university and the beauty of the campus. Creighton's investment in redevelopment and east campus expansion has been part of the renaissance of downtown

Omaha. These changes have enhanced the living and learning experience of Creighton's 6,800 students.

A graduate of St. Louis University with a BA in philosophy and classics (1969) and an MA in political science (1970), he also earned a theology degree from the University of London (1973) and a doctorate from Oxford University in international relations (1977).

Wehnona Stabler, MPH

Wehnona Stabler is an enrolled member of the Omaha Tribe. She is a daughter, wife, mother, and new grandmother. She is also a member of the Buffalo clan and her Omaha name is Mi-texi', meaning sacred moon.

Ms. Stabler is currently the Omaha tribal health director and CEO of the Carl T. Curtis Health Education Center in Macy, Nebraska. She has worked in the Indian Health Service or in tribal health programs since 1981.

Ms. Stabler has a bachelor of science degree in social work from Morningside College in Sioux City, Iowa, and a masters in public health administration from the University of Hawaii in Manoa. She has also completed an injury prevention fellowship with the Indian Health Service.

John R. Stone, MD, PhD

Dr. John R. Stone is adjunct professor at the Center for Health Policy and Ethics, Creighton University Medical Center. He is a physician and philosopher, whose focus is social justice and other ethical issues related to inequalities in health and health care associated with race, ethnicity, and socioeconomic status. He received a BA from Emory University in 1963, an MD from the Johns Hopkins University School of Medicine in 1967, and a PhD in philosophy from Brown University in 2001. Dr. Stone has been with Creighton's Center for Health Policy and Ethics since August 2006. Prior to that, he was associate professor with the Tuskegee University National Center for Bioethics in Research and Health Care, Tuskegee, Alabama, for seven years. Previously, Dr. Stone practiced cardiology for many years in Missoula, Montana. There he co-founded an Institute of Medicine and Humanities between St. Patrick Hospital and the University of Montana.

Dr. Stone has written or co-authored several articles in the *Cambridge Quarterly of Healthcare Ethics*, *Family & Community Health*, *Theoretical Medicine and Bioethics*, and the *Hastings Center Report*.

Chutima Suraratdecha, MBA, PhD

Dr. Chutima Suraratdecha is a health policy and economics officer at PATH in Seattle, Washington. She received a BS degree in food technology and biotechnology from Chulalongkorn University (Thailand) and an MBA and PhD, with a concentration on health and pharmaceutical economics, from the University of Memphis. Dr. Suraratdecha has extensive experience in teaching and research on various topics internationally, and with policy makers, government officials, nongovernmental organizations, donors, bilateral organizations, and academic institutions. In particular, her work has focused on the economics of health and pharmaceutical care, including economic evaluations of health programs and health interventions, health expenditure and health financing mechanisms, adoption and use of health technologies, demand assessment, and access to care. Dr. Suraratdecha has worked in Cambodia, China, India, Indonesia, Philippines, Sri Lanka, Myanmar, Thailand, the United States, and Vietnam.

Ethel Williams, PhD

Dr. Ethel Williams is an associate professor and chair of the Master of Public Administration Program at the University of Nebraska at Omaha. She holds a doctorate in political science, with an emphasis in public administration and public policy from the University of Nebraska–Lincoln, and a master's degree in public administration from the Graduate School of Public and International Affairs at the University of Pittsburgh.

Her areas of specialization include human resource management and public policy. Dr. Williams's current research interests focus on succession planning and health disparities among African Americans.

M. Roy Wilson, MD, MS

Dr. M. Roy Wilson began serving as chancellor of the University of Colorado Denver (UCD) in July 2006. UCD consists of a general academic campus with seven schools and colleges and a health sciences campus with Schools of Medicine, Nursing, Pharmacy, and Dentistry, as well as the Graduate School of Biomedical Sciences. He is an elected member of the Institutes of Medicine of the National Academy of Sciences, the American Ophthalmological Society, and the Glaucoma Research Society.

Dr. Wilson was an initial Advisory Council member of the National Center on Minority Health and Health Disparities of the National Institutes of Health (NIH) and served four years as chair of its Strategic Plan subcommittee. He currently serves on the Advisory Council of the National Center for Research Resources of NIH.

Dr. Wilson received his medical degree from Harvard Medical School and his master's of science in epidemiology at the University of California–Los Angeles (UCLA) School of Public Health. He performed both his ophthalmology residency and glaucoma fellowship at the Massachusetts Eye and Ear Infirmary, Harvard Medical School. Dr. Wilson was named president of the Texas Tech University Health Sciences Center in 2003. In 1998, he was appointed dean of the School of Medicine at Creighton University, and then served as both dean and vice president for Health Sciences from 1999 to 2003. Prior to that time, he was professor of ophthalmology both at the Jules Stein Eye Institute of UCLA and Charles R. Drew University of Medicine & Science.

Dr. Wilson's major scientific contributions have been in bridging the fields of epidemiology and ophthalmology. He received the Association of American Medical College's Herbert W. Nickens Award in November 2007. Dr. Wilson is married to Suzanne and has two children, Yoshio and Presley.

Anthony Zhang, MA

Anthony Zhang is currently serving as health surveillance specialist for the Nebraska Department of Health and Human Services, Office of Minority Health. He received his master's degree in health education from University of Nebraska–Lincoln. Before coming to America, Mr. Zhang was the research director of Gallup-China, where he established research policies and procedures, directed all project aspects, and shared in management development of this market research firm. Mr. Zhang was also an assistant professor at the Renmin University of China and Tianjin University.

Index

Page numbers followed by *f* denote figures; those followed by *t* denote tables